Respiratory Medicine

Editor

VLADIMÍR JEKL

VETERINARY CLINICS OF NORTH AMERICA: EXOTIC ANIMAL PRACTICE

www.vetexotic.theclinics.com

Consulting Editor
JÖRG MAYER

May 2021 • Volume 24 • Number 2

ELSEVIER

1600 John F. Kennedy Boulevard ● Suite 1800 ● Philadelphia, Pennsylvania, 19103-2899
http://www.vetexotic.theclinics.com

**VETERINARY CLINICS OF NORTH AMERICA: EXOTIC ANIMAL PRACTICE Volume 24, Number 2
May 2021 ISSN 1094-9194, ISBN-13: 978-0-323-77849-7**

Editor: Stacy Eastman
Developmental Editor: Axell Ivan Jade M. Purificacion

Veterinary Clinics of North America: Exotic Animal Practice (ISSN 1094-9194) is published in January, May, and September by Elsevier, Inc., 360 Park Avenue South, New York, NY 10010-1710. Subscription prices are $290.00 per year for US individuals, $687.00 per year for US institutions, $100.00 per year for US students and residents, $338.00 per year for Canadian individuals, $735.00 per year for Canadian institutions, $352.00 per year for international individuals, $735.00 per year for international institutions, $100.00 per year Canadian students/residents, and $165.00 per year for international students/residents. To receive student/resident rate, orders must be accompanied by name of affiliated institution, date of term, and the *signature* of program/residency coordinator on institution letterhead. Orders will be billed at individual rate until proof of status is received. Foreign air speed delivery is included in all *Clinics* subscription prices. All prices are subject to change without notice. **POSTMASTER:** Send address changes to *Veterinary Clinics of North America: Exotic Animal Practice*, Elsevier Health Sciences Division, Subscription Customer Service, 3251 Riverport Lane, Maryland Heights, MO 63043. **Customer Service: Telephone: 1-800-654-2452** (U.S. and Canada); **1-314-447-8871** (outside U.S. and Canada). **Fax: 1-314-447-8029. E-mail: journalscustomerservice-usa@elsevier.com (for print support); journalsonlinesupport-usa@elsevier.com (for online support).**

Reprints. For copies of 100 or more of articles in this publication, please contact the Commercial Reprints Department, Elsevier Inc., 360 Park Avenue South, New York, New York 10010-1710. Tel.: 212-633-3874; Fax: 212-633-3820; E-mail: reprints@elsevier.com.

Veterinary Clinics of North America: Exotic Animal Practice is covered in *MEDLINE/PubMed (Index Medicus).*

Contributors

CONSULTING EDITOR

JÖRG MAYER, Dr med vet, MSc
Diplomate, American Board of Veterinary Practitioners (Exotic Companion Mammals); Diplomate, European College of Zoological Medicine (Small Mammals); Diplomate, American College of Zoological Medicine; Associate Professor of Zoological Medicine, Department of Small Animal Medicine and Surgery, University of Georgia College of Veterinary Medicine, Athens, Georgia, USA

EDITOR

VLADIMÍR JEKL, DVM, PhD
Diplomate, European College of Zoological Medicine (Small Mammal); Associate Professor, Department of Pharmacology and Pharmacy, Faculty of Veterinary Medicine, University of Veterinary and Pharmaceutical Sciences Brno, Brno, Czech Republic

AUTHORS

ANDRÉS MONTESINOS BARCELÓ, LV, MSc, PhD
Centro Veterinario Los Sauces, Associated Professor of Exotic Animals Medicine and Surgery, Department of Animal Medicine and Surgery, Veterinary Faculty, Universidad Complutense de Madrid, Madrid, Spain

JESSICA R. COMOLLI, DVM
Resident of Zoological Medicine, Department of Small Animal Medicine and Surgery, College of Veterinary Medicine, University of Georgia, Athens, Georgia, USA

LORENZO CROSTA, DVM, PhD, GP Cert (Exotic Animal)
Diplomate, European College of Zoological Medicine (EBVS European Veterinary Specialist in Zoo Health Management); Associate Professor of Avian and Zoological Medicine, Faculty of Science, Sydney School of Veterinary Science, University Veterinary Teaching Hospital Camden, Director, Avian, Reptile and Exotic Pet Hospital, Camden, New South Wales, Australia

NICOLA DI GIROLAMO, DVM, MSc(EBHC), PhD
Diplomate, European College of Zoological Medicine (Herp); Diplomate, American College of Zoological Medicine; Oklahoma State University, Center for Veterinary Health Sciences, Stillwater, Oklahoma, USA

STEPHEN J. DIVERS, BVetMed, FRCVS
Diploma in Zoological Medicine; Diplomate, European College of Zoological Medicine (Herpetology, Zoo Health Management); Diplomate, American College of Zoological Medicine; Professor of Zoological Medicine, Department of Small Animal Medicine and Surgery, College of Veterinary Medicine, University of Georgia, Athens, Georgia, USA

MARÍA ARDIACA GARCÍA, LV
Veterinarian, Centro Veterinario Los Sauces, Madrid, Spain

MICHAELA GUMPENBERGER, DVM
Assistant Professor, Diagnostic Imaging, Department for Companion Animals and Horses, University of Veterinary Medicine Vienna, Austria

VLADIMÍR JEKL, DMV, PhD
Diplomate, European College of Zoological Medicine (Small Mammal); Associate Professor, Department of Pharmacology and Pharmacy, Faculty of Veterinary Medicine, University of Veterinary and Pharmaceutical Sciences Brno, Brno, Czech Republic

ANGELA M. LENNOX, DVM
Diplomate, American Board of Veterinary Practitioners (Exotic Companion Mammals, Avian); Diplomate, European College of Zoological Medicine (Small Mammals); Avian and Exotic Animal Clinic, Indianapolis, Indiana, USA

RACHEL E. MARSCHANG, PD, Dr med vet
FTÄ Mikrobiologie, Diplomate, European College of Zoological Medicine (Herpetology); Laboklin GmbH & Co KG, Bad Kissingen, Germany

CRISTINA BONVEHÍ NADEU, LV
Veterinarian, Centro Veterinario Los Sauces, Madrid, Spain

LADISLAV NOVOTNY, MVDr, MSc, PhD, FRCPath, MRCVS
Finn Pathologists, CVS Group plc, Norfolk, United Kingdom; Novopath Ltd, Ceperka, Czech Republic

MICHAEL PEES, Dr med vet
Diplomate, European College of Zoological Medicine (Avian); Diplomate, European College of Zoological Medicine (Herpetology); Professor, Department for Birds and Reptiles, University Veterinary Teaching Hospital, University of Leipzig, Clinic for Birds and Reptiles, Leipzig, Germany

EKATERINA SALZMANN, Dr med vet
Laboklin GmbH & Co KG, Bad Kissingen, Germany

KELSEA STUDER, DVM
Oklahoma State University, Center for Veterinary Health Sciences, Stillwater, Oklahoma, USA

Contents

 Video content accompanies this article at http://www.vetexotic. theclinics.com.

> The piscine respiratory system is represented by gills. Gill diseases are extremely common and may be caused by a large variety of etiologic agents. The gills are in direct contact with water and reflect its quality, for example, pollution, and they also must face the presence of biotic agents, such as viruses, bacteria, fungi, and parasites. Evolution has established many defense mechanisms to combat these agents. Failure of these mechanisms is life-threatening for the fish, due to impaired respiration. Gills are relatively easily accessible for clinical examination and sampling, which facilitates intravital diagnosis.

> Detailed information is given about technique and image interpretation of radiography and computed tomography of the respiratory tract in reptiles. MRI and sonography are mentioned when supporting differential diagnoses. Various diseases and imaging pitfalls are described with multiple figures and graphics. One focus is on lung compression in chelonians, which may be misinterpreted as pneumonia in dyspneic patients without the help of imaging tools.

> Respiratory abnormalities in snakes are a common clinical presentation in zoologic medical practice. There are often compounding issues involving translocation and substandard husbandry that can predispose to infectious and noninfectious causes of respiratory disease. Endoscopic evaluation of the respiratory tract and the collection of biopsies for histopathology and microbiology is preferred but may only be available from the specialist. Alternatively, transtracheal lavage for cytology and microbiology is a practical method for most practitioners. A variety of bacterial, fungal, viral, and parasitic infections, as well as noninfectious diseases have been reported. Accurate diagnosis dictates specific therapy, which increases the likelihood of successful treatment.

Respiratory tract disease in chelonians can be difficult to treat and as such proper diagnostics are paramount. Infectious agents that can affect the respiratory tract of chelonians include viral, bacterial, fungal, and parasitic organisms. Noninfectious diseases can also develop. Because chelonians lack a proper diaphragm, changes in size of celomic organs can cause compression of the respiratory system. These conditions result in clinical signs that could be attributed to the respiratory system, such as open-mouth breathing. In this article, anatomy, physiology, and current standards for diagnostics and treatments of major diseases of the respiratory tract in chelonians are discussed.

Methods for the detection of pathogens associated with respiratory disease in reptiles, including viruses, bacteria, fungi, and parasites, are constantly evolving as is the understanding of the specific roles played by various pathogens in disease processes. Some are known to be primary pathogens with high prevalence in captive reptiles, for example, serpentoviruses in pythons or mycoplasma in tortoises. Others are very commonly found in reptiles with respiratory disease but are most often considered secondary, for example, gram-negative bacteria. Detection methods as well as specific pathogens associated with upper- and lower-respiratory disease are discussed.

This article is aimed to help the reader to understand better how to diagnose and treat different respiratory diseases in Psittaciformes (parrot-like birds). The article starts from a review of avian respiratory anatomy and physiology, and then moves forward into diagnostic techniques, most common diseases, split in species and anatomic location, and common treatment regimens.

The diagnosis and treatment of respiratory disease in pet guinea pigs, chinchillas, and degus still face profoundly serious challenges owing to their relatively small size, conspicuous clinical signs, difficulty for sampling, and insufficient scientific evidence to correlate signs and particular pathologies. This article is intended to summarize the available information on the relevant anatomy, physiology, and respiratory pathology in these species.

Vladimír Jekl

Respiratory disorders are very common in rabbits. Rabbits are obligate nasal breathers, so "simple" rhinitis can cause severe respiratory distress and patient collapse. Causes of dyspnea could be of primary origin or secondary, whereby diseases primarily affecting other organs can result in respiratory embarrassment even if the respiratory system is healthy (eg, anemia, cardiac disease). Diagnosis is based on radiography, ultrasonography, endoscopy, computed tomography, and/or pathogen isolation. Once the diagnosis has been completed, treatment options should be discussed with the owner. The article describes the anatomy of the respiratory tract, diagnostics, and therapy for selected respiratory disorders in rabbits.

Angela M. Lennox

Ferrets are susceptible to many disorders affecting the respiratory tract including both primary diseases and diseases of other body systems secondarily affecting the respiratory tract. Some primary respiratory diseases are shared with other mammal species including humans; potentially zoonotic diseases include important pathogens such as influenza and SARS-CoV-2. Other diseases include infections (bacterial, parasitic, and fungal) and neoplasia. A thorough workup is important to identify exact causes in order to formulate a treatment plan. Infectious diseases include bacterial, fungal, parasitic, and viral.

VETERINARY CLINICS OF NORTH AMERICA: EXOTIC ANIMAL PRACTICE

SERIES OF RELATED INTEREST

Veterinary Clinics of North America: Small Animal Practice
Available at: https://www.vetsmall.theclinics.com/

THE CLINICS ARE NOW AVAILABLE ONLINE!
Access your subscription at:
www.theclinics.com

Preface

Respiratory Medicine

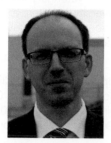

Vladimír Jekl, DVM, PhD, DECZM
Editor

It is indeed an honor and a pleasure to introduce the new issue of *Veterinary Clinics North America: Exotic Animal Practice*. This issue focuses on respiratory disorders of fishes, reptiles, avian, and exotic companion mammals.

Within the past few years, quality research has evolved, especially in the area of molecular diagnostics of new viruses, especially in the reptile species.

This issue intended to review the most current and up-to-date knowledge about respiratory tract anatomy, physiology, diagnostics, and respiratory tract diseases of fish and exotic companion animals (eg, reptiles, parrots, guinea pigs, chinchillas, degus, rabbits, and ferrets).

I sincerely thank the authors, who are specialists with considerable routine experience with the animal species they write about, for sharing their knowledge and valuable time. I hope the amount and depth of information, supplemented with high-quality images, will be of interest and value to practitioners, researchers, veterinary students. All information is given in an easy-to-read style and can be readily applicable in the clinical and zoologic practice. I would also like to thank Nicole Congleton and Axell Ivan Jade M. Purificacion, Editors, for their great assistance during preparation of this issue.

Vet Clin Exot Anim 24 (2021) ix–x
https://doi.org/10.1016/j.cvex.2021.02.003
1094-9194/21/© 2021 Published by Elsevier Inc.

vetexotic.theclinics.com

I would like to also wish you good health, especially in this time of the coronavirus pandemic.

Vladimír Jekl, DVM, PhD, DECZM
Department of Pharmacology and Pharmacy
Faculty of Veterinary Medicine
University of Veterinary and
Pharmaceutical Sciences Brno
Palackeho tr. 1, 61242 Brno
Czech Republic

Jekl & Hauptman Veterinary Clinic–
Focused on Exotic Companion Mammal Care
Mojmirovo Namesti 1305/6a
61200 Brno, Czech Republic

E-mail addresses:
VladimirJekl@gmail.com; jeklv@vfu.cz

Respiratory Tract Disorders in Fishes

Ladislav Novotny, MVDr, MSc, PhD, FRCPath, MRCVS[a,b,]*

KEYWORDS

- Branchitis • Ichthyopathology • Parasites • Gill illness

KEY POINTS

- Main respiratory organ in fish is gills.
- Gills are important organ of osmoregulation and metabolism.
- Microscopy of fresh wet mounts of gills are often diagnostic for parasitic diseases (eg, *Ichthyophthirius, Ichthyobodo, monogeneans*).
- Gill tissue is an entrance for many infectious diseases and serious damage of gills is frequent cause of death.
- Gills are main target of water pollution.

 Video content accompanies this article at http://www.vetexotic.theclinics.com.

INTRODUCTION

Fish are the most diverse group of ectothermic vertebrates, containing approximately 34,000 species. Taxonomically it is a paraphyletic group of aquatic tetrapods bearing gills all their life. This group includes hagfish, lampreys, and cartilaginous and bony fish. The gill, as the main respiratory organ, is thus the most typical structure determining this group. Gill disease is probably the most important branch of fish medicine. Normal function of gills is crucial in gas exchange and also in excretion of metabolites and ions to maintain homeostasis. Gills are in direct contact with the aquatic environment, hence the common entrance of abiotic and biotic pathogens. Some fish species (eg, labyrinth fish) have accessory organs/tissue adaptations for gas exchange using atmospheric air, such as lung, gas bladder, the buccal, branchial and opercular cavities, esophagus, pneumatic duct, intestine, and skin. This article focuses on bony fish (Teleostei) gill diseases.

GILL MORPHOLOGY AND PHYSIOLOGY

The gills (*branchiae*) are bilateral respiratory organs situated on either side of pharynx in the opercular cavity covered by the gill lid (*operculum*). The gills are composed of 4

[a] Finn Pathologists, CVS Group plc, Norfolk, UK; [b] Novopath Ltd, Ceperka, Czech Republic
* Finn Pathologists, One Eyed Lane, Weybread IP21 5TT, UK.
E-mail address: Ladislav.Novotny@finnpathologists.com

osteochondral arches providing support for soft gill filaments (primary lamellae). Every gill arch bears a holobranch, which is composed of 2 hemibranchs (**Figs. 1** and **2**). Teleosts also possess a pseudobranch, which is a reduced hemibranch of the first gill arch, usually situated on the inner surface of the opercle.[1] The pseudobranch does not function in gas exchange and its function is still unclear, but it seems to be an osmoregulatory organ.[2] Every hemibranch possesses rows of filaments (primary lamellae) subdivided into multiple secondary lamellae covered by respiratory epithelial cells, supported by pillar cells among which are blood capillaries (see **Fig. 2**). At the base of secondary lamellae, there are also other types of cells: goblet cells, neuroepithelial cells, chloride cells, and undifferentiated cells. Chloride cells play an important role in excretion of chlorides and other ions. The mucous cells secrete a protective layer of mucus acting as a physical, chemical, and immunologic barrier. In addition to these main cell types, there are also eosinophilic granule cells (EGCs) resembling mast cells in mammals, containing immune active substances (eg, lysozyme, peroxidase, alkaline phosphatase, piscidins, serotonin and histamine).[3] Blood flow in the capillaries is opposite to the water flow, ensuring the most effective gas exchange between blood and water through the respiratory epithelium. Afferent arteries bring the venous blood from the ventral aorta to the capillaries of the secondary lamellae, where it is oxygenated and returns through the efferent arteries into the dorsal aorta. Ventilation is regulated by oxygen and carbon dioxide receptors and mechanoreceptors, which respond to water flow.

The delicate structure of the gill makes it very vulnerable, and many biotic and abiotic agents may impair its function, leading to respiratory failure and death.

CLINICAL EXAMINATION OF GILLS

The gills and branchial cavity are relatively easily accessible for clinical, gross, and microscopic examination in most fish species. First, observation and counting of opercular movement should be done on unstressed fish in the tank. Respiratory rate (number of opercular movements) depends mainly on water temperature and saturation by oxygen and mostly ranges between 20 to 60 opercular movements. Short-term

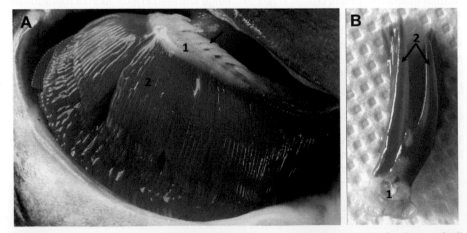

Fig. 1. Anatomy of gills of common carp. (*A*) Gills in situ, operculum removed. 1, bone of gill arch with gill rakers (*arrow*). 2, primary lamellae. (*B*) Transverse section of one holobranch, 1, bearing 2 hemibranchs with rows of primary lamellae, 2.

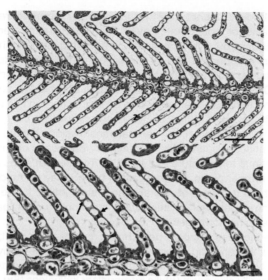

Fig. 2. Normal gill histology. 1, primary lamella; 2; secondary lamella; black arrow, pillar cells; green arrow, epithelial cell; asterisk, blood capillary in secondary lamellae. Hematoxylin-eosin stain.

anesthesia or sedation should be used for further examination. Drugs that can be used for short-term anesthesia are, for example, clove oil (eugenol) in dose 0.06 to 0.10 mL/L or 2-phenoxyethanol in dose 100 to 400 µL/L for 2 to 4 minutes.[4] The branchial cavity should be closely examined after sedation. Normal gills are bright red with no excessive mucus or any discoloration. The samples of gill tissue for wet mount, polymerase chain reaction (PCR), or histopathology can be taken using either scissors or surgical curette. Biopsy sample of 1 or 2 gill filaments in length approximately of 1 cm is usually sufficient for both histopathology and PCR. The bleeding from the gill tissue is usually mild to moderate and can be stopped by gentle compression using mosquito forceps. Swabbing for bacterial culture should be done before sedation/anesthesia (anaesthetics may influence the bacterial growth).

SELECTED RESPIRATORY PATHOGENS IN FISH
Viral Diseases

Koi herpes virus diseases
Koi herpesvirus disease (KHVD) is a worldwide viral disease of common carp (Cyprinus carpio), but viral DNA has been also isolated from other species, not showing clinical signs of infection, for example, tench (Tinca tinca), Atlantic sturgeon (Acipenser oxyrinchus), blue back ide (Leuciscus idus), common roach (Rutilus rutilus), Euraseas ruffe (Gymnocephalus cernuus), European perch (Perca fluviatilis), rainbow trout (Oncorhynchus mykiss), Russian sturgeon (Acipenser gueldenstaedtii), silver carp (Hypophthalmichthys molitrix), stone loach (Barbatula barbatula), scud (Gammarus pulex), swan mussel (Anodonta cygnea). KHVD causes large-scale mortalities, up to 100%, especially in ornamental variants of common carp.[5]

Etiology and pathogenesis
KHVD is caused by koi herpesvirus (KHV), which belongs to the family Alloherpesviridae and is classified as cyprinid herpesvirus-3 (CyHV-3).[6,7] KHV remains active in

water for at least 4 hours, but not for 21 hours, at water temperatures of 23 to 25°C,[8] but infectivity remains for more than 7 days.[9] The virus is inactivated by UV radiation and temperatures above 50°C for 1 minute. The following disinfectants are also effective for inactivation: iodophor at 200 mg/L for 20 minutes, benzalkonium chloride at 60 mg/L for 20 minutes, ethyl alcohol at 30% for 20 minutes, and sodium hypochlorite at 200 mg/L for 30 seconds, all at 15°C. Disinfection of fish eggs can be achieved by iodophor treatment. KHV has been shown to be inactivated on fish eggs by iodophor at 200 mg/L for 30 seconds at 15°C.[10] Virus enters the fish via gills or/and skin.[11] Transmission of KHV is horizontal, but vertical transmission cannot be ruled out. Virus is shed via feces, urine, gills, and skin mucus. KHV outbreaks occur at temperatures over 16°C with optimal temperatures 23 to 25°C. The clinical signs usually appear in 3 days in optimal temperatures, but incubation period may be much longer in lower temperatures. Fish up to 1 year of age are more susceptible to the disease. Clinical signs include lethargic behavior, erratic swimming, sunken eyes, pale gills and skin, gill necrosis, and skin hemorrhages.[12,13]

Gross pathology includes necrosis, petechial hemorrhage, and inflammation of gills, kidney and liver, which are also enlarged. Histopathology shows hyperplasia and/or necrosis of gills, swelling of nuclei of respiratory epithelial cells, margination of chromatin, and occasionally also eosinophilic intranuclear inclusions (**Fig. 3**). Inflammation,

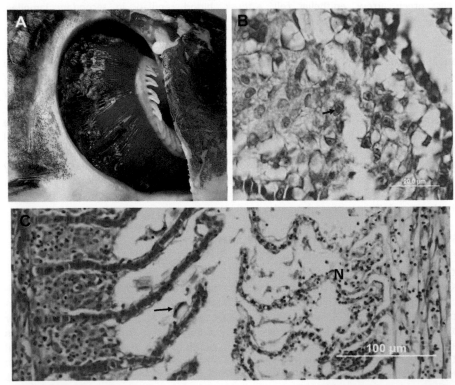

Fig. 3. KHVD. (*A*) Koi carp (bronze nezu ogon) with severe gill necrosis and secondary growth of green algae. (*B*) Histopathology of gills with hyperplasia and edema of gill epithelium with intranuclear herpesviral inclusion (*arrow*). (*C*) Histopathology of 2 primary gill primary lamellae. One is completely necrotic (N) and the contralateral shows hyperplasia of basal epithelium with inflammatory infiltrate comprising small lymphocytes, macrophages, and EGCs and also secondary infection with *Trichodina* (*arrow*).

necrosis, and intranuclear inclusions have been observed also in other organs (kidney, spleen, pancreas, liver, brain, gut, and oral epithelium). Secondary infections by skin and gill protozoal parasites, monogeneans, as well as fungi and bacteria are common.

Final diagnosis must be done by PCR detection of viral DNA or virus isolation and identification.

Moribund or freshly dead carp displaying typical clinical disease signs are suitable for testing. Whole alive or euthanized fish or collected organ (gill, kidney, and spleen) samples should be sent to the laboratory in sealed aseptic containers on ice. Small samples of tissue in alcohol (eg, 80%–100% ethanol) also may be submitted for PCR-based testing. Fish carcasses showing advanced autolysis are not suitable for testing.

There is no treatment for KHV. Fish that survive the disease may carry the virus and act as a source of infection for a very long time. Commercial vaccine is currently not available but has been proven experimentally to protect fish for at least 8 months.[14] The only available live attenuated immersion vaccine is commercialized and used exclusively in Israel (KV3, Phibro Animal Health Corporation, Teaneck, NJ, USA).

Carp edema virus disease/koi sleepy disease

The disease was first reported in Japan in the 1970s. Nowadays it is spread worldwide and may cause high morbidity and mortality in common carp and its ornamental varieties.

Etiology and pathogenesis

Carp edema virus (CEV) is a poxvirus infecting mainly juvenile stressed koi carps. Mortality in naïve koi or common carp exposed by bath challenge to CEV begins as early as day 6 and continues until day 16 postinfection. It is likely that virus shedding into the water occurs from gill and skin lesions of sick fish. Vertical transmission has not been confirmed. Optimal water temperature for development of clinical signs is between 15°C and 25°C,[15,16] but outbreaks have been observed in wild common carp at much lower water temperatures, between 6°C and 9°C.[17] Decreased morbidity and mortality has been observed in temperature over 28°C.

Clinical signs include that fish typically lie motionless on the bottom of the pond and die within 2 weeks. Affected animals are lethargic, hanging just under the surface of the water, have sunken eyes (enophthalmos), erosive or hemorrhagic skin lesions with edema (especially in juvenile fish), and pale swollen gills.[18]

Histopathology shows hyperplasia or "clubbing" of secondary lamellae,[19,20] inflammation and gill necrosis, skin ulcerations, and edema. Secondary infections by skin and gill protozoal parasites, monogeneans, as well as fungi and bacteria are common.[19,20]

Definitive diagnosis is made by isolation of the virus or by PCR detection. Gill biopsy in live fish or samples of gills, skin lesions, spleen, and kidney are suitable for virus detection.

There is no treatment for CEV, but some measures may be applicable, such as 0.5% salt bath, which helps to prevent the disease.[17,20,21] The salt does not treat infection, but decreases the amount of nitrates that can cause methemoglobinemia, which is a predisposing factor for infection. Immediate isolation and testing of sick fish showing suspect clinical signs is recommended, as well as removal of dead fish from ponds to minimize disease transmission. Freshly arrived koi carp should be quarantined at a temperature between 15°C and 25°C for at least 30 days.

Bacterial Diseases

Bacteria are a normal component of the aquatic environment and usually cause clinically apparent disease only in certain circumstances. Stress is the most important factor for establishment of bacterial infection, due to impairment of the immune system. The main stress factors are overcrowding, transport/handling, hypoxia, high ammonia and nitrates, and inappropriate temperature for the fish species. The gills are a common target of bacterial infection and present a point of entry for systemic bacteremia. Clinical signs are similar for many bacterial species and bacterial culture or molecular biology techniques, such as PCR or matrix assisted laser desorption ionization-time of flight mass spectrometry, are generally required to identify bacteria specifically. The most important bacteria in ornamental fish are gram-negative bacteria from genera *Aeromonas*, *Flavobacterium*, *Citrobacter,* and *Pseudomonas*. Gram-positive bacteria are less common and include mainly genera *Streptococcus*, *Lactococcus*, *Enterococcus*, and *Vagococcus*.[22]

Flavobacterium columnare (formerly *Flexibacter/Cytophaga columnaris)* and motile aeromonads, most importantly *Aeromonas hydrophylla*, are gram-negative bacteria causing gill and skin infections in temperate and tropical fish, including many ornamental fish. Infected fish show gill necrosis, skin erosions, and ulcerations and fin rot if the infection is only superficial. Superficial infection may progress to systemic disease, leading to bacteremia, septic shock, and death.[23] Typical signs of systemic involvement are ascites (dropsy), renal and splenic necrosis, and multifocal skeletal muscle hemorrhage. Presumptive diagnosis of bacterial infection can be made by microscopy of gill and skin scrapes. Large numbers of rod bacteria are often seen at medium and high-power magnification. *F columnare* often forms typical haystacklike colonies (**Fig. 4**).

Treatment
Treatment includes correcting any water quality problems or removing stressors in the environment. Introduction of UV light and salt bath (0.5% salt bath) also often helps to combat bacterial infections. Antibiotic treatment should always be based on culture and testing of sensitivity of the strain to specific antibiotics. Many antibiotics have been shown to have activity against bacteria affecting fish (eg, enrofloxacin, chloramphenicol, erythromycin, furazolidone, kanamycin, lincomycin, nalidixic acid, oxytetracycline, florfenicol, nitrofurazone, trimethoprim-sulfamethoxazole, and streptomycin).[24] Nowadays, multiresistant bacterial strains are seen and antibiotic treatment is often very difficult. Antibiotics can be administered by injection, mixed in feed, or in a bath treatment. Pharmacokinetics differ in different types of antibiotics

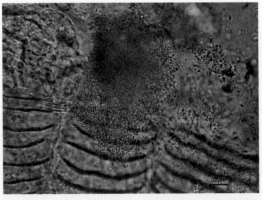

Fig. 4. *Flavobacterium columnare,* skin scrape, typical haystack like colonies of rods on a scale.

and depend on fish species and water temperature. The goal is to reach minimal inhibitory concentration (MIC) in the blood and therefore in tissues. The dose of antibiotics is often not based on extensive experimental work in ornamental fish, but has been known from clinical experience and approximated from farm fish. Injection is the most effective method of administration, but is time-consuming and applicable only in larger individuals. Intramuscular and intraperitoneal route of administration is recommended. Oral administration is possible only in fish that are still eating. The antibiotics may be mixed into the feed in the factory during feed processing (premix) or added after production. Ideal is a dry feed with high absorbing capacity. Some amount of antibiotic is washed out in water so the feed should be eaten very quickly after immersion. Medicated bath is less effective and requires a high dose of antibiotics to reach MIC. High dose of antibiotics in water often harms bacterial filters and may cause life-threatening worsening of water parameters. Daily major water changes are often necessary. For the dosages of antibiotics, see Noga,[4] Stoskopf,[25] and Carpenter and colleagues.[26]

Mycobacteriosis

Mycobacteriosis in fish is a chronic progressive ubiquitous disease caused mainly by *Mycobacterium marinum*, *Mycobacterium gordonae*, and *Mycobacterium fortuitum*.[27] Usually it is a systemic disease causing granulomatous type of inflammation in many organs and tissues, mainly in kidney, liver, skin, and mesenteric adipose tissue. Gills are less commonly affected.

Lethargy and emaciation are the main clinical signs. Compression fresh tissue preparations and histopathology show multiple granulomas in the infected tissues and Ziehl-Neelsen stain highlights myriad of acid-fast rods (**Fig. 5**). Definitive diagnosis is made by culture in specific media (Lowenstein-Jensen) and/or PCR.

Treatment is very difficult and is generally not attempted in practice; sick fish should be euthanized. Mycobacterium has great resistance to disinfectants and requires long contact times for most disinfectants to be effective; 5% phenol, 1% sodium hypochlorite, iodine solutions, glutaraldehyde, and formaldehyde are usually effective.

Fish mycobacteriosis has zoonotic potential, mainly in immunocompromised humans (fish tank granuloma on fingers to severe systemic illness leading to death).

Nocardiosis

Nocardiosis is caused by several species of *Nocardia* in fish (*Nocardia asteroides*, *Nocardia seriolae*, *Nocardia salmonicida*, and *Nocardia crassostreae*).This branching filamentous bacterium causes a granulomatous inflammation and may be Ziehl-Neelsen positive, which makes this disease a main differential diagnosis for mycobacteriosis.

Clinical signs include erratic swimming, anorexia, emaciation, and abdominal distension with grossly apparent white granulomas (nodules). Granulomas are seen on compression smears from gills and other organs. Definitive diagnosis is made by PCR.[28]

Treatment with doxycycline, sulfamethoxazole, and minocycline has been successful in history, but antibiotics are not generally used to treat this infection. Administration of interleukin-12 and vaccines seems to be effective.[29]

Epitheliocystis

Epitheliocystis is a disease of the gills and skin of both marine and freshwater fish cause by chlamydialike organisms (several *Candidatus* species), characterized by the presence of cystic structures in the epithelial cells. This infection may cause severe respiratory distress and mortality.[30,31]

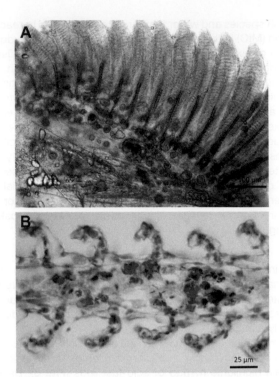

Fig. 5. Branchitis, granulomatous, severe. (*A*) Wet mount of gills from *Betta splendens* with mycobacteriosis with myriad of granulomas. (*B*) Histopathology of gill mycobacteriosis with numerous acid-fast rods within the granulomatous inflammation of primary lamellae and in blood vessel. Ziehl-Neelsen stain.

Clinically, the fish exhibit tachypnea, gasping, and lethargy. Grossly, there are multiple white nodules on the gills. Wet mounts reveal large numbers of bacteria in cystic structures. Histopathology confirms the presence of cystic structures filled with basophilic bacteria and usually also hyperplasia and/or necrosis of respiratory epithelium (**Fig. 6**). Mortality depends on the severity of infection and can range from 4% to 100%.[32]

Epitheliocystis has typical microscopic morphology (see **Fig. 6**), sufficient to make a definitive diagnosis, but it should be confirmed by PCR sequencing.

Data about treatment of epitheliocystis are limited. Oxytetracycline has been used in dosage of 25 ppm twice a day for 3 days.[33] Alternatively, nonantibiotic treatment has been used: formalin (30 ppm), salt (2 ppt), benzalkonium chloride (2 ppm), and potassium permanganate (4 ppm).[34]

Fungal Diseases

Mycotic disease in fish is often secondary, seen in immunosuppressed individuals often complicating bacterial and parasitic infections and also following skin trauma. Fungi belonging to the genus *Saprolegnia* or *Achlya* are the most commonly observed species. A gross presentation of *Saprolegnia/Achlya* infection would be fluffy white growths on the skin or gills (cotton wool disease).[35] Microscopically, typical fungal hyphae are found (**Fig. 7**). Treatment includes mechanical removal of the mycelia and

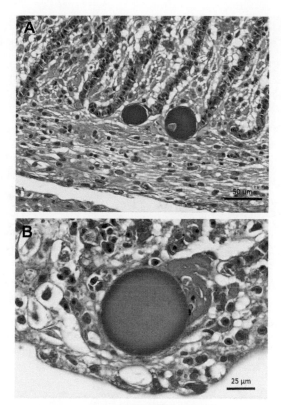

Fig. 6. Epitheliocystis. (*A*) Histopathology of gills with 2 cysts at the base of secondary lamellae and severe hyperplasia of the epithelium with fusion of secondary lamellae. (*B*) Detail of the cyst containing fine granular content.

medicated bath. These fungi are susceptible to several compounds including formaldehyde (1 mL/40 L for 2 hours), malachite green (1 mg/L for 1 hour) and salt (0.3%).

Gills can be primarily infected with *Branchiomyces sanguinis* or *Branchiomyces demigrans* (gill rot) causing ischemic gill necrosis, typically in cyprinid fish. This fungus grows in blood vessels and causes thrombosis. The infection occurs mainly in higher temperatures, in overcrowded ponds/tanks with high levels of ammonia or nitrate. Clinical signs include gasping and mottled or necrotic gills tissue. The diagnosis is made by histopathology confirming the presence of sporulating hyphae, with intrahyphal round bodies, within the blood vessels (**Fig. 8**). There is no reliable treatment and infected fish usually die.

Protozoan Diseases

White spot disease (Ich)
White spot disease in probably the most common protozoan skin and gill disease in ornamental fish. It is caused by the ciliated protozoan parasite *Ichthyophthirius multifiliis*. This parasite has a direct life cycle including the trophonts found on fish, a reproducing stage called tomont and motile, fish-seeking theront. The length of the life cycle depends on temperature. In warm water (25°C) it lasts 3 to 6 days. The parasite is highly infective and can cause severe mortality reaching 100%.[36]

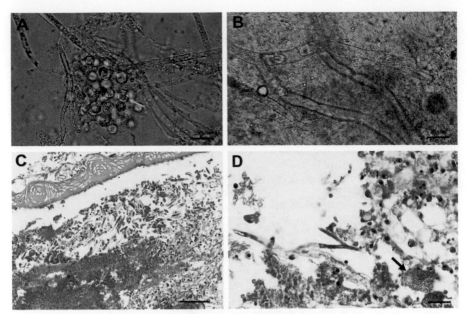

Fig. 7. Saprolegniasis. (*A*) Gill scrape with *Saprolegnia* hyphae with multiple oospores (*arrow*). (*B*) Dichotomous branching of hyphae. (*C*) Histopathology of severe gill necrosis with myriad of hyphae. (*D*). Detail of dichotomous branching of hyphae and bacterial colonies (*arrow*).

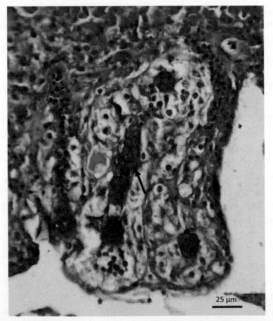

Fig. 8. Histopathology of Branchiomycosis. Gill of Koi carp with hyphae full of spores of *Branchiomyces sanguinis* occluding blood capillaries of secondary lamellae (*arrow*). Hematoxylin-eosin stain.

The disease presents as small white spots on the skin (**Fig. 9**A) and changes in behavior caused by irritation, such as flashing, gasping, and lethargy. The infection may be limited only to gills.

The diagnosis is made by clinical signs and microscopic examination of wet mounts of skin and gill scrapes, containing typical large, round to pear-shaped, slow motile ciliates with typical horseshoe nucleus and slow movement (**Fig. 9**B, C, Video 1) or by histopathology (**Fig. 9**D, E).

Treatment should follow immediately after diagnosis and consists of moving the fish to a quarantine tank, increasing water temperature to 28 to 30°C, and adding noniodized salt 1 to 5 g/L for 5 days. Some fish cannot tolerate high water temperature and in such cases the salt treatment should be prolonged to 7 to 8 days. In fish reared in low temperature, the increase of temperature should be slow, 1 °C per hour to reach maximum temperature tolerated by the fish species. The level of ammonia and nitrates should be checked every day during the treatment. If bath treatment is not possible (eg, in a pond with large koi carp) oral metronidazole in dose 25 mg/kg for 5 to 10 days can be used. Another possibility is prolonged bath in formalin at dosage 0.015 to 0.025 mL/L every other day for 3 treatments.[37]

Marine white spot disease

The marine counterpart of ichthyophthiriosis is *Cryptocaryon irritans*. The life cycle and symptoms are very similar to those of *I multifiliis*. Obviously we cannot use salt for

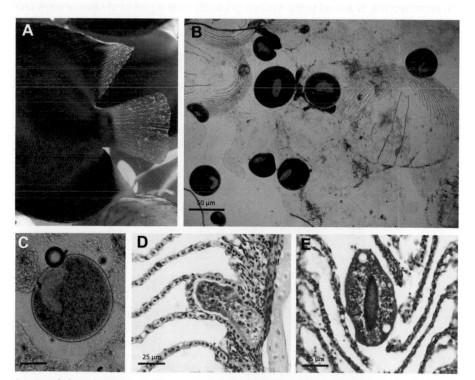

Fig. 9. *Ichthyophthirius multifilis.* (A) Discus (*Symphysodon aequifasciatus*) with large amount of tiny white dots on caudal and dorsal fin consistent with *I multifiliis*. (*B, C*) Wet mount of skin and gill scrapes with typical *I multifiliis* organisms. (*D, E*) Histopathology of gills with *I multifiliis* buried in the basal epithelium of secondary lamellae and free among the secondary lamellae. Hematoxylin-eosin stain.

treatment, and it is usually treated by formalin 25 ppm every other day for 2 weeks with a complete water change on alternate days.[38]

Oodiniosis

Oodiniosis, also known as velvet disease, is caused by the dinoflagellates *Piscinoodinium pillulare* and *Piscinoodinnium limneticum* in freshwater fish and *Amyloodinium ocellatum* in marine fish. Trophonts are attached to the gill or epidermal epithelium by an attachment disc comprising nail-like organelles, the rhizocysts. Head-parts of the rhizocysts are inverted in separate compartments, rhizothecas, in the sole of the disc, while their long shafts are firmly embedded in the cytoplasm of cells. *Piscinoodinium* has well-developed chloroplasts visible under the microscope. The adult stages of the parasites are known as trophonts and are able to feed on adult fish. In the second stage, the parasites develop into tomonts, detach from the host, and begin developing motile dinospores. The dinospores may remain infective for as long as 15 days in the absence of a fish host.[39]

Clinical signs include a dense white dusting on the skin, dyspnea, lethargy, and death.[40] Diagnosis is made by microscopic examination of skin and gill scrapes with typical appearance of parasites (**Fig. 10**).

The most effective treatment in freshwater is increasing water temperature to 25° to 28° C and prolonged salt bath (noniodized salt 1 to 5 g/L for 5 days).

In marine species, the treatment of choice is copper. The copper, as a copper sulfate pentahydrate, is added to the system gradually over a period of several days until

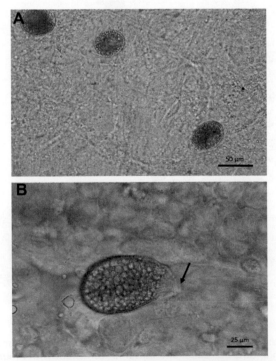

Fig. 10. *Piscinoodinium pillulare* in gill wet mount. (*B*) Detail of trophont of *P pillulare* attached to gill epithelial cell via an attachment disc (*arrow*) and large numbers of chloroplasts in the cytoplasm.

the free copper ion is at a concentration of 0.2 mg/L; this level is then maintained for up to 3 weeks. This treatment can kill all invertebrates and some fish species.[41]

Other common gill protozoan parasites are listed in **Table 1**. Generally, all the protozoan ectoparasitic infections usually respond well to salt treatment 0.3% for 3 to 5 days or formalin (35%–38%) in dose 0.1 to 0.2 mL/L for 30 minutes or 0.01 to 0.02 mL/L for 24 to 48 hours with extensive oxygenation of water. There may be differing individual responses to both salt and formalin and pretreatment testing on a low number of individuals should be performed.

Microsporidia

Microsporidians are obligate, spore-forming intracellular parasites, now belonging to fungi. A characteristic feature of microsporidia is the polar tube or polar filament found in the spore used to infiltrate host cells (**Fig. 16**). There are approximately 1400 described species of microsporidia. The microsporidian life cycle consists of a proliferative phase (merogony), the spore production phase (sporogony), and the mature spore or infective phase. Infected cells are markedly hypertrophic and may form grossly visible structures called xenomas. The most important genera infecting gills are *Glugea, Loma,* and *Heterosporis.*

Spores are typically very tenacious and can often survive for more than 1 year in the environment. Most microsporidian infections are very difficult to treat. Fumagillin and albendazol showed some effect to slow infection.[42]

Metazoan Diseases

Myxozoa

Myxozoa are primitive metazoan parasites characterized by spores, called myxospores, containing a polar capsule with polar filament (**Fig. 17**). These parasites may infect various tissues, including gills. Many freshwater fish myxozoans have an indirect life cycle, which involves asexual reproduction in the vertebrate (fish) host and sexual reproduction in an invertebrate host (oligochaete, polychaete, or bryozoan). Genera most commonly infecting gills are *Myxobolus, Henneguya, Thelohanellus,* and *Sphaerospora.* Diagnosis is usually easily made by microscopic examination of wet mounts of affected tissue with presence of myriad of typical myxospores or via histopathology with Giemsa stain (see **Fig. 17D**).

Treatment is difficult and usually not applied. Prevention of infection is the best approach in management of this infection.

Monogenean trematodes (flukes)

Monogenean trematodes are common skin and gill parasites with a direct life cycle in both marine and freshwater fish and can cause considerable damage to the host when

Table 1	
List of common freshwater and marine gill protozoan parasites	
Freshwater	**Marine**
Tetrahymena, *Chilodonella piscicola* (**Fig. 11**), *Chilodonella hexasticha,* Trichodina (**Fig. 12**), Trichodinella, Trichophrya, Tripartiella, Dipartiella, Paratrichodina, Hemitrichodina, Vauchomia, Apiosoma, Riboscyphidia, Ambiphrya, Epistylis (**Fig. 13**)	*Brooklynella hostilis,* Scuticociliatosis (**Fig. 15**) (eg, *Uronema marinum, Miamiensis avidus*)
Ichthyobodo necator (form. *Costia necatrix,* **Fig. 14**), *Cryptobia branchialis.*	

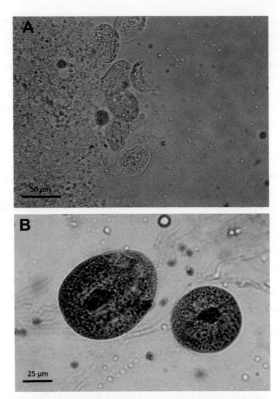

Fig. 11. *Chilodonella* sp. Wet mount of gill scrape (*A*) and after adding Giemsa stain (*B*).

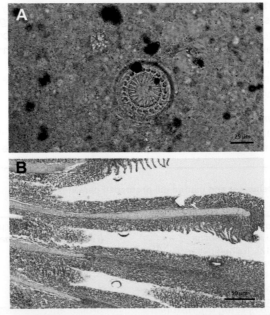

Fig. 12. *Trichodina* sp. (*A*) Gill scrape with individual *Trichodina* sp with obvious denticle ring. (*B*) Histopathology of gills with cross sections through the 3 individual *Trichodina* organisms among the secondary gill lamellae with severe proliferative branchitis.

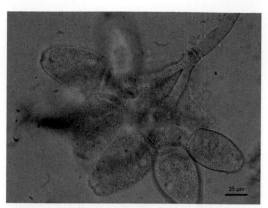

Fig. 13. Gill scrape with colony of *Epistylis* sp: stalk with 5 zoites.

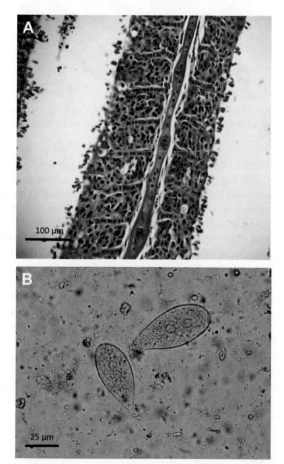

Fig. 14. *Ichthyobodo necator.* (*A*). Histopathology of proliferative branchitis with myriad of *I necator* attached. Hematoxylin-eosin. (*B*). Trophozoite of *I necator* from gill scrape stained with methylene blue.

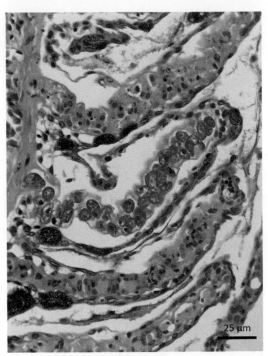

25 μm

Fig. 15. Histopathology of *Scuticociliatosis*. Gills of zebra shark (*Stegostoma fasciatum*) with intravascular pyriform ciliated protozoa-probable *Philasterides dicentrarchi*. Hematoxylin-eosin.

present in higher numbers. Approximately 4000 species of these parasites are known. Some species live also in the esophagus, stomach, ureters, and even kidney. The best known genera in freshwater fish are *Dactylogyrus* and *Gyrodactylus*, and in marine fish *Benedenia* and *Neobenedenia* (Capsalidae). The flukes possess a multiple-hooked attachment organ called an opisthaptor, damaging skin and gills. They can be oviparous or viviparous and may complete their entire life cycle on a single host. In some viviparous species, the cycle may be as short as 24 hours, if all environmental conditions are optimal. Generally families with eye spots (eg, *Dactylogyrus*) lay eggs. *Eudiplozoon nipponicum*, an oviparous, strict gill parasite of common carp has quite unusual morphology, forming fused sexually immature, post-oncomiracidial stages with interconnection of their nervous systems (permanent copula) (**Fig. 18**). Free-swimming ciliated larvae (oncomiracidia) hatch in water temperature of approximately 25 °C in a few days; in cold water (about 10°C) it can take weeks to hatch. Poor environmental conditions, crowding, and other stress factors predispose fish to infection. Transmission is by direct contact.[43]

Clinical signs include lethargy, pale mucous membranes (anemia), decreased appetite, flashing (rubbing against objects in the pond/aquarium), and excessive mucus production. Typical skin lesions are erythema, scale loss, white to gray irregular patches, erosions, and ulceration. Gills are swollen and pale. Diagnosis is made by microscopic examination of wet mount/scrapes from gills and skin or by histopathology (**Fig. 19**, Video 2).

Treatment. Most freshwater monogeneans can be killed quickly with a 3-minute to 5-minute saltwater bath (0.3%). Another possibility is formalin bath 0.2 mL/L for

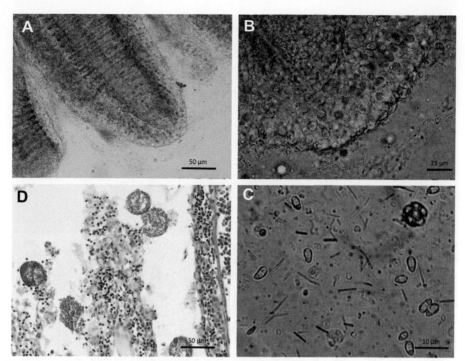

Fig. 16. Microsporidia. (*A, B*) Wet mount of gills with myriad of sporophorous vesicles with large numbers of spores. (*D*) Histopathology of gills with multiple sporophorous vesicles with large numbers of spores, hematoxylin-eosin. (*C*) Detail of ruptured sporophorous vesicle with individual spores typical of microsporidia, genus *Glugea*.

60 minutes every other day for 3 days. Praziquantel baths have also proved to be effective at dosage of 2 to 5 mg/L in a prolonged bath for 2 to 3 weeks. Praziquantel may also be given orally by mixing it into feed at the rate of 40 mg/kg of body weight per day; the praziquantel-medicated feed should be administered for 11 days. Alternative to praziquantel is fenbendazole at dose 25 mg/kg for 12 hours. In marine systems, copper treatments applied at 0.2 mg/L active copper ion for up to 3 weeks, but some fish species may not tolerate this treatment. Salinities less than 20 ppt may significantly reduce numbers of monogeneans in marine fish. Two 40-hour baths (48 hours apart) in 5 mg/L praziquantel in seawater were required to remove all parasites from branchial and nasal tissues.[44]

Digenean trematodes

Most digenean fluke problems appear to be primarily aesthetic in nature among tropical fish. Fish commonly serve as an intermediate host for these parasites, which frequently have a complex life cycle. Not many digenean parasites are found on gills. One of these is *Centrocestus formosanus* originating in Asia. Metacercariae of this parasite live in the gills of freshwater fish, the adult stage inhabiting the small intestine of birds and mammals.[45] An intermediate host is an aquatic snail *Melanoides tuberculatus*. The metacercariae induce a reactive chondroplasia in the gills. Diagnosis is made by microscopy of wet mounts from gill tissue. Treatment is difficult and management is focused on eradication of the intermediate host.

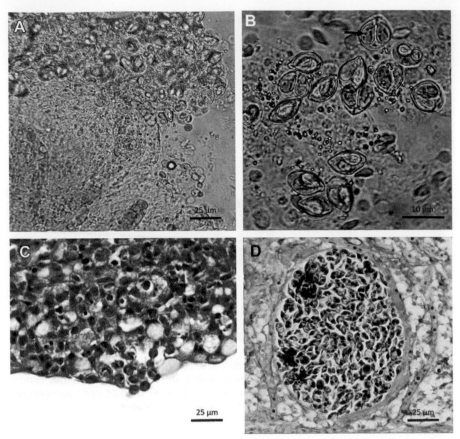

Fig. 17. Myxosporea (A) and (B) gill wet mounts with *Myxobolus koi* from a Koi carp with (B) detail of typical myxosporan spores with 2 polar capsules (*arrow*) containing polar filament. (C) Histopathology of a Koi carp with *Sphaerospora molnari* infection. Hematoxylin-eosin. (D) Histopathology of gills of bream (*Abramis brama*) with spherical pseudocyst containing spores of *Myxobolus* (probable *M parviformis*).

Crustacean Diseases

Copepods

Copepods are parasites of both marine and freshwater fish. They may attach to gill arches, oral cavity, or skin and cause erosion and/or ulceration. The most important genera are *Ergasilus, Laernea, Caligus, Pseudocaligus, Lepeophtheirus, Salmincola,* and *Achtheres*. The life cycle of copepods usually comprises 1 to 5 free-living nauplius stages, 1 to 5 free-living or parasitic copepodid stages, 1 pre - adult, and the adult stage. Gill copepods have a single median eye on their head and antennae. The second antennae are modified into prehensile pincers. In low numbers they cause only minor harm, but severe infections can cause severe damage to gills due to the parasites feeding on the delicate tissue of the gill lamellae or on the blood circulating within the lamellar capillaries, resulting in respiratory impairment and increased risk of secondary infections, with consequent stress and osmoregulatory failure.[46,47]

The parasites are grossly observed on the gills or on the operculum. Treatment may be difficult and is based on bathing in organophosphates or feeding avermectins. The

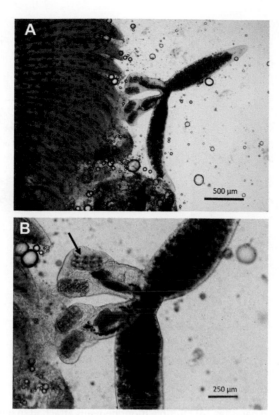

Fig. 18. Monogenean parasite *Eudiplozoon nipponicum* from the gills of a koi carp, wet mount. Two individuals form a permanent copula (*A*). Each individual bears both male and female gonads. Parasite is attached to gills via a haptor (*B, arrow*).

organophosphate diflubenzuron bath (also known as Dimilin) can be used at a dose of 0.066 mg diflubenzuron/l. The licensed product SLICE (MSD Animal Health) contains emamectin and is fed in a dosage 50 μg emamectin benzoate/kg body weight for 7 days.[48] Treatment with lufenuron (Program; Novartis) may be also effective at a dosage of 0.1 mg/L once per week for 5 weeks.[49] Fish can also be removed from the system for 7 days to break the life cycle.

Quarantine in fish to prevent infections
Quarantine is a crucial measure to prevent viral, bacterial, and parasitic infection of tank/pond. *All newly arrived fish should be considered as infected.* The fish should be quarantined for at least 21 days before they are placed into the main tank or a pond. New fish should be carefully examined clinically and by microscopic examination of skin and gill scrapes. Ideally, in the case of small ornamental fish, 1 to 3 individual should be killed and complete examination of fresh mounts of internal organs and/or histopathology should be performed. Any identified infections should be specifically treated. The design of a quarantine system should be very simple (glass, water, and fish) so that fish are readily accessible for observation and handling and so that water can be easily changed and treatments easily administered. Basic water parameters (temperature, pH, ammonium, nitrate, nitrites) should be daily measured.

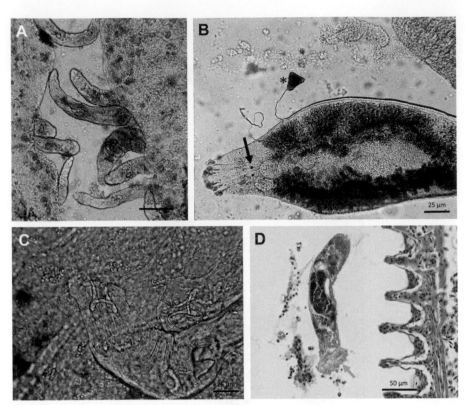

Fig. 19. Monogenean parasites. (*A*) Multiple monogeneans attached to gills, wet mount. (*B*) Detail of the oviparous monogenean (*Dactylogyrus* sp) with 4 eye spots (*arrow*) and an egg (***) with a fine filament. (*C*) Detail of the anchors (*orange arrow*) of the opisthohaptor, wet mount. (*D*) Histopathology of fluke gill infection with one monogenean with typical opisthohaptor (*green arrow*), hematoxylin-eosin.

NONINFECTIOUS DISEASES
Neoplasms

Gill neoplasms are rare, with only a few recorded cases, mostly of primary, spontaneous tumors, such as branchioblastoma (**Fig. 20**), branchial chondroma, osteochondroma, and osteosarcoma. There are also virally induced tumors, most often caused by retro viruses such as lymphoma and sarcomas (eg, fibrosarcoma, leiomyosarcoma). Main differential diagnosis of neoplastic proliferation is chronic inflammation, including parasitic granulomas and xenomas.

Environmental Diseases

Hypoxia

The amount of dissolved oxygen (DO) in water depends mainly on water temperature, but salinity and altitude also play a role. Damage of gill respiratory epithelium disables gas exchange and causes secondary hypoxia. There are 2 sources of DO in water: diffusion of atmospheric oxygen and photosynthesis of water plants. The concentration of DO can fluctuate diurnally, typically in ponds, with the lowest DO just before sunrise and highest level just before dusk. Oxygen is used by all living organisms in the pond or tank, including algae and bacteria. The pond with large numbers of fish, large

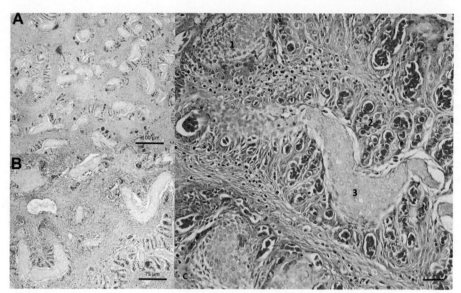

Fig. 20. Barnchioblastoma in Koi carp. Neoplastic mass is composed of 3 haphazardly inter-mingled cellular populations embedded in small amounts of dense fibrous stroma. Structure of neoplasm in low (A), medium (B), and high (C) power. These cell populations consist of dense aggregates of basophilic blastemal cells (1), polygonal to cuboidal epithelial cells formed into secondary lamellaelike structure (2) and islands of cartilage (3). Photograph courtesy of Chris Knott.

amounts of algae, and organic detritus decomposed by bacteria is highly susceptible to hypoxia, especially in high water temperatures in summer. Minimal concentration of DO for most fish species is 5.0 mg/L. Some species have accessory organs to absorb atmospheric oxygen in case of low DO such as labyrinthine organ in suprabranchial chamber (Betta, Gourami) or modified gut mucosa (Callichthys, Hypostomus).

Hypoxia may be acute or chronic. Acute hypoxia is usually caused by failure of aeration or oxygen generators in aquaria or closed aquaculture systems, usually due to a power cut. Subacute hypoxia or suffocation is observed in ponds with large amounts of aquatic plants and/or algae, which are the major producers, albeit consumers of DO, and with no additional mechanical aeration. This event happens in early morning when the concentration of DO is lowest. Chronic hypoxia, due to long exposure to suboptimal concentration of DO, is observed in overcrowded tanks with low numbers of water plants.

Clinical signs of acute hypoxia are crowding of fish near the water surface or near the water source, piping, and tachypnea. Fish that have died from asphyxia have wide open mouth and flared opercula. Chronic hypoxia causes anorexia, slow growth and reproduction, and higher susceptibility to infections. Definitive diagnosis is made by measuring the concentration of DO.

Treatment of acute hypoxia includes intensive mechanical aeration and major water exchange if possible. Hydrogen peroxide can increase DO short term by spraying of 3% solution into water.[50]

Ammonia, nitrite, and nitrate intoxication

All organic matter in water is decomposed by bacterial oxidation of ammonia (NH_3 and ionized NH_4) to nitrite (NO_2) and nitrate (NO_3). Ammonia is the primary degradation product of nitrogenous compounds and is consumed by denitrifying bacteria and algae. It is highly toxic for fish with lethal concentration ≥ 1.00 mg/L. Un-ionized NH_3 is more toxic than ionized forms. Chronic exposure to sublethal concentration (≥ 0.05 mg/L) causes chronic stress.[51,52] If the bacterial degradation of ammonia or consumption by algae are impaired, the concentration rapidly rises. The amount of ammonia depends also on pH and water temperature, with highest concentrations in alkaline hot water. The causes of rising of ammonia are lack of denitrifying bacteria and/or algae, large amount of decaying organic substrate, and increase in pH or temperature. In fish, ammonia is the main product of protein catabolism and it is eliminated by diffusion through the gill epithelium. Accelerated protein catabolism or damage to the gill epithelium may lead to hyperammonemia and ammonia autointoxication.[53]

Acute ammonia intoxication displays clinically as anorexia, hyperexcitability, convulsion, and death probably due to displacement of K^+ by elevated $NH4^+$ and depolarization of neurons, causing an influx of excessive Ca^{2+} and subsequent neuron death.[54] Chronic ammonia intoxication is associated with gill hyperplasia, high mortality, and decreased feed intake.[55]

Nitrite intoxication occurs when nitrite oxidizing bacteria (eg, *Nitrobacter*) do not efficiently convert nitrite to nitrate. Nitrate enters the bloodstream via gills and oxidizes the hemoglobin to methemoglobin, which leads to methemoglobinemia (brown blood disease). Methemoglobin cannot bind oxygen properly, leading to tissue hypoxia. Clinical signs include dyspnea, light tan to brown gills and tan to chocolate brown blood. Some fish species (eg, Centrarchids) are fairly resistant to increased levels of nitrite in the water so clinical signs may differ in the fish tank with different fish species. Treatment should include a major water change if possible, adding salt (sodium chloride 1–2 g/L), because chlorine ions competitively inhibit nitrite absorption through the gills[56,57]; and removal of organic debris (slime).

Nitrate has relatively low toxicity due to the low permeability of gills for nitrate. Nitrate level usually rises in ponds/tanks with absence of water plants, which usually absorb nitrate from water. The pathogenesis of intoxication is similar to that with nitrite, that is, oxidation of hemoglobin to methemoglobin. Susceptibility of fish to levels of nitrate is species dependent.[58] We usually see subacute to chronic cases with symptoms such as lethargy, slow growth, increased susceptibility to diseases, delayed wound healing, dilated blood vessels, gill hyperplasia (environmental branchitis) and skin hyperemia. Chronic exposure to nitrates may lead to goiter (mainly in sharks) due to competition of nitrate and iodine for the same ion uptake system.[59] The treatment is similar to treatment of nitrite intoxications.

Gas bubble disease (supersaturation)

Gas bubble disease (GBD) is caused by supersaturated levels of total dissolved gas in the water and creates gas emboli in capillaries and small blood vessels. Gas supersaturation occurs in tanks when gas is injected into the water under pressure or when air bubbles are developed at great depth. Fish with GBD often exhibit loss of equilibrium, abnormal buoyancy, and may float at the water surface. Fish may also exhibit skin hemorrhage, blindness, convulsions, and bubbles in subcutis (emphysema), exophthalmos, and gas bubbles in the anterior ocular chamber.[60]

SUMMARY

Successful treatment of gill diseases in fish requires a systematic approach, including analysis of water environment, husbandry, and epidemiology. Some gill diseases are relatively easily treatable, but in many cases a cure is unavailable and only establishing the correct diagnosis can ensure proper management of disease. Absence of quarantine is a frequent reason for spread of infectious diseases from newly acquired fish to well-established and prosperous fish tank or pond, hence to prevent extensive and often very expensive and problematic treatment it is crucial to isolate all new fish. This article provides a review of the most common gill diseases in fish, and their diagnostics, therapy, and prevention.

CLINICS CARE POINTS

- Environmental (eg, poor water quality) and social (eg, overcrowding) stress are frequent inciting factors of infectious gill diseases.
- Bacterial infections in fish are often secondary and antibiotic treatment may be unsuccessful if the primary cause (parasites, poor water quality) is not eliminated.
- Many bacterial strains show multiresistance to antibiotics, so targeted therapy based on bacteriology and antibiotic sensitivity testing is crucial.
- All koi carps should be tested for KHVD and CEV if there is a mortality in the pond and during a quarantine.
- All newly acquired fish should be taken as infectious and go through a quarantine.

ACKNOWLEDGMENTS

I wish to thank Jan Misik for providing an excellent technical assistance and Chris Knott for correction of this manuscript and microphotographs of branchioblastoma.

DISCLOSURE

There are not any commercial or financial conflicts of interest and any funding sources.

SUPPLEMENTARY DATA

Supplementary data related to this article can be found online at https://doi.org/10.1016/j.cvex.2021.01.001.

REFERENCES

1. Laurent P, Dunel-Erb S. The pseudobranch: morphology and function. In: Hoar W, editor. Fish physiology. Oxford (UK): Academic Press; 1984. p. 285–323.
2. Yang SH, Kang CK, Hu YC, et al. Comparisons of two types of teleostean pseudobranchs, silver moony (*Monodactylus argenteus*) and tilapia (*Oreochromis mossambicus*), with salinity-dependent morphology and ion transporter expression. J Comp Physiol B 2015;185(6):677–93.
3. Sfacteria A, Brines M, Blank U. The mast cell plays a central role in the immune system of teleost fish. Mol Immunol 2015;63(1):3–8.
4. Noga EJ. Pharmacopoeia. In: Noga EJ, editor. Fish disease: diagnosis and treatment. Hoboken (NJ): John Wiley & Sons; 2010. p. 375–420.
5. Kielpinski M, Kempter J, Panicz R, et al. Detection of KHV in freshwater mussels and crustaceans from ponds with KHV history in common carp (Cyprinus carpio). Isr J Aquac 2010;62(1):28–37.
6. Haramoto E, Kitajima M, Katayama H, et al. Detection of koi herpesvirus DNA in river water in Japan. J Fish Dis 2007;30(1):59–61.

7. Waltzek TB, Kelley GO, Alfaro ME, et al. Phylogenetic relationships in the family Alloherpesviridae. Dis Aquat Org 2009;84:179–94.

8. Perelberg A, Smirnov M, Hutoran M, et al. Epidemilogical description of a new viral disease afflicting cultured Cyprinus carpio in Israel. Isr J Aquac 2003; 55:5–12.

9. Shimizu T, Yoshida N, Kasai H, et al. Evaluation of survival of koi herpesvirus in environmental water. Fish Pathol 2006;41:153–7.

10. Kasai H, Muto Y, Yoshimizu M. Virucidal effects of ultraviolet, heat treatment and disinfectants against koi herpesvirus (KHV). Fish Pathol 2005;40(3):137–8.

11. Costes B, Raj VS, Michel B, et al. The major portal of entry of koi herpesvirus in Cyprinus carpio is the skin. J Virol 2009;83(7):2819–30.

12. Bretzinger ACHIM, Fischer-Scherl T, Oumouna M, et al. Mass mortalities in koi carp, Cyprinus carpio, associated with gill and skin disease. Bull Eur Assoc Fish Pathol 1999;19(5):182–5.

13. Hedrick RP, Waltzek TB, McDowell T. Susceptibility of koi carp, common carp, goldfish, and goldfish× common carp hybrids to cyprinid herpesvirus-2 and herpesvirus-3. J Aquat Anim Health 2016;18(1):26-34.

14. Ilouze M, Davidovich M, Diamant A, et al. The outbreak of carp disease caused by CyHV-3 as a model for new emerging viral diseases in aquaculture: a review. Ecol Res 2011;26(5):885–92.

15. Oyamatsu T, Hata N, Yamada K, et al. An etiological study on mass mortality of cultured colorcarp juveniles showing edema. Fish Pathol 1997;32:81–8.

16. Oyamatsu T, Matoyama HN, Yamamoto K, et al. A trial for the detection of Carp Edema Virus by using polymerase chain reaction. Suisanzoshoku 1997;45: 247–51.

17. Way K, Stone D. Emergence of carp edema virus-like (CEV-like) disease in the UK. Finfish News 2013;15:32–5.

18. Lewisch E, Gorgoglione B, Way K, et al. Carp edema virus/Koi sleepy disease: An emerging disease in Central-East Europe. Transbound Emerg Dis 2015; 62(1):6–12.

19. Ono SI, Nagai A, Sugai N. A histopathological study on juvenile colorcarp Cyprinus carpio, showing edema. Fish Pathol 1986;21:167–75.

20. Miyazaki T, Isshiki T, Katsuyuki H. Histopathological and electron microscopy studies on sleepy disease of koi Cyprinus carpio koi in Japan. Dis Aquat Organ 2005;65:197–207.

21. Seno R, Hata N, Oyamatsu T, et al. Curative effect of 0.5% salt water treatment on Carp, Cyprinus carpio, infected with Carp Edema Virus (CEV) results mainly from reviving the physiological condition of the host. Suisan Zoshoku 2003;51:123–4.

22. Lewbart GA. Bacteria and ornamental fish. In: Fudge AM, editor. Seminars in Avian and exotic pet medicine. Philadelphia (PA): WB Saunders; 2001. p. 48–56.

23. Walczak N, Puk K, Guz L. Bacterial flora associated with diseased freshwater ornamental fish. J Vet Res 2017;61(4):445–9.

24. Decostere A, Haesebrouck F, Devriese LA. Characterization of four Flavobacterium columnare (Flexibacter columnaris) strains isolated from tropical fish. Vet Microbiol 1998;62(1):35–45.

25. Stoskopf MK. Chemotherapeutics. In: Stoskopf MK, editor. Fish medicine. Philadelphia (PA): W.B. Saunders Co.; 1993. p. 832–9.

26. Carpenter JW, Mashima TY, Rupiper DJ. Exotic animal formulary. Manhattan (KS): Greystone Publications; 1996. p. 310.

27. Novotny L, Halouzka R, Matlova L, et al. Morphology and distribution of granulomatous inflammation in freshwater ornamental fish infected with mycobacteria. J Fish Dis 2010;33(12):947–55.

28. Xia L, Zhang H, Lu Y, et al. Development of a loop-mediated isothermal amplification assay for rapid detection of *Nocardia salmonicida*, the causative agent of nocardiosis in fish. J Microbiol Biotechnol 2015;25:321–7.

29. Matsumoto M, Araki K, Hayashi K, et al. Adjuvant effect of recombinant interleukin-12 in the Nocardiosis formalin-killed vaccine of the amberjack *Seriola dumerili*. Fish Shellfish Immunol 2017;67:263–9.

30. Stride MC, Polkinghorne A, Nowak BF. Chlamydial infections of fish: diverse pathogens and emerging causes of disease in aquaculture species. Vet Microbiol 2014;170(1–2):19–27.

31. Blandford MI, Taylor-Brown A, Schlacher TA, et al. Epitheliocystis in fish: an emerging aquaculture disease with a global impact. Transbound Emerg Dis 2018;65(6):1436–46.

32. Nowak BF, LaPatra SE. Epitheliocystis in fish. J Fish Dis 2006;29(10):573–88.

33. Goodwin AE, Park E, Nowak BF. Successful treatment of largemouth bass, *Micropterus salmoides* (L.), with epitheliocystis hyperinfection. J Fish Dis 2005;28(10):623–5.

34. Somridhivej B, Taveekijakarn P, Me-anan C, et al. Treatment of epitheliocystis in juvenile tilapia. In Proceedings of the 47th Kasetsart University Annual Conference, 2009 Kasetsart, March 17-20, 2009. Subject: Fisheries (pp. 1-8).

35. Khoo L. Fungal diseases in fish. In: owers L, editor. Seminars in avian and exotic pet medicine. Philadelphia (PA): WB Saunders; 2000. p. 102–11.

36. Wang Q, Yu Y, Zhang X, et al. Responses of fish to *Ichthyophthirius multifiliis* (Ich): a model for understanding immunity against protozoan parasites. Dev Comp Immunol 2019;93.93–102.

37. Gratzek JB, Blasiola G. Checklists, quarantine procedures, and calculations of particular use in fish health management. In: Gratzek JB, Matthews JR, editors. Aquariology: the science of fish health management. Morris plains (NJ): Tetra press; 1992. p. 301–15.

38. Dickerson HW, Dawe DL. *Ichthyophthirius multifiliis* and *Cryptocaryon irritans* (phylum Ciliophora). In: Fish diseases and disorders. Wallingford (England): CABI; 2006. p. 116–53.

39. Martins ML, Moraes JRE, Andrade PM, et al. *Piscinoodinium pillulare* (Schäperclaus, 1954) Lom, 1981 (Dinoflagellida) infection in cultivated freshwater fish from the Northeast region of São Paulo State, Brazil: parasitological and pathological aspects. Braz J Biol 2001;61(4):639–44.

40. Levy MG, Litaker RW, Goldstein RJ, et al. Piscinoodinium, a fish-ectoparasitic dinoflagellate, is a member of the class Dinophyceae, subclass Gymnodiniphycidae: convergent evolution with Amyloodinium. J Parasitol 2007;93(5):1006–15.

41. Reed PA, Francis-Floyd R. Amyloodinium infections of marine fish. Fact Sheet VM-90, a series of the College of Veterinary medicine, Florida Cooperative extension Service. Gainesville (FL): Institute of Food and Agricultural Sciences, University of Florida; 1994.

42. Speare DJ, Athanassopoulou F, Daley J, et al. A preliminary investigation of alternatives to fumagillin for the treatment of *Loma salmonae* infection in rainbow trout. J Comp Pathol 1999;121(3):241–8.

43. Buchmann K, Bresciani J. Monogenea (Phylum Platyhelminthes). Fish diseases and disorders. Wallingford (England): CABI; 2006. p. 297–344.

44. Chisholm LA, Whittington ID. Efficacy of praziquantel bath treatments for monogenean infections of the Rhinobatos typus. J Aquat Anim Health 2002;14(3): 230–4.
45. Han ET, Shin EH, Phommakorn S, et al. *Centrocestus formosanus* (Digenea: Heterophyidae) encysted in the freshwater fish, *Puntius brevis*, from Lao PDR. Korean J Parasitol 2008;46(1):49.
46. Lester RJG, Hayward CJ. Phylum Arthropoda. In: Woo PTK, editor. Fish diseases and disorders vol 1: Protozoan and Metazoan infections. London: CAB international; 2006. p. 466–565.
47. Vinoth R, Ajith Kumar TT, Ravichandran S, et al. Infestation of Copepod parasites in the food fishes of Vellar estuary, Southeast coast of India. Acta Parasitol Globalis 2010;1(1):1–5.
48. Hakalahti T, Lankinen Y, Valtonen ET. Efficacy of emamectin benzoate in the control of *Argulus coregoni* (Crustacea: Branchiura) on rainbow trout Oncorhynchus mykiss. Dis Aquat Organ 2004;60(3):197–204.
49. Mayer J, Hensel P, Mejia-Fava J, et al. The use of Lufenuron to treat fish lice (*Argulus* sp) in Koi (*Cyprinus carpio*). J Exot Pet Med 2013;22(1):65–9.
50. Taylor NI, Ross LG. The use of hydrogen peroxide as a source of oxygen for the transportation of live fish. Aquaculture 1988;70(1–2):183–92.
51. Arillo A, Margiocco C, Melodia F, et al. Ammonia toxicity mechanism in fish: studies on rainbow trout (*Salmo gairdneri* Rich.). Ecotoxicol Environ Saf 1981; 5(3):316–28.
52. Person-Le Ruyet J, Chartois H, Quemener L. Comparative acute ammonia toxicity in marine fish and plasma ammonia response. Aquaculture 1995;136(1–2): 81–194.
53. Smutna M, Vorlova L, Svobodova Z. Pathobiochemistry of ammonia in the internal environment of fish. Acta Vet Brno 2002;71(2):169–81.
54. Ip YK, Chew SF, Randall DJ. Ammonia toxicity, tolerance, and excretion. Fish Physiol 2001;20:109–48.
55. Wajsbrot N, Gasith A, Diamant A, et al. Chronic toxicity of ammonia to juvenile gilthead seabream *Sparus aurata* and related histopathological effects. J Fish Biol 1993;42(3):321–8.
56. Lewis Jr WM, Morris DP. Toxicity of nitrite to fish: a review. Trans Am Fish Soc 1986;115(2):183–95.
57. Tomasso JR. Toxicity of nitrogenous wastes to aquaculture animals. Rev Fish Sci 1994;2(4):291–314.
58. Svobodova Z, Machova J, Poleszczuk G, et al. Nitrite poisoning of fish in aquaculture facilities with water-recirculating systems. Acta Vet Brno 2005;74(1): 129–37.
59. Morris AL, Hamlin HJ, Francis-Floyd R, et al. Nitrate-induced goiter in captive whitespotted bamboo sharks Chiloscyllium plagiosum. J Aquat Anim Health 2011;23(2):92–9.
60. Speare DJ. Endothelial lesions associated with gas bubble disease in fish. J Comp Pathol 1991;104(3):327–35.

Diagnostic Imaging of the Respiratory Tract of the Reptile Patient

Michaela Gumpenberger, DVM*

KEYWORDS

- Diagnostic imaging • Radiography • CT • Respiratory tract • Reptile • Pneumonia
- Lung compression • Mass effect

KEY POINTS

- Diagnostic imaging (preferably radiography and/or computed tomography [CT]) should always be included in the clinical examination in any dyspneic reptile, especially in chelonians.
- For proper radiographic evaluation, 2 orthogonal radiographs are needed. In lizards and snakes dorsoventral and lateral views are used, whereas in chelonians an additional craniocaudal view is performed. Although the respiratory tract is less differentiable on a dorsoventral radiograph in chelonians, it can provide additional valuable informations.
- Lateral radiographs should be performed in horizontal beam technique.
- Exposure settings (for radiographs and CTs, respectively) may be adapted from protocols of the head of dogs for chelonians, whereas protocols of the thorax or abdomen of small mammals, cats or dogs may be adapted for similar sized lizards and snakes.
- Multiple figures will demonstrate the advantages of the different imaging techniques as well as the appearance of different respiratory diseases. The focus will be laid on chelonians, as they are less accessible for clinical examination.

SHORT INTRODUCTION TO IMAGING TECHNIQUES
Radiographic Technique and Positioning

Laterolateral (LL) and craniocaudal (CC, to compare right and left side) views are the basic and most important views for evaluation of the respiratory tract, especially the lungs, in *chelonians*. The radiographs should be performed with horizontal beam technique with the patient placed on an—ideally—radiolucent, stabile device or pedestal that is able to bear the weight and movement of the reptiles (**Fig. 1**). The legs should be extended as much as possible to minimize superimposition. For the same reason,

Diagnostic Imaging, Department for Companion Animals and Horses, University of Veterinary Medicine Vienna, Austria
* Diagnostic Imaging, vetmeduni Vienna, Veterinärplatz 1, Vienna 1210, Austria.
E-mail address: Michaela.Gumpenberger@vetmeduni.ac.at

Vet Clin Exot Anim 24 (2021) 293–320
https://doi.org/10.1016/j.cvex.2021.01.002
1094-9194/21/© 2021 Elsevier Inc. All rights reserved.

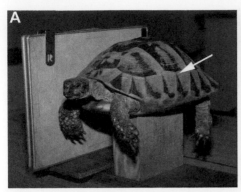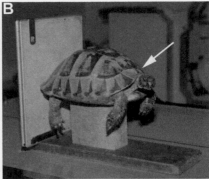

Fig. 1. Radiographic technique: lateral (*A*) and craniocaudal (*B*) views should be performed with horizontal beam technique in chelonians. The animals should retract the head and legs from the shell to reduce organ compression and superimposition. The beam is centered between the costal and marginal shields or on the nuchal shield (*arrow*), respectively. The pedestal should be high and small enough so that the patient cannot flee from the setup.

the head should be extracted and lowered for CC views. An additional dorsoventral (DV) view performed in table-top technique in perpendicular beam supports interpretation of the trachea or bronchi as well as all other organ systems that may influence lung capacity.[1] Some investigators point out the value of horizontal beam radiographs with chelonians in upright position when the benefit of gravity helps to detect larger free fluid accumulations.[2] It is not recommended to perform LL views in perpendicular beam with the animal, for example, taped to a device, as this will cause a shift of the coelomic organs and undesired superimposition of organ contours and is therefore prone to misinterpretation.[3]

Larger iguanas and *lizards* may be handled similarly to cats or dogs, whereas smaller species can be placed in a plastic box to perform standard DV and LL views

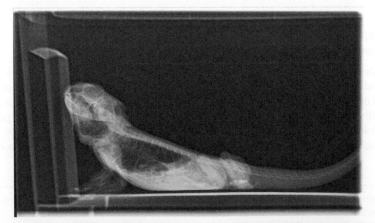

Fig. 2. Radiographic technique: lateral views may be performed with horizontal beam technique in lizards as well. Manual restraint can be avoided when using small translucent plastic boxes or tubes for positioning. Although images may be partially superimposed by the extremities, usually good to fair results are achieved. In this example a bearded dragon (*Pogona vitticeps*) was placed in a storage box. The normal lungs are clearly seen.

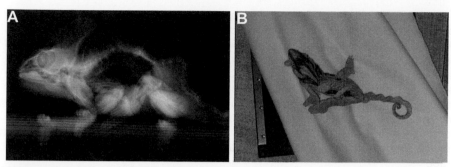

Fig. 3. Radiographic technique: lateral views (A) may be performed with horizontal beam technique without manual restrain in chameleons as well. A short branch or stick is used as a climbing device. For dorsoventral views (B) a paper towel is placed on the cassette to comfort the patient and avoid slipping.

(**Fig. 2**). The latter should be done in horizontal beam technique as described earlier. Smaller lizards can be manipulated with a Q-tip. Rübel and colleagues[4] used a stockinette tubing to immobilize some patients. Be aware that some species have a very delicate skin. *Chameleons* may be offered any climbing device for performing LL images in horizontal plane. These animals feel also more comfortable with some paper-towels to grab for DV radiographs (**Fig. 3**) in order to avoid manual restraint. However, this will result in some superimposition of the extremities. In case of disturbing superimposition, chameleons need to be stretched and positioned similarly to iguanas. Although manual restraint is done quickly and easily, it may not be allowed in all countries due to radiation safety regulations. Therefore, sedation may be needed when, for example, taping or tying the animal on the cassette or on the table. At the author's clinic alfaxalon, 7 mg/kg body weight (BW) intravenously or 10 mg/kg BW intramuscularly is used for sedation in reptiles. In chelonians intramuscular administration of midazolam (0.5 mg/kg BW) may be added.

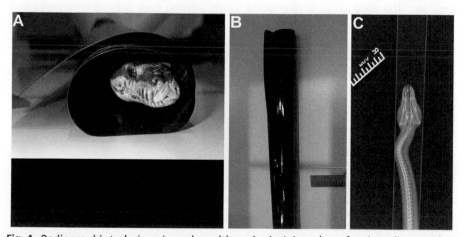

Fig. 4. Radiographic technique in snakes: although plexiglas tubes of various diameter (see **Fig. 6**) may act as positioning device, a cheaper tool of adaptable diameter is a rolled up old radiographic film (A, B). Exposed films have the advantage of being black, which is preferred by the snakes. The film causes no artifacts that would hinder image interpretation (C).

A meaningful *snake* radiograph can only be fabricated with an extended, properly positioned animal and when performing 2 orthogonal planes, namely DV and LL views. A long plastic tube (which has to be cleaned after each patient) or a coiled recycled old radiographic film (**Fig. 4**) can be used as positioning device in conscious patients. The latter is simple and cheap and can be replaced easily. In addition, dark tubes invite snakes to move in. A prewarmed table or cassette may comfort the snake or any other reptile as well. Lateral views performed in horizontal beam technique in inspiration provide better radiographs than in vertical beam in expiration. However, diagnostic value for mild-to-moderate lung changes is low in snake radiography. Furthermore, recent feeding may compromise pulmonary inflation due to distension of the gastrointestinal tract.

GENERAL TECHNICAL RECOMMENDATIONS FOR RADIOGRAPHIC EXAMINATIONS

A R/L marker should be used for any radiograph to ensure identification of the proper side affected. Usually there is rarely need for anesthesia to take overview radiographs of reptiles. Good radiographs are mostly achieved—after preparing the whole imaging setup—with quick positioning and some patience. If digital systems (cassette system, detector, or dental radiographic units) are used, increased milliampere-seconds (mAs) (in comparison to analogue settings) will prevent quantum noise and provide higher image resolution (**Fig. 5**). However, be aware of "chronic" overexposure and check the exposure index for adequate settings. Algorithm, kV, and mAs used for radiographs of the skull of cats or dogs should be adaptable for chelonians, those of the abdomen of smaller mammals for smaller lizards and smaller snakes, and those of the abdomen of cats or middle-sized dogs for larger iguanas and larger snakes, respectively. If analogue technique is used, high-resolution film-screen or even mammography and dental systems should be used, especially for smaller species. For example, at the authors clinic, a digital Fuji cassette and detector system is used when exposing 0.5 to 3 kg BW chelonians with 55 to 65 kV and 2.6 to 5.6 mAs with a film focus distance of 60 to 70 cm.

One advantage of digital radiography is the "postprocessing" opportunity on the computer. The wide range of gray scale allows altering contrast and brightness and

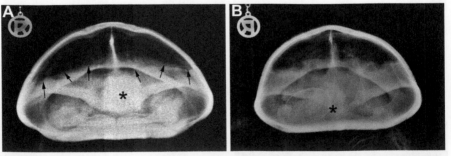

Fig. 5. Craniocaudal radiograph of 2 different Herman's tortoises (*Testudo hermanni*) in horizontal beam technique. The beam is centered on the nuchal shield. The head (*asterisk*) of the animals is lowered to hinder superimposition with the dorsally positioned lung fields (*arrows*). Note the mottled appearance of the soft tissues ventral to the lung border in (*A*). This is quantum noise due to insufficient exposure settings, usually mAs. The aerated lung is not influenced in this case. The animal in (*B*) is exposed with proper exposure setting. Note the eggs in (*B*). However, the craniocaudal view is not particularly useful in evaluating dystocia.

therefore adaption of the different soft tissues. Pathologic changes may also be highlighted by inverting the image or using high-resolution filters. Yet, one should be aware that improper positioning of the animal and poor exposure settings cannot be compensated with a computer.

Computed Tomography

Computed tomography (CT) is a cross-sectional imaging technique that provides sufficient resolution images without any superimposition for easier diagnostic and therapeutic approach (eg, carapacial osteotomy for sample taking or intrapulmonic therapy in chelonians). Depending on the mobility and temperament of the patient, CT examination can be performed in the unrestrained animal in a radiolucent box. Be aware that metallic hinges or locks of some boxes will cause beam hardening artifacts. The extremities of chelonians may be taped in physiologic position into their shell (**Fig. 6**A). However, this compromises the lung volume.[3] Otherwise, chelonians may be mounted on a box or wooden cube that is smaller than the plastron to prevent escaping from the scene (**Fig. 6**B). Depending on the indication for CT, movement of the head and extremities may not affect the diagnosis. Snakes can be placed into a tube similar as in radiographic examinations (**Fig. 6**C). Some animals can be

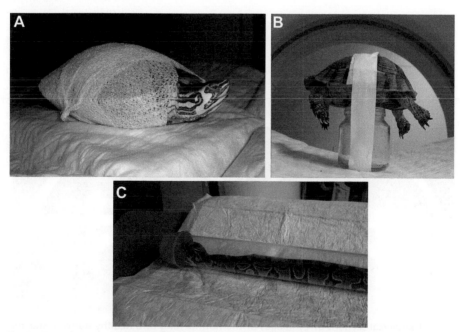

Fig. 6. CT technique: most animals are put in a box without further restraint. The legs are taped into the shell in physiologic position in some chelonians (*A*), whereas others are placed on a stabile for example, wooden block (*B*), depending on the temperament of the patient. Some snakes (*C*, placed in a tube) or lizards may need anesthesia to guarantee meaningful high-quality images. Symmetric images in not perfectly aligned patients are gained with multislice helical CT and modern software that allows multiplanar reconstruction (MPR) in any desired plane. Standard image interpretation includes sagittal, transversal, and coronal planes, whereas some disorders may profit from plane alignment along the trachea or bronchus.

calmed by blindfolding them. Mobile or agitated patients need to be sedated to receive images free of motion artifacts.[5]

At the authors clinic, CT scans (with a 16-slice helical CT) of chelonians and most other reptiles are performed with the following technical parameters: 100 to 130 kV, eff. 80 to 200 mAs, rotation time 0.6 sec, pitch 0.8, slice thickness 0.75 mm, and reconstruction increment 0.5 mm. As already suggested for digital radiography, processing programs can be adapted from small mammals, cats and dogs. The author prefers a high-resolution bony algorithm to interpret the respiratory tract as well as the skeleton, complemented by a soft tissue algorithm. It is essential to reconstruct various windows instead of manually shifting the window settings in a soft tissue window to mock a bony window. Good image quality depends on proper algorithms **(Fig. 7)**.

Densitometry (done in Hounsfield units, HU) enables further evaluation of tissues. Zero Hounsfield unit equals water whereas 20 to 100 HU represent different soft tissues. Cancellous bone measures more than 350 HU, whereas bone cortex or corticalis reach up to 2000 HU. Fat has a density of 0 HU to minus 100 HU and air minus 1000 HU. Therefore, densitometry supports, for example, diagnosis of hepatic lipidosis or infiltrations, which indicate pneumonia.[6]

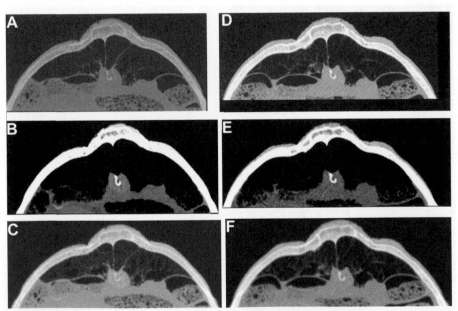

Fig. 7. Transversal sections of CT images of the normal lung of a healthy Burmese star tortoise (Geochelone platynota) demonstrating the importance of variable algorithm and exposure settings. (A) and (D) show a high detailed bony algorithm while (B) and (E) are a routine soft tissue window. Note the loss of pulmonary and bony detail in (D) and the increase of quantum noise in (D) and (E). The scans in (D), (E) and (F) were taken with only 50mAs and 80kV while (A), (B) and (C) were performed with 150mAs and 130kV. (C) and (F) demonstrate the poorer image quality of the soft tissue windows from (B) and (E) after manually shifting the window width and level to a bony window. It is important to recalculate different windows instead of pretending a bony window by adapting a soft tissue window.

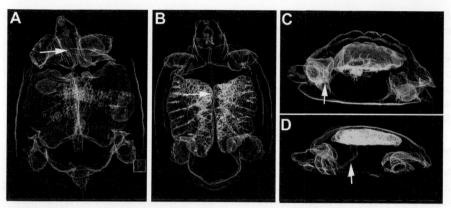

Fig. 8. A three-dimensional (3D) model of the CT of the respiratory tract (dorsoventral and lateral view) of a Herman's tortoise (*Testudo hermanni*) (*A, C*) and red-eared slider turtle (*Trachemys scripta elegans*) (*B, D*). These models demonstrate the situs of the tracheal bifurcation (*arrows*) as well as of the paired lungs. The trachea is shorter in terrestrial species and the bifurcation is therefore located more cranially than in most aquatic species.

Multiplanar reconstruction (MPR) facilitates correct interpretation due to better understanding of the spatial sense and easier illustration of pathologies. Mapping of some pathologies is only possible when viewed in at least 2 orthogonal planes, as in radiography. The imaging plane may be adapted as well, along the trachea or one bronchus for instance. Three-dimensional models are used to demonstrate anatomy as well as pathologic findings (**Figs. 8** and **9**). Curved MPR may ease interpretation in coiled snakes.[7] As a curved MPR may be hampered by artifacts and due to some lung distortion, the author prefers snakes being stretched out when possible.

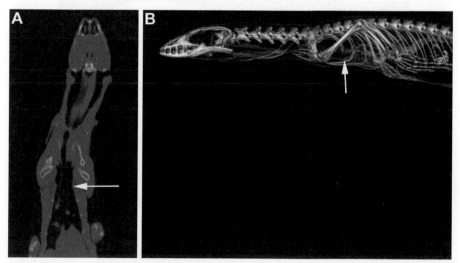

Fig. 9. Coronary CT (modified bony window [*A*] and lateral 3D model [*B*] of the cranial body and the respiratory tract of a blue spotted tree monitor (*Varanus macraei*). The position of the tracheal bifurcation (*arrow*) varies between species but is important to know especially for intubation. Note that the MPR of the coronary CT (*A*) is aligned along the trachea and bronchi.

Virtual endoscopy is often included into the software package of most CT machines and may be useful for further evaluation of trachea and bronchi.

Note that in case of a single slice CT it is important to place the animals as symmetrically as possible in the gantry. Although modern software allows MPR of any image package, the quality may not be sufficient, especially in smaller species. The author preferred sagittal scans of chelonians when no MPR was available because they corresponded to lateral radiographs. If necessary, smaller patients may be placed in each desired plane in the gantry in older machines to obtain robust diagnoses.

Magnetic Resonance Imaging

Another cross-sectional imaging technique is MRI. It is able to differentiate between various soft tissues much better than CT. However, any patient movement influences each single image of a sequence. Therefore, usually general anesthesia is mandatory. Some investigators[8] state that taping the head and limbs into the shell is sufficient to mechanically immobilize chelonians to perform MRI. In our experience, most animals, especially anxious or agile patients, will still struggle and cause artifacts that hinder adequate diagnosis.

Several sequences must be performed to gain sufficient tissue information (soft tissues—fat—fluid/liquor—blood), which means that MRI lasts much longer than CT. Given that most animals recommended to diagnostic imaging of the respiratory tract suffer from dyspnea or are in a poor condition, one would prefer a quick examination that does not require anesthesia. In addition, it has a lower resolution than CT or radiography, which may limit differentiation of tiny structures in delicate patients. Different coils are needed to support imaging of different animal's size and shape, which makes MRI even more expensive and less affordable (**Fig. 10**).

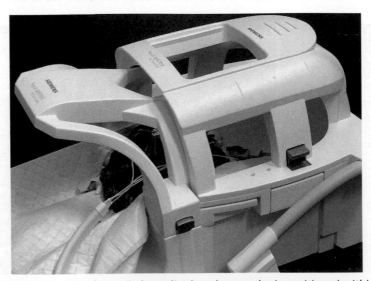

Fig. 10. Radiated tortoise (*Astrochelys radiata*) under anesthesia positioned within a combined head and neck coil to undergo an MRI. Any movement will compromise image quality and is therefore to be prevented by sedation. Although CT examinations with modern multi-slice helical machines take only few seconds to minutes, a basic MR lasts minimally 15 to 30 minutes, depending on the animal size and desired sequences.

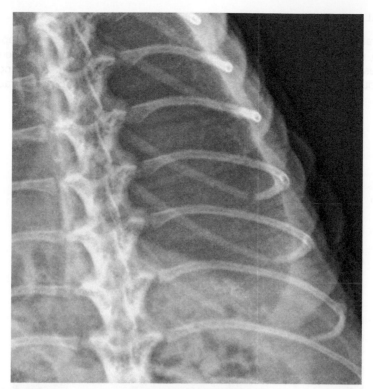

Fig. 11. Magnification of a dorsoventral radiograph of the caudal left lung of a black and white tegu (*Salvator merianae*). Note the superimposing scutes throughout the whole lung. They should not be misinterpreted as pathologic lung pattern.

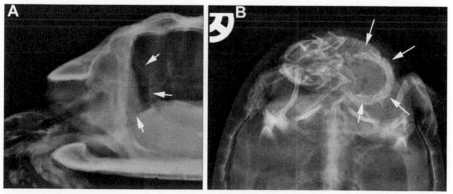

Fig. 12. Sections of lateral (*A*) and dorsoventral (*B*) radiographs of a Herman's tortoise (*Testudo hermanni*) and a Gibba turtle (*Hrynops gibbus*), respectively. The 2 images compare the situs of the cervical spine (*arrows*) and trachea of a hidden-neck turtle or Cryptodira (*A*) and side-neck turtle or Pleurodira (*B*). The retracted head of a hidden-neck turtle may be misinterpreted on lateral radiographs as a pathologic lung pattern (especially when fully retracted).

GENERAL RECOMMENDATIONS FOR IMAGE INTERPRETATION

In general, CT is the gold standard for imaging of the respiratory tract in all reptiles. In addition, reading CT images helps to improve radiographic interpretation. The various examples given later will point out the importance of especially lateral radiographs. One should not neglect or underestimate a basic set of "classic" radiographs, as

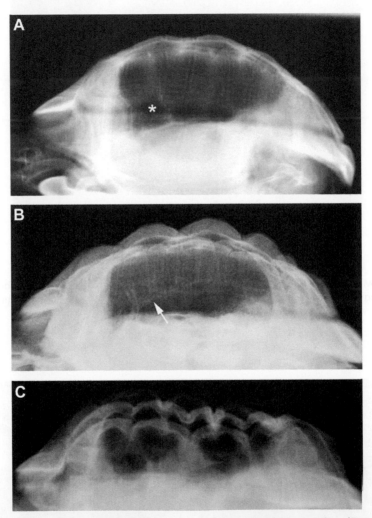

Fig. 13. Sections of lateral radiographs of 3 different Herman's tortoises (*Testudo hermanni*). Growth lines of the shell superimpose the lung fields (*A*) and may be misinterpreted as "interstitial lung pattern" by veterinarians who are not familiar with reptiles. The radiolucent line (*asterisk*) is visible in perfectly horizontally performed images and represents the suture line between costal and marginal bony plates and shields. The tortoises in (*B*) and (*C*) suffer from various grades of metabolic bone disease. The spongy bony plates (*B*) may be misinterpreted as bronchial lung pattern (although only 2 main stem bronchi exist in chelonians), whereas the sunken carapace with the pyramidal shaped bony plates may superimpose with and therefore hide pathologic lung patterns (*C*). The arrow indicates pulmonary vessels.

CT is not as globally available as radiography is. Furthermore, a CT is much more expensive and may therefore not be affordable for each owner.

In *film reading or image interpretation* of radiographs or CTs, respectively, a standard hierarchy should be maintained, independent from the requested organ or disease. First, image orientation should always follow the international standard for radiographs, CT, or MRI images because it eases identification of pathologic changes and comparison of literature: the head of the patient points to the left in lateral or sagittal views and to the top in DV/ventrodorsal (VD) radiographs or coronal planes. The right side of the animal on DV or VD views points always to the left of the image. A side marker prevents misunderstandings, especially when planning surgical procedures.

The author prefers the following *order and evaluation criteria* apart from image quality verification:

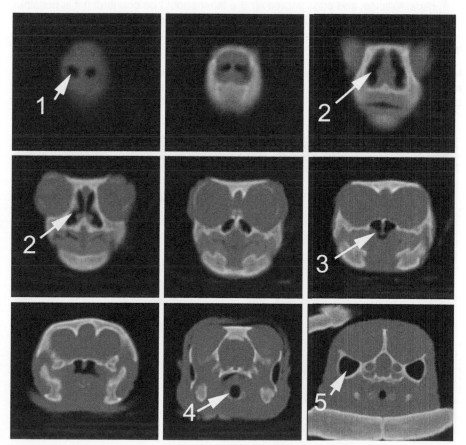

Fig. 14. Selected images of a transversal CT (bony window) of the head of a normal red-eared slider turtle (*Trachemys scripta elegans*): (1) nares/nasal cavity, (2) simple conchae, (3) choana, (4) glottis/trachea, (5) bulla tympanica. Note the simple architecture with a septum dividing the right from the left nasal chamber, although these chambers lack turbinates and sinuses.

- General body composition (obesity, cachexia)
- Skeleton: position and shape of single bones, overall density, bony plate thickness of the shell in chelonians, structure, periosteal reactions, local soft tissue swellings (especially in extremities and tail)
- *Respiratory tract:* nose, choana, glottis, larynx, trachea, mainstem bronchi, and lung as well as air sacs (if present) for position, wall thickness and density, size or diameter and shape, opacification of lumen or changes of structure. Abnormalities are categorized according to their location (uni- or bilateral, cranial, caudal, dorsal, ventral, peribronchial), extent, and density. Asymmetry of the lungs should be evaluated as well. Note that each species holds variable anatomic features (eg, a multicameral lung in chelonians or varanidae, a paucicameral type in chameleons, or a unicameral type in most lizards and snakes).
- All other coelomic organs are evaluated for position, size/diameter, shape, density (in comparison to muscles), margins, contents, wall structure and wall thickness of hollow organs, inner architecture of parenchymal organs or eggs: heart, liver and gall bladder, spleen, gastrointestinal tract, kidney, urinary bladder, gonads, follicles, and eggs (moreover the latter should be counted) if it is possible.
- Head (including eyes, ears, brain, maxilla, mandibula, teeth), thyroid

IMAGE INTERPRETATION OF THE NORMAL RESPIRATORY TRACT

Motion artifacts caused by breathing are usually barely visible due to the slow respiratory rate. *Radiographically* the nasal cavity is aerated, and glottis and trachea or bronchi appear as radiolucent tubular structures that may be bordered by a

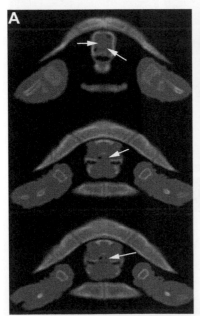
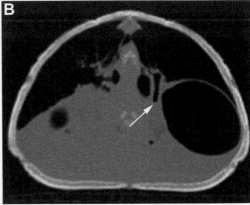

Fig. 15. Selected images of a transversal CT (bony window) of the head and cranial lung of a Leopard tortoise (*Stigmochelys pardalis*) suffering from severe rhinitis (*A, arrows*). The whole nasal cavity is obstructed by soft tissue dense material (compare **Fig. 14**). In addition, the left bronchus (*B*) shows an abrupt blunted end (*arrow*), which indicates most likely more secret accumulation.

mineralized, thin wall. Depending on the species the lung (and air sac, if present) is an elongated to oval radiolucent area. The size of the lungs depends on the status of inspiration or expiration, as the expandability is influenced by the surrounding organs, especially the digestive tract.[1,2] Positive pressure ventilation influences the lung appearance most prominently in snakes and lizards. Pulmonary artery (dorsal) and vein (ventral) bordering the primary bronchus may be differentiable within the lung field, especially in chelonians (see **Fig. 5**). The delicate honeycomb-like network of faveolae and ediculae in chelonians (note the more complex, parenchyma-rich architecture in sea turtles[1]) and more primitive lizards or the more vascularized anterior part of the lungs in snakes[9] are only seen when thickened or of increased density. Note that most coelomic organs cannot be differentiated properly on plain radiographs in reptiles due to the lack of internal fat between the coelomic organs. Nevertheless, gas and mineralized ingesta provide "natural contrast media" for gastrointestinal tract evaluation and identification. Per oral or intravenous contrast media (barium sulfate suspension or iodinated contrast media, respectively) can be used to highlight some organs further.

Be aware that bony plates, osteoderms, and scutes (especially in pine cone lizards *Tiliqua rugosa* or crocodiles; **Fig. 11**) as well as the shell, the spine, or ribs superimpose the lung fields and may be misinterpreted as pathologic lung pattern, especially in veterinarians who are less familiar with reptile anatomy (**Figs. 12** and **13**).

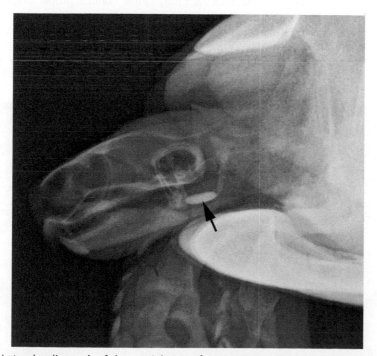

Fig. 16. Lateral radiograph of the cranial part of a Herman's tortoise (*Testudo hermanni*). A flat stone is locked immediately caudal to the glottis (*arrow*). Loud respiratory noise made a foreign body or stenosis the most likely differential diagnosis. Although a CT may provide additional information, plain radiographs are usually sufficient to localize radiodense foreign bodies in the neck region.

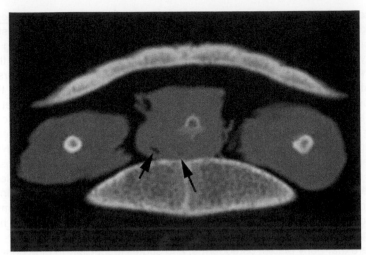

Fig. 17. Transversal CT (bony window) of a Herman's tortoise (*Testudo hermanni*) suffering from bilateral severe bronchial collapse (*arrows*, more severe on the left side). This rare disorder has only recently been described in literature[17] and can hardly be detected on radiographs. Note the thickened spongy demineralized bony plates (of the plastron) indicating metabolic bone disease that may have aggravated the collapse.

Meteorized parts of the gastrointestinal tract may further confuse proper lung differentiation, especially in chelonians.

CT on the other hand allows precise visualization not only of the upper respiratory tract[10] (**Fig. 14**) but especially of the variable delicate architecture of the lungs in the different species, especially in (adapted) lung or bony windows (see **Fig. 7**). The tracheal rings (especially when even mildly mineralized) as well as the exact location

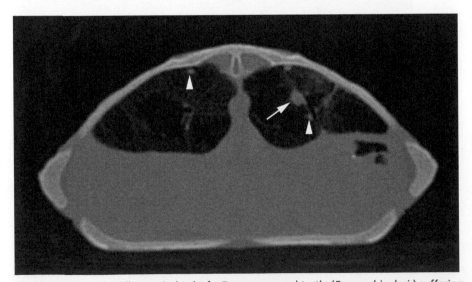

Fig. 18. Transversal CT (lung window) of a European pond turtle (*Emys orbicularis*) suffering from unilateral (left side) bronchitis (*arrow*) and bronchial obstruction (most likely due to mucus or exudate) as well as mild pneumonia on the left side. Arrowheads indicate pulmonary vessels.

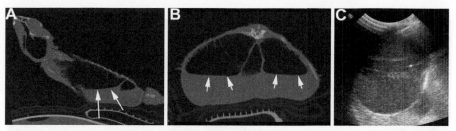

Fig. 19. Sagittal (*A*) and transversal (*B*) CT images of a Bearded dragon (*Pogona vitticeps*) suffering from severe dyspnea. The animal was placed in a plastic box to perform the CT. No restraint or anesthesia was used due to the poor clinical condition. Movement artifacts were therefore accepted. The animal sat in a very upright position to maintain breathing. The ventral half of the lung was fluid filled bilaterally. The fluid created a horizonal level (*arrows*). The dorsal half of the lung showed the typically small rim of respiratory epithelium or parenchyma, whereas most of the lung consisted of a large untextured air bubble. Although sonography (*C*) is not typically used as an imaging tool in lung disorders in reptiles, it helped to localize and aspirate the jellylike fluid. Cytology of the effusion was diagnostic for a septic, massive exudative pneumonia (Graphics by © Michi Gumpenberger). Note the more simple, peripherally situated parenchyma of this Bearded dragon, whereas the Savanna monitor in **Fig. 26** has a much more complex architecture.

of the bifurcation or lumen of the bronchi are seen. In chelonians the arrangement of the air chambers, the various ridges, and septae, which create the sponge-like appearance, can be depicted easily.[5,11–13] However, the *septum horizontale* or pleuroperitoneal membrane cannot be differentiated in healthy animals. In lizards and

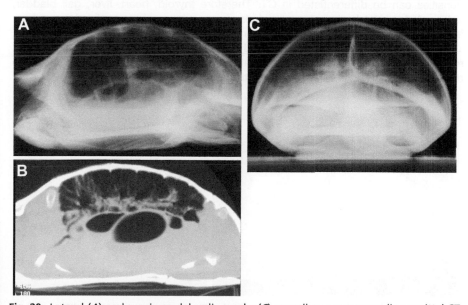

Fig. 20. Lateral (*A*) and craniocaudal radiographs (*C*) as well as a corresponding sagittal CT (modified lung window, *B*) of a Herman's tortoise (*Testudo hermanni*) suffering from bilateral moderate, exudative pneumonia. On the craniocaudal view heterogeneous opacifications are seen ventromedially in both lung fields (more severe on the right side). On lateral view the pathologic pattern is distributed in the caudoventral half of the lung. CT images reveal the full extent along the whole central bronchi bilaterally. Cranially the whole parenchyma has an increased density. The easily and quickly performed CT represents the gold standard for lung evaluation in reptiles.

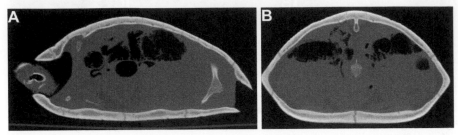

Fig. 21. Sagittal (*A*) and transversal (*B*) CT (lung window) of a Florida red-bellied cooter (*Pseudemys nelsoni*) suffering from bilateral severe bacterial pneumonia. Especially the dorsal lung parenchyma shows a massive increased density. The central air chambers seem compressed and partially opacified. The caudal half of the lung is less affected than the cranial half.

chameleons the different types of lungs (more saclike vs more complex architecture) are accessible as is the elongated, ring-like tissue with the central air chamber in snakes.[14] Even minimal mineralization can be depicted using densitometry. Recently, a detailed paper pointed out the similarity of the pulmonary anatomy of alligators and avians in CT.[15] Bronchi were identified in alligators that equal the avian entrobronchi, laterobronchi, and dorsobronchi, as well as regions of the lung hypothesized to be homologous to the avian air sacs.

Although there is no fat between the coelomic organs the slightly different soft tissue densities can be differentiated in CT. Therefore thyroid, heart, liver, gall bladder, spleen, kidney, fat body, urinary bladder, or gonads can be visualized apart from the gastrointestinal tract, even on plain images.

A private collection of radiographs and CTs of various species with an unaffected respiratory tract will serve as a kind of atlas, as the available literature is unable to document all different reptile species. Although sufficient information is provided for

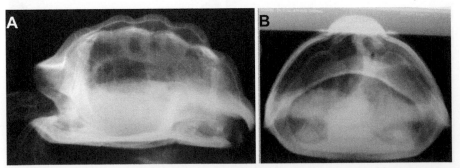

Fig. 22. Lateral (*A*) and craniocaudal radiographs (*B*) of a Herman's tortoise (*Testudo hermanni*) suffering from unilateral moderate-to-severe interstitial pneumonia (*left*). Severe heterogeneous opacification of the lung can even be seen on both views. On the craniocaudal view the unilateral lung affection (*left*) and contralateral mild emphysema (*right*), causing some midline shift to the left, is seen. Especially, the lateral view demonstrates that mostly the parenchyma seems to be affected with centrally aerated chambers. Therefore, severe fluid accumulation is less likely. Only a CT (or MRI) examination would be able to visualize mild fluid accumulations.

common species, rarer species should always receive radiographs in 2 (lizard, snake) or 3 (chelonians) views to serve as reference models.

IMAGE INTERPRETATION IN THE DISEASED REPTILE RESPIRATORY TRACT
Nasal Cavity

Rhinitis or severe epistaxis (usually caused by trauma or in context with lung hemorrhage) present as more or less homogeneous opacification of one or both *nasal cavities* (**Fig. 15**).

Trachea and Bronchi

The most common pathologic radiographical findings of the *trachea* are luminal opacifications that most likely resemble either secret accumulations, foreign bodies (**Fig. 16**), or masses, such as fungal granulomas. Recently, a rare case of a tracheal T-cell lymphoma was documented radiographically and in CT in a boa constrictor.[16]

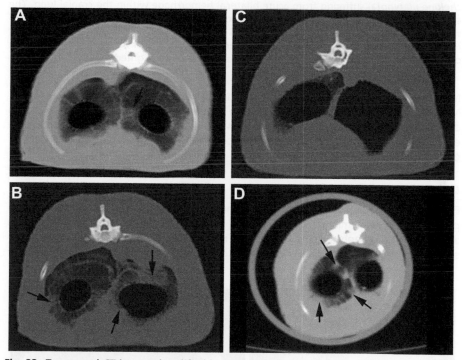

Fig. 23. Transversal CT images (modified bony window) of 2 different Indian rock pythons (*Python molurus*) suffering from bilateral pneumonia. The cranial part of the lung nearly seemed normal (*A*) in the first snake. The circular lung parenchyma looks like the iris of an eye, whereas the central chamber is airfilled and free of any structures. The increased density and patchy infiltration (exemplary *black arrows*) of the parenchyma began in the middle part of the lung and became severer the more caudally (*B*) the scan proceeded. The caudal part of the lung (*C*) in snakes is nonrespiratory and mainly functions as an air sac (left lung; at the right lung remnants of the lung parenchyma are visible). Therefore, no "irislike" structure is seen there. The second snake (*D*) was placed in a plexiglas tube. The more severe patchy infiltrates are pointed out (*arrows*). Note the more blurred images: this is due to a poor reconstruction algorithm: a soft tissue algorithm was manually adapted to fit a lung window.

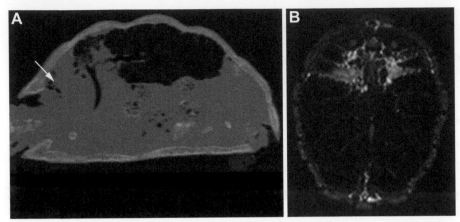

Fig. 24. Paramedian sagittal CT (*A*) and coronal T2W-MRI (*B*) of a Burmese star tortoise (*Geochelone platynota*) suffering from acute bilateral hemorrhage within the cranial lung. The clinical history (intended injection into the dorsal sinus, bloody smear from the nostrils) as well as the local emphysema (*arrow*) ventral to the nuchal shield prove that bleeding instead of pneumonia caused the increased densities/signal. However, most common cause of hemorrhage within the lung are shell fractures. T2W, T2-weighted.

Mild mucosal swelling that indicates tracheitis will not be visible radiographically. Meyer[17] illustrated a tortoise suffering from tracheal and *bronchial collapse* (**Fig. 17**) due to chondromalacia. This was first shown in a CT and then proved in pathologic examination. Bronchial obstruction and bronchial wall thickening can be easily depicted on CT as well (**Fig. 18**).

Lungs

Frye[18] listed aspiration pneumonia, bronchopneumonia, chronic granulomatous pneumonia, and verminous pneumonia as the most common respiratory disorders in reptiles. Radiographically the veterinarian is only able to differentiate increased densities that suggest pathologies within the *lung*.[19] These changes may be classified and

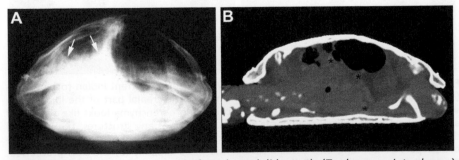

Fig. 25. Craniocaudal radiograph (*A*) of a red eared slider turtle (*Trachemys scripta elegans*). The ventrolateral part of the right lung field (*white arrows*) shows a soft tissue density, indicating a fluid filled lung suspicious for pneumonia. A sagittal CT (soft tissue window, *B*) demonstrates multiple hyperdense nodules in the cranial lung. These granulomas could not be differentiated radiographically but aggravate the diagnosis. More granulomas were outspread in the whole coelomic cavity (exemplary *black asterisk*).

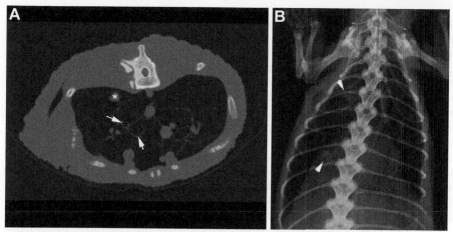

Fig. 26. Transversal CT (modified lung window) of a Savanna monitor (*Varanus exanthematicus, A*). The animal suffered from multiple oral abscesses as well as a sarcoma of an intestine wall. Two nodules (*asterisk*) were found in the honeycomb like parenchyma of the lung. All other round structures in this plane represent transsections of vessels. The most likely differential diagnoses were granuloma, but metastases cannot be ruled out, certainly (*arrows—*bronchi). These changes were barely visible radiographically (*arrowhead, B*). Nodules or masses that are localized in the periphery of the lung may be approached by ultrasound for sampling. Note the quite complex multichambered lung architecture of this animal, whereas the Bearded dragon in **Fig. 19** shows the more typical, hollow, sac-like lizard lung with only a peripheral rim of respiratory tissue.

described as unilateral or bilateral, diffuse (entire lung involved), regional or local (only part of the lung affected), homogeneous or heterogeneous, and well or poorly demarcated.

Radiographically severe, more exudative *pneumonia* or lung consolidation is seen as a more or less homogeneous soft tissue opacification of the usually ventral parts of the lung.[20] Poor ciliary clearance and inability to cough aggravate disease.

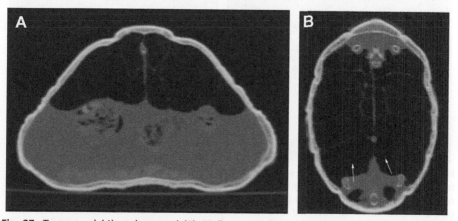

Fig. 27. Transversal (*A*) and coronal (*B*) CT (lung window) of a Herman's tortoise (*Testudo hermanni*). The faveoli are thinned and the air chambers widened. In the caudal part some septae are missing (*arrow*). These findings were interpreted as emphysema, most likely originating from an experienced and healed pneumonia.

Especially in chelonians and lizards one can follow the gravity-dependent horizontal line of fluid accumulation (**Figs. 19–21**; compare **Fig. 25**). However, this very obvious finding is missing in a more interstitial pneumonia when only the faveoli or septae become thickened and denser (**Figs. 22** and **23**) without massive fluid accumulation in the air chambers.[1,9] Poor definition of pulmonary vasculature helps to identify pulmonary infiltrates and enhanced reticular pattern. Depending on the severity of these infiltrates they may be superimposed and obscured on plain radiographs and therefore overlooked, whereas in CT any delicate changes will be detected. Nevertheless, some authors found it even easier to depict an interstitial or honeycomb pattern in DV instead of CC radiographs in cold-stunned sea turtles suffering from pneumonia.[1] In MRI, fluid accumulations will appear hyperintense in T2W images (**Fig. 24**). In case of equivocal signals, a fat suppression sequence should be performed, whereas T1W sequences demonstrate anatomic details further. Similar findings are present in marine turtles suffering from saltwater aspiration and near drowning.

Lim[21] described a generalized, diffuse unstructured interstitial lung pattern with thickened pulmonary septae on whole-body radiographs of a leopard tortoise. In CT, the lungs seemed emphysematous with irregularly thickened pulmonary septae,

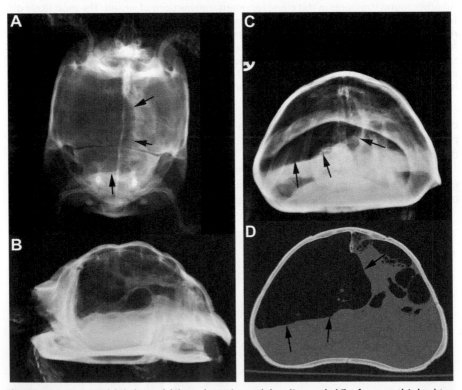

Fig. 28. Dorsoventral (*A*), lateral (*B*), and craniocaudal radiograph (*C*) of a spur-thighed tortoise (*Testudo graeca*) suffering from unilateral pneumonia (left side) and contralateral compensatory lung emphysema (*arrows*) or overinflation. Severe unilateral opacification of the lung can even be detected on dorsoventral views but should always be further investigated with additional "lung-specific" views. A corresponding transversal CT image (*D*) demonstrates the opacification of the air chambers, thickening of the septae, and reduced lung volume on the left side, whereas the normally configured aerated right lung causes some midline shift (*arrows*) to the left.

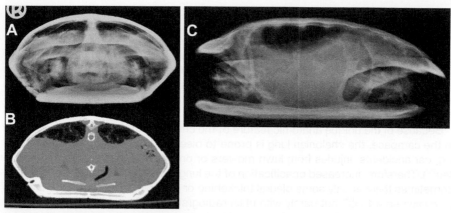

Fig. 29. Craniocaudal (*A*) and lateral (*C*) radiographs of a red-eared slider turtle (*Trachemys scripta elegans*) in horizontal beam technique. The lungs are compressed by the large opacification of the coelomic organs (sonographically identified as follicles) and the retracted head and extremities. A corresponding transversal CT (*B*) demonstrates how the faveoli and septae of the multichambered lung become thicker and denser due to compression. This pattern is homogenously distributed throughout the whole lung. There is no fluid accumulation in the air chambers. This is in contrary to pneumonia where the lung parenchyma usually increases more heterogeneously in density or the air chambers are even filled with liquid.

diffuse ground-glass opacity, and toward the periphery of the lungs several smaller areas of pulmonary honeycombing. These changes differed markedly from the reticular pattern described in normal tortoises and were compatible with chronic, extensive interstitial *pulmonary fibrosis*. Hyperattenuating lines within a quite normal lung parenchyma were interpreted as fibrosis as well.[22]

Accumulation of *granulomas* may seem similar to a less complicated exudative pneumonia radiographically (**Fig. 25**). Multiple radiopaque nodules throughout the lung that were differentiable even on DV radiography were described in cases of fibropapillomatosis and neoplasia (myxomas) in sea turtle.[23,24] Focal, more ill-defined areas of lung consolidation may be more commonly identified in other chelonians

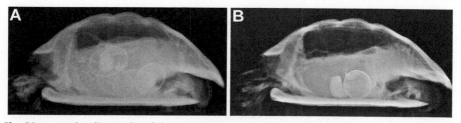

Fig. 30. Lateral radiographs of the same Herman's tortoise (*Testudo hermanni*) in horizontal beam technique in a 16-day interval. Development of multiple follicles as well as of eggs (*A*) caused physiologic compression of the lung fields. Note the change of the size of the lungs as soon as part of the eggs were disposed (*B*). Note the mineralized structure cranial to the eggs. This is feces in the caecum and transverse colon.

and lizards.[2] Most likely differential diagnoses for nodular lung pattern are granulomas, abscesses, and rarely neoplasia (**Fig. 26**).[5]

One should be aware that the different causes of pneumonia (eg, bacterial/viral/mycotic/verminous, foreign body due to force feeding, near-drowning etc.) can usually not be differentiated with imaging methods (apart from differentiable foreign bodies such as fishhooks). On the other hand, multiplanar reconstruction enables precise planning for transcarapacial sampling in chelonians or site for transcutaneous pulmoscopy in snakes, for example.

Because of the unique anatomic feature of the chelonian lung that adheres dorsally to the carapace, the chelonian lung is prone to bleeding in any cause of shell *trauma* (eg, car accidents, injuries from lawn mowers or propeller of motor boats in sea turtles[22]). Therefore, increased opacification of the lung is visible close to a shell fracture. Sometimes there is only some pleural thickening or extrapleural hemorrhage that can be evaluated with CT but barely with plain radiography.

Epistaxis and hemoptysis may be caused by fractured mineralized lung vessels originating from hypercalcemia.[25] The mineralized vessels can be easily depicted radiographically or with CT. Local hemorrhage will appear as increased density within the lungs, similar to pneumonia. It is therefore crucial to interpret any image in the light

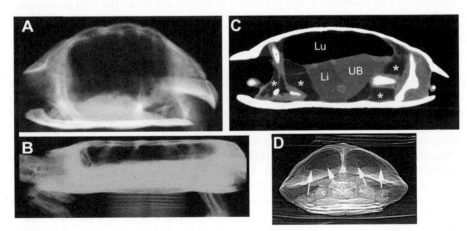

Fig. 31. Lateral radiograph of a Herman's tortoise (*Testudo hermanni*, *A*), a pancake tortoise (*Malacochersus tornieri*, *B*), and sagittal CT (*C*, soft tissue window) as well as the axial topogram of the CT (*D*) of a red-eared slider turtle (*Trachemys scripta elegans*). The radiograph of the first animal was taken after hibernation when the patient had fasted for months. The soft tissue opacification of the coelomic organs should usually occupy 50% of the height of the shell and should be leveled horizontally. This is true for most chelonians, even for a pancake tortoise (*B*). An anorectic patient or an animal with an empty GIT shows an obvious reduced shadow of coelomic organs. Controversially the red-eared slider turtle was obese with huge fat accumulations (*asterisk*) along the inner contour of the shell and around the extremities. (LU, lung; LI, hypodense liver with lipidosis; UB, urinary bladder). Although fat can be clearly differentiated on radiographs of dogs or cats due to its darker gray it is barely distinguishable in chelonians. Reptiles do not have fat in between the single coelomic organs. The lungs are compressed by those huge amounts of fat, therefore raising the horizontal border of the coelomic organs. Note that there is no lung parenchyma differentiable in this soft tissue window. Instead, the lung appears black. The topogram (in the absence of a radiograph) shows the lung compression (*arrows*) likewise.

of clinical signs and physical examination. *Pulmonary edema* from cardiac or hepatic disease may seem similar to pneumonia as well.[25]

Decompression sickness happens in marine turtles when caught in trawls and gill-nets. Although the already complex lungs are partially collapsed and show increased density, gas embolism can be found in the heart, major vessels, hepatic venous system, or even nervous system.[26]

Emphysema may be more likely seen in CT than radiography and mostly results not only in overinflation and enlargement of the lung but also in disruption of septae and confluence of air chambers[21] (**Figs. 27** and **28**). It may be observed with severe unilateral pneumonia in the contralateral lung. Emphysematous pulmonary *bullae* were described in marine turtles.[22,24]

Pulmonary *parasitism* was documented in snakes with positive contrast bronchography.[2] Aerosolized tantalum powder was used as contrast medium. The pentastomides appeared as radiolucent linear structures within the contrast-enhanced lungs.

Schachner[11] provides a detailed pulmonary anatomic and CT study in a rare case of unilateral *aplasia* of the lung in a common snapping turtle (*Chelydra serpentina*).

Lung Compression

The veterinarian should not only focus on imaging the respiratory tract in dyspneic patients. Especially chelonians live in a kind of bony box, which limits the space for the inner organs. Therefore, the abnormal or even physiologic (eg, pregnancy; **Figs. 29** and **30**) enlargement of single organs will influence all others, which may lead to significant *lung compression*.[27] Lung compression due to severe adipositas (**Fig. 31**), may also result in severe respiratory distress, which can be misinterpreted as a primary lung disorder such as pneumonia. In addition, reptilian patients with pneumonia

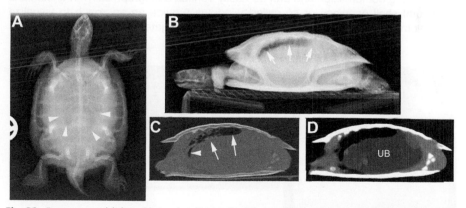

Fig. 32. Dorsoventral (*A*) and lateral radiographs (*B*) as well as corresponding sagittal CT (lung (*C*) and soft tissue window (*D*)) of a yellow-bellied slider (*Trachemys scripta scripta*) suffering from severe urinary bladder (UB) distension. The urine accumulation displaced all other coelomic organs craniodorsally and therefore caused severe lung compression (*arrows*). Even the bronchus was deviated cranially (in *C*, *arrowhead*). On the dorsoventral radiograph the compressed lungs can be seen (*arrow heads*) bilaterally. The CT images confirmed what was suspected on the radiographs: the lung compression from caudoventrally was most likely caused by severe urinary bladder distension or superovulation. In addition, this example proves again the importance of lateral radiographs. Because of open-mouth breathing this patient was treated for several weeks with antibiotics to fight the actually not existing pneumonia. To the author's opinion, a clinical examination, especially in a dyspnoeic chelonian, is incomplete without performing radiographs or ideally a CT.

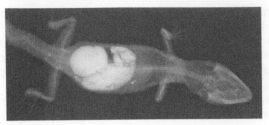

Fig. 33. A slim dyspneic leopard gecko (*Eublepharis macularius*) was suspected to suffer from dystocia on palpation. A dorsoventral radiograph revealed severe obstipation with mineralized material that caused additionally lung compression. It can be expected that on a thorough physical examination the obstipation would be palpated.

are typically systemically ill.[19] The clinical examination in a dyspneic reptile without the use of any additional imaging technique is incomplete and may lead to a wrong and even fatal diagnosis (**Figs. 32** and **33**). Besides, it is said that turtles show asymmetric swimming and floating as a typical clinical sign for pneumonia or that open-mouth breathing indicates pneumonia. However, fractures of the shoulder girdle or spine[22] as well as any unilateral mass or gas accumulation can also cause asymmetric swimming,[18,19,23] or severe pain may be responsible for open-mouth breathing. A more common reason for open-mouth breathing is severe lung compression, which may be accompanied by pale mucosal surfaces. On radiographs, organ displacement may give an indirect information for organ enlargement due to the so-called mass-effect[28] (**Figs. 34** and **35**). **Fig. 36** provides a schematic overview that may help to identify the origin of lung compression in chelonians. Severe urine retention is a common cause of lung compression and can be easily verified sonographically. In chelonians the natural shell openings or so-called windows provide an approach to visualize the coelomic organs. All other reptiles may be investigated similar to cats or dogs

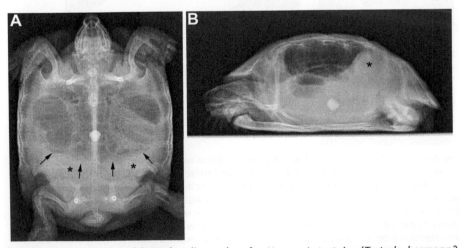

Fig. 34. Dorsoventral and lateral radiographs of a Herman's tortoise (*Testudo hermanni*) suffering from severe renomegaly (pathologically proven as gout, *asterisk*). A soft tissue dense mass is bulging into the lung fields caudoventrally (*B*). This massive lung deformation is even seen on a dorsoventral view (*arrows, A*). The stomach is gas-filled. A small pebble lies in a bowel loop.

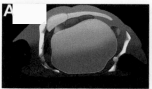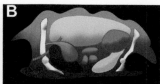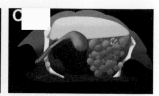

Fig. 35. Organ displacement and mass-effect in chelonians; lateral view: head is to the left. (*A*) Severe urinary retention displaces all organs to cranial and dorsal and therefore causes usually the most severe lung compression. Sonographically a severely enlarged urinary bladder may be confused with ascites. However, ascites does not displace organs. (*B*) Renomegaly results in a typical caudoventral impression or superimposition of the lung. Accompanying metabolic bone disease (as indicated here by the bumpy carapace) suggests kidney gout as the most likely reason for kidney enlargement. (*C*) A more evenly increase of the soft tissue level of the coelomic organs is caused in cases of very severe hepatomegaly or synchronous hepatomegaly and clutch development or hepatomegaly and enlarged urinary bladder, respectively. In case of obstipation or distended bowel loops the gastrointestinal tract is usually identified due to its contents. Note that the stomach is displaced (caudo-) dorsally, and the bronchi are displaced cranially by the enlarged liver. Red—heart, brown—liver, green—GIT, orange—kidney, dark yellow—urinary bladder, blue—bronchus and lung, gray—shell, bright yellow—shoulder and pelvic girdle (*circle* marks the shoulder and coxofemoral joints, respectively). (Graphics by © Michi Gumpenberger & Martina Konecny.)

with attachment of the transducer at the region of interest. This may be of great use to confirm the diagnosis or for sample collection (see **Fig. 19**).

In conclusion, each dyspneic patient should receive a thorough clinical examination in combination with appropriate diagnostic imaging. In all reptiles, at least 2 orthogonal radiographs should be performed. The lateral view should be done with horizontal

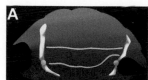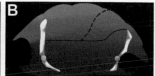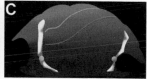

Fig. 36. The course of the usually horizontal line between lungs and coelomic organs as usually seen on lateral radiographs (head is to the left) performed in horizontal beam technique in (mediterranean) chelonians: (*A*) Normally the lungs occupy approximately 50% of the height of the shell in a healthy, feeding chelonian (*yellow line*). Chelonians after hibernation, very active males in breeding season or anorectic patients, have a relatively larger lung volume (*green line*). (*B*) Kidney enlargement creates a bump into the caudoventral lung field. The size of the indention depends on the degree of renomegaly (*broken line*—severe enlargement). (*C*) Urinary bladder enlargement or development of larger numbers of follicles or eggs (*pink line*) cause a more continuous rise of the horizontal line from cranially to caudodorsally. It seemingly tends to be more cranial convex if caused by a severely enlarged urinary bladder (*blue line*). Concurrent renomegaly will be superimposed in such cases. Simultaneous hepatomegaly will rise the cranial part of this level as well. In severe cases the lung is compressed exceptionally to craniodorsally and respiration will therefore be severely compromised. Note that performing lateral views in perpendicular beam will cause some organ shift and may therefore obscure the above-described situs! (Graphics by © Michi Gumpenberger & Martina Konecny.)

beam technique, especially in chelonians. However, CT is the gold standard to evaluate the entire respiratory tract.

ACKNOWLEDGMENTS

The author would like to thank the whole team of the service of avian and reptile medicine, division of the Clinic of Small Animal Internal Medicine, Department for Companion Animals and Horses, University of Veterinary Medicine Vienna, Austria for providing the patients and the great cooperation. Dr Martina Konecny has helped in drawing **Figs. 35** and **36**.

CLINICS CARE POINTS

- Severely dyspneic animals should be manipulated as quickly and carefully as possible. Therefore horizontal beam technique (if neccessary with the use of a box for restraint) should be used instead of lateral recumbency for lateral radiographs.

- Symmetric positioning is mandatory to gain meaningful radiographs. This is especially true in chelonians when the level and course of the soft tissues is interpreted in lateral views (done in horizontal beam technique).

- CT is superior to radiography in imaging the respiratory tract in reptiles. However, a properly performed full set of radiographs will support diagnosis frequently.

- Lung compression, especially in chelonians, causes dyspnea which may be misinterpreted as pneumonia without the use of diagnostic imaging tools.

DISCLOSURE

The author has nothing to disclose.

REFERENCES

1. Stockman J, Innis CJ, Solano M, et al. Prevalence, distribution, and progression of radiographic abnormalities in the lungs of cold-stunned Kemp's ridley sea turtles (Lepidochelys kempii): 89 cases (2002–2005). JAVMA 2013;242(5):675–81.
2. Silverman S. Diagnostic Imaging. In: Mader DR, editor. Reptile medicine and surgery. 2nd edition. St Louis (MO): Saunders; 2006. p. 471–89.
3. Mans C, Drees R, Sladky KK, et al. Effects of body position and extension of the neck and extremities on lung volume measured via computed tomography in red-eared slider turtles (Trachemys scripta elegans). JAVMA 2013;243(8):1190–6.
4. Rübel A, Kuoni W, Frye FL. Radiology and Imaging. In: Frye FL, editor.). Reptile care, an atlas of diseases and treatment, vol. I. Neptun City (NJ: T.F.H. Publications; 1991. p. 185–208.
5. Gumpenberger M. Chelonians. In: Schwarz TSJ, West S, editors. Veterinary computed tomography. UK: Wiley-Blackwell; 2011. p. 533–44.
6. Gumpenberger MR, B; Kübber-Heiß, A. CT as a quick non invasive imaging tool for diagnosing hepatic lipidosis in reptiles. Proceedings WSAVA FESAVA March 5–9, 2013; Auckland, NZ.
7. Hedley J, Eatwell K, Schwarz T. Computed tomography of ball pythons (Python regius) in curled recumbency. Vet Radiol Ultrasound 2014;55(4):380–6.
8. Straub J, Jurina K. Magnetic resonance imaging in chelonians. Sem Avian Exot Pet Med 2001;10(4):181–6.

9. Pees M, Kiefer I, Oechtering G, et al. Computed tomography for the diagnosis and treatment monitoring of bacterial pneumonia in Indian pythons (Python molurus). Vet Rec 2008;163(5):152–6.

10. Yamaguchi Y, Kitayama C, Tanaka S, et al. Computed tomographic analysis of internal structures within the nasal cavities of green, loggerhead and leatherback sea turtles. Anat Rec 2020;1–7. https://doi.org/10.1002/ar.24469.

11. Schachner ER, Sedlmayr JC, Schott R, et al. Pulmonary anatomy and a case of unilateral aplasia in a common snapping turtle (Chelydra serpentina): developmental perspectives on cryptodiran lungs. JAnat 2017;231(6):835–48.

12. Da Silva ICC, Bonelli MDA, Rameh-de-Albuquerque LC, et al. Computed tomography of the lungs of healthy captive red-footed tortoises (Chelonoidis carbonaria). J Exot Pet Med 2020;34:27–31.

13. Polanco JBA, Mamprim MJ, Silva JP, et al. Computed tomographic and radiologic anatomy of the lower respiratory tract in the red-foot tortoise (Chelonoidis carbonaria). Pesquisa Veterinária Brasileira 2020;40:637–46.

14. Pees M, Kiefer I, Thielebein J, et al. Computed tomography of the lung of healthy snakes of the spiecies Python regius, Boa constrlctor, Python reticulatus, Morelia viridis, Epicrates cenchria and Morelia spilota. Vet Radiol Ultrasound 2009;50(5): 487–91.

15. Sanders RK, Farmer CG. The pulmonary anatomy of alligator mississippiensis and its similarity to the avian respiratory system. Anat Rec 2012;295(4):699–714.

16. Summa NM, Guzman DS-M, Hawkins MG, et al. Tracheal and Colonic Resection and Anastomosis in a Boa Constrictor (Boa constrictor) with T-Cell Lymphoma. JHMS 2015;25(3–4):87–99.

17. Meyer J, Richter B, Gressl H. Bilateral Bronchial Collapse in a Hermann's Tortoise (Testudo hermanni boettgeri). JHMS 2012;22(1–2):17–21.

18. Frye F. Common pathologic lesions & disease processes. In: Frye FL, editor. Reptile care, an atlas of diseases and treatment, vol. II. Neptun City (NJ): T.F.H. Publications; 1991. p. 529–619.

19. Murray MJ. Section VII: Specific Diseases and Clinical Conditions: Pneumonia and Lower Respiratory Tract Disease. In: Mader DR, editor. Reptile medicine and surgery. 2nd edition. St Louis (MO): Saunders Elsevier; 2006. p. 865–77.

20. Gumpenberger M. Diagnostic imaging of dyspnoic chelonians. In: Seybold J, Chimaira, MF, ed. Proceedings of the 7 th International Symposium on Pathology and Medicine in Reptiles and Amphibians (Berlin 2004). 2007:217–22.

21. Lim CK, Kirberger RM, Lane EP, et al. Computed tomography imaging of a leopard tortoise (Geochelone pardalis pardalis) with confirmed pulmonary fibrosis: a case report. Acta Vet Scand 2013;55(1):1–6.

22. Oraze JS, Beltran E, Thornton SM, et al. Neurologic and computed tomography findings in sea turtles with history of traumatic injury. J Zoo Wildl Med 2019; 50(2):350–61.

23. Wyneken J, Mader D, Weber ES, et al. Medical Care of Seaturtles. In: Mader DR, editor. Reptile medicine and surgery. 2nd ediiton. St Louis (MO): Saunders Elsevier; 2006. p. 972–1007.

24. Boylan SM, Valente ALS, Innis ChJ, et al. Chapter 12: respiratory system. In: Manire CA, Norton TM, Stacy BA, et al, editors. Sea Turtle - health & rehabilitation. Florida: Ross Publishing; 2017. p. 315–35.

25. Barten SL. Section VI: Differential Diagnoses by Symptoms: Lizards. In: Mader DR, editor. Reptile medicine and surgery. 2nd edition. St Louis (MO): Saunders Elsevier; 2006. p. 683–95.

26. García-Párraga D, Crespo-Picazo JL, Bernaldo de Quirós Y, et al. Decompression sickness ('the bends') in sea turtles. Dis Aquat Org 2014;111(3):191–205.
27. Chitty J. Respiratory System. In: Girling SJ, Raiti P, editors. BSAVA manual of reptiles. 3nd edition. Gloucester: British Small Animal Veterinary Association; 2019. p. 309–22.
28. Root CR. Chapter 36: Abdominal Masses. In: Thrall DE, editor. Textbook of veterinary diagnostic radiology, vol. xiii. Philadelphie: W.B. Saunders Company; 1998. p. 621, 417–441.

Respiratory Diseases of Snakes

Jessica R. Comolli, DVM,
Stephen J. Divers, BVetMed, DZooMed, DECZM(Herpetology, Zoo Health Management), DACZM, FRCVS*

KEYWORDS

- Reptile • Snake • Respiratory disease • Pneumonia • Endoscopy

KEY POINTS

- Snakes possess a unique respiratory system composed of nares, rhinarium, choana, larynx, trachea, bronchus/bronchi, and vascular and saccular lungs.
- Disease diagnosis requires more than just identification of a potential pathogen by culture or polymerase chain reaction. Demonstration of a host pathologic response is also important.
- Clinical signs of respiratory disease include abnormal posturing with head and neck elevated, forced nasal exhalation, dyspnea including open-mouth breathing, swollen or distended throat, nasal/oral/choanal/laryngeal discharge, and increased respiratory sounds.
- Potentially valuable diagnostic techniques include hematology, serology, radiography/computed tomography, and endoscopy (or tracheal lavage). Precise diagnosis will improve therapeutic success.
- If a bacterial pneumonia is suspected, first-line antimicrobials should be used after the collection of material for cytology/histopathology and microbiology (ie, endoscopy or transtracheal lung lavage). The routine use of advanced, broad spectrum antimicrobials implies a low level of skill or expertise on the part of the practitioner.

INTRODUCTION

The respiratory tract of snakes includes the nares, rhinarium, choana, larynx, trachea, bronchus/bronchi, and lungs. Recent importation, movement through the pet trade, parasitism, malnutrition, and suboptimal temperatures are all stressors that can predispose to primary or secondary respiratory disease. This text represents an abbreviated version (limited to snakes) of more extensive, recent reviews.[1-4]

Department of Small Animal Medicine and Surgery, College of Veterinary Medicine, University of Georgia, 2200 College Station Road, Athens, GA 30677, USA
* Corresponding author.
E-mail address: sdivers@uga.edu

Vet Clin Exot Anim 24 (2021) 321–340
https://doi.org/10.1016/j.cvex.2021.01.003
1094-9194/21/© 2021 Elsevier Inc. All rights reserved.

ANATOMY

A basic understanding of the normal anatomy and physiology of the serpentine respiratory tract is important for successful diagnosis and management. The respiratory tract of Serpentes (Order Squamata) is anatomically and physiologically different from other reptilian orders.[5-7]

The upper respiratory tract consists of the rhinarium and includes the external nares, vestibulum nasi, *cavum nasi proprium*, conchae (turbinates), *ductus nasopharyngeus*, vomeronasal organ, and the choanae.[8] Snakes typically breathe in air through the external nares with their mouth closed. The nasolacrimal ducts typically open within the vomeronasal organ (olfaction) and drains from the medial canthus of the eye. Air enters the relatively short vestibulum and passes across the conchae in the nasal chamber and then enters the pharynx via the choanae, which are in close anatomic association with the larynx. The primary function of the larynx is to protect the lower airways by closing on mechanical stimulation. Snakes have one of the most specialized laryngeal structures, with a muscular hyoid-type attachment allowing forward movement of the upper trachea pulling the larynx forward. The larynx is situated rostrally in the oral cavity. It opens in the floor of the mouth caudal to the lingual sheath opening and is generally easily visualized. The larynx consists of 2 small vertical arytenoid cartilages laterally, connected by a large azygous and rounded, ventral cricoid cartilage.[5] The glottis is the opening to the trachea and controls airflow and permits hissing. A preglottal keel is obvious in some species (eg, *Pituophis spp.*). The cranial part of the trachea, or glottal tube, is composed of 3 to 16 fused cartilaginous rings and can, during large prey ingestion, be pushed craniolateral to maintain ventilation. The glottis is actively opened and closed by the dilator and sphincter laryngeal muscles, respectively. Excluding the glottal tube, the trachea is composed of 70 (*Thamnophis*) to 1120 (*Hydrophis*) incomplete cartilaginous rings; however, there are exceptions with *Crotalus viridis* and *Python molurus* having up to 25 and 30 complete cartilaginous rings following the glottal tube. All the remaining rings are incomplete and possess a significant dorsal ligament, which is thin and composed of collagenous and elastic connective tissue, but lacking muscle fibers (**Fig. 1**). This dorsal tracheal membrane proliferates to form a tracheal lung and is particularly common in the Elapidae, Viperidae, Hydrophiidae and Colubridae. Tracheal lungs facilitate additional gas exchange and can be used to inflate the neck (but not to spread the hood of cobras). The trachea normally courses ventrad or dextrolaterad to the esophagus and either dorsal or left of the heart. The trachea enters the right lung in 2 distinct ways (although intermediate variations exist): (1) *subterminal*—the trachea enters the medial side of the lung, caudal to the anterior tip or lobe (eg, boids [boas and pythons]); and (2) *terminal*—the trachea enters the most cranial portion of the lung and an anterior lobe is absent.[1] In most snakes with a single lung, the trachea becomes an intrapulmonary bronchus on entry into the right lung; however, in boids, the differentiation is at the level of the bifurcation. The bronchus terminates proximally within the faveolar region but can extend far caudally in some species.[5] The epithelium has relatively fewer cilia, which diminishes the ability to remove foreign material from the respiratory tract. A poorly developed mucociliary escalator in the airways reduces the ability of the reptile to clear discharges.

All snakes have a right lung, located dorsal to the liver and lateral to the stomach, which typically measures 25% to 60% of the total snout-to-vent length (SVL) (**Fig. 2**). The left lung is generally smaller or absent, except in boids where it may be equal to the right (**Fig. 3**). In all snakes (except some typhlopids) the lung is unicameral (single chamber). The right lung (and left lung of boids) is divided into a thick-walled,

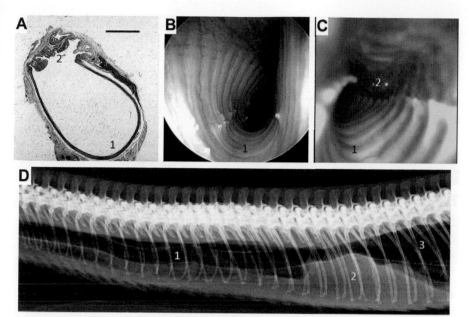

Fig. 1. Snake trachea. (*A*) Histologic cross-section of a trachea demonstrating the incomplete cartilaginous ring (1) and dorsal ligament expansion into the tracheal lung (2) of a colubrid (bar = 1 mm). (*B*) Endoscopic view within a boid trachea demonstrating the incomplete tracheal rings (1) and dorsal ligament (2). (*C*) Endoscopic view within a colubrid trachea demonstrating the incomplete tracheal rings (1) and expanded dorsal ligament expansion into the dorsal lung (2). (*D*) Lateral radiograph (horizontal beam) of a boid snake illustrating the trachea (1) coursing dorsal over the heart (2) and terminating in the vascular lung (3). (*Courtesy of* Stephen Divers.)

highly vascular, respiratory portion (vascular lung) and a thin-walled, transparent, avascular, nonrespiratory portion (air sac or saccular lung), which are variably demarcated by a transitional zone (semisaccular lung). This air sac may act as an oxygen reservoir during periods of apnea and as a buoyancy organ in aquatic snakes.[5]

Three different types of reptilian lung parenchyma have been described: (1) *trabecular,* consisting of a single layer of low-relief branching muscular structures (trabeculae); (2) *edicular,* composed of a single layer of trabeculae with raised walls or septa that form cubicles (ediculae) that are wider than they are deep; and (3) *Faveolar,* single- or multiple-layered faviform parenchyma, the compartments (faveoli) of which are deeper than wide and have a honeycomb appearance (see **Fig. 2C–F**).[1]

The vascular lung is typically located starting at 20% to 30% SVL and ending approximately 40% to 60% SVL.[9] This respiratory region is rich in faveolar parenchyma, heavily perfused, and red in color and can easily be distinguished from the reduced vascularization of the grey-white air sac. This saccular portion extends caudally for a variable length, depending on species.[5] These 2 clearly defined regions are separated by a transitional zone of varying magnitude in which the parenchyma gradually becomes less concentrated and the faveoli exhibit larger diameters, lower and thinner walls, and fewer horizontal tiers.[5] In some snake species (*Gonyosoma* sp., *Naja* sp., *Boiga* sp., and other arboreal colubrids) the transition from the vascular lung to the avascular air sac is abrupt. The air sac may constrict to 10% to 20% of its cranial diameter and continue to its tip as a very slender tail. The position of the air sac

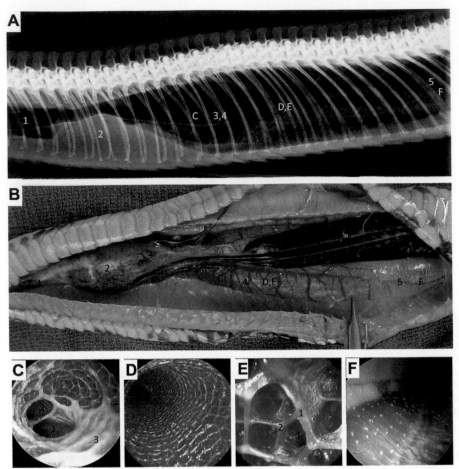

Fig. 2. Python (*Python regius*) lungs. Radiographic (*A*), courtesy of Stephen Divers, and anatomic (*B*) courtesy of Scott Stahl, views of the distal trachea (1), heart (2), vascular left (3) and right (4) lungs, and semisaccular right lung (4). The location of endoscopic images C–F are also indicated. (*C*) Endoscopic view of the anterior right lung illustrating the distal trachea (1), anterior lobe (2), and intrapulmonary bronchus (3). (*D*) Endoscopic view of the entire right vascular lung. (*E*) Close-up endoscopic view of the faveolar parenchyma illustrating the primary (1), secondary (2), and tertiary (3) divisions. (*F*) Endoscopic view of the right saccular lung. Note how the liver is visible through the transparent membrane. (*Courtesy of* Stephen Divers.)

tip is sexually dimorphic in most species of snakes, with the tip more caudally placed in males than in females.[5]

The respiratory cycle of the snake involves both active and passive components. Elevation of the ribs, caused by contraction of levator costarum and retractor costarum muscles, decreases intrapulmonary pressure, resulting in the active component of inspiration. Expiration is controlled by dorsolateral (transverse dorsal and superior internal intercostal) and ventrolateral (transverse abdominal and internal abdominal oblique) muscles. Relaxation of the expiratory muscles results in initial passive inspiration, whereas limited passive expiration occurs as a result of relaxation of the inspiratory muscles.[1–3]

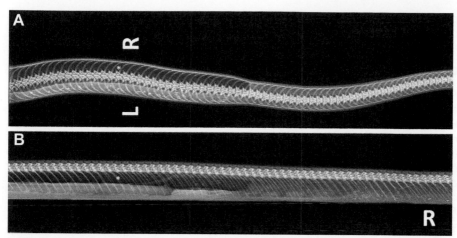

Fig. 3. Dorsoventral (*A*) and horizontal right lateral (*B*) radiographs of a cornsnake (*Pantherophis guttatus*, 50%–85% snout to vent) demonstrating the single, right lung (*asterisk*) typical of most snakes. Several healed fractures are visible. (*Courtesy of* Stephen Divers.)

PHYSIOLOGY

The following is a summary of a more detailed explanation of respiratory function that has been previously published.[7] Although most gas exchange is pulmonary, it is important to appreciate that cutaneous (skin, gular, cloacal) gas exchange may be significant. Cutaneous gas exchange can be significant in many terrestrial species (5%–15% of total gas exchange) but is most used in aquatic species where it can account for up to 35% of total gas exchange. During periods of inactivity, especially hibernation at low temperatures, it is possible for all gas exchange requirements to be met through nonpulmonary routes.

The arrhythmic breathing pattern of snakes may seem abnormal compared with mammals. Reptile metabolism and hence needs for oxygen and carbon dioxide exchange are reduced, and it is more energy efficient to maintain a normal inspiratory/expiratory breathing pattern (largely based on the intrinsic elasticity of lungs and associated tissues) with nonventilatory periods. Nevertheless, as other reptiles, snakes are tolerant of greater variations in blood pH and are capable of prolonged periods of anoxia or asphyxia.

Increasing inspired CO_2 or decreased O_2 results in less or shortened nonventilatory periods. In general, hypercapnia causes an increase in tidal volume (due to suppression of pulmonary stretch receptors), whereas hypoxia acts to increase breathing frequency (due to arterial and pulmonary chemoreceptors). However, exceptions exist, and acute hypercapnia can result in sudden breath holding. These effects are also significantly affected by temperature, with more robust responses to hypercapnia and hypoxia at higher temperatures.[7]

Most (nonaquatic) snakes seem to be more sensitive to hypercapnia than hypoxia. For most, $Paco_2$ values range between 15 and 35 mm Hg and should be maintained during anesthesia.[7]

Arterial Pco_2 is predominantly determined by pulmonary ventilation, and plasma pH shows only minor deviations among reptiles and other vertebrates, provided comparisons are made at identical temperatures. In general, arterial pH decreases consistently with increasing temperature predominantly from an increase in arterial Pco_2

production (due to relative decrease in pulmonary ventilation relative to CO_2 production).[7]

CLINICAL INVESTIGATION

A presumptive diagnosis of respiratory tract disease may be made based on historical analysis, physical examination, and a variety of ancillary diagnostic techniques.[8–11] However, a definitive diagnosis requires demonstration of both a host pathologic response (cytology, histopathology, paired rising titers) and the causative agent (microbiology, parasitology, toxicology, paired rising titers). The mere identification of a bacterial, fungal, or even viral agent should not be considered definitive for disease.

Predisposing Factors

The historical data collected from owners can often confirm significant deficiencies in husbandry and/or nutrition. Optimal temperature and humidity regimens are often overlooked. Excessively high (often at the expense of ventilation) or low humidity may result in bacterial and fungal proliferations with heavy environmental exposure predisposing to pneumonia. The culture of keeping snakes in small, glass vivaria or stacking systems is unacceptable in most cases. Nutritional imbalances that are commonly hypothesized to predispose to respiratory disease (eg, hypovitaminosis A) are probably less important in snakes fed whole vertebrate prey. Significant ecto-parasite loads are often associated with poor environmental hygiene. Snake mites (*Ophionyssus natricis*) have been implicated as a vector of several infectious causes of pneumonia, including aeromoniasis.[12,13] Lack of appropriate quarantine is a common cause of infectious disease outbreaks.

Clinical Signs

Increased respiratory rate or respiratory noise associated with acute disturbance, shedding, or defensive hissing should be differentiated from a disease presentation. Blocked nares from shed, debris, discharge, or trauma will result in open-mouth breathing. Nasal-choanal examination can help differentiate between upper and lower respiratory tract disease. Abnormal respiratory signs in snakes may include abnormal posturing with head and neck elevated, forced nasal exhalation, dyspnea including open-mouth breathing, swollen or distended throat, nasal/oral/choanal/laryngeal discharge, and increased respiratory sounds. Inflammatory debris may accumulate within vascular or saccular portions of the lung. Infectious material can persist within the lower respiratory tract because the saccular lung is minimally vascularized and there is poor ability to forcibly cough. Many snakes with respiratory illness are anorectic and lethargic.

Hematology, Biochemistry, and Serology

Collection of blood for routine hematology and plasma chemistry profiles before starting therapy can be informative, although seldom specific. Infectious disease may result in leukocytosis, often characterized by heterophilia and monocytosis (including azurophilia). Eosinophilia may be expected but is not invariably associated with verminous pneumonia. Most snakes with pneumonia are critically ill and evaluation of hydration, as well as renal and hepatic function is necessary before initiating specific treatment. Serologic assays (enzyme-linked immunosorbent assay) and polymerase chain reaction (PCR) for ophidian paramyxovirus are available in some countries.

Radiography

Radiographic evaluation of the respiratory tract requires dorsoventral (vertical beam) and lateral (horizontal beam) views to detect fluid lines and avoid organ displacement (**Fig. 4**). Quality radiographs permit the clinician to evaluate the trachea and bronchi in the cervical region and as they enter the lungs in the cranial coelom, often near the heart (**Fig. 5**). As in other reptiles, because the structures of the snake lungs (faveolar and saccular) differs greatly from mammals, the standard radiographic patterns (ie, alveolar, interstitial, bronchial, pleural) used to describe the mammalian lung are not applicable. Increased pulmonary opacity, either focal, multifocal, or diffuse suggests exudate or increased tissue presence that can be consistent with infection or tissue proliferation. Radiographic appreciation of respiratory disease may be limited, however, as changes may not become obvious until advanced. Further examination with advanced imaging or endoscopy may be indicated for snakes with less-advanced disease.[2]

Computed Tomography and Magnetic Resonance Imaging

Computed tomography (CT) scans and less commonly, MRI, are useful techniques for evaluating the lungs and localizing pulmonary lesions (see **Fig. 5**B,C).[10–12] Snakes are best sedated or anesthetized to ensure the necessary immobility for proper positioning during image acquisition. CT, including pre- and postcontrast image acquisition is most useful for evaluating soft tissue and air interfaces, generally at higher resolutions compared with MRI. Postprocessing software allows for the reconstruction of the cross-sectional image series into a complete 3-dimensional respiratory tract; however, consultation with a diagnostic imaging specialist is strongly recommended to avoid misinterpretation.

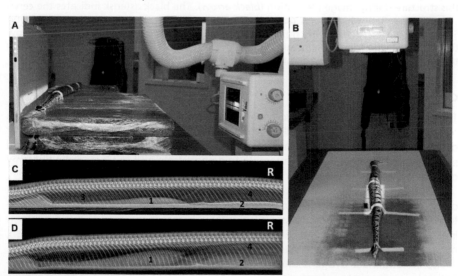

Fig. 4. Positioning and corresponding horizontal beam (*A, C*) and vertical beam (*B, D*) right lateral radiographs of an anesthetized ball python (*Python regius*, 25%–65% snout to vent length). Note the displacement of the liver (1) and stomach (2), which has resulted in an apparent reduction in the size of the vascular (3) and saccular lungs (4). Visceral displacement and an inability to detect fluid lines are the primary reasons for recommending horizontal beam lateral views over the more usual vertical beam technique used in small animal practice. (*Courtesy of* Stephen Divers.)

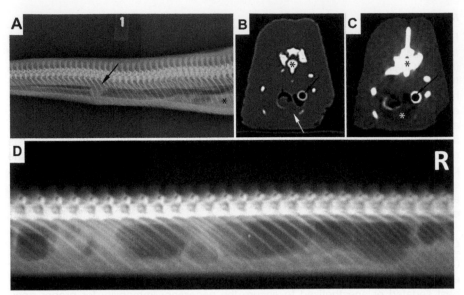

Fig. 5. (A) Right lateral radiograph of the tracheal region of an 8-year-old boa constrictor (*Boa constrictor*). A round, soft-tissue mass (*black arrow*) is invading the tracheal lumen at the level of the midtrachea, cranial to the heart (*asterisk*). Transverse computed tomography images of the cervical area of a boa constrictor in a lung algorithm (*B*) and soft-tissue algorithm (*C*) revealed a soft tissue mass partially obstructing the tracheal lumen (*white asterisk*). The mass extends ventrally and medially beyond the tracheal wall (*white arrow*), close to the esophagus (*black arrow*). A rubber tube has been inserted into the esophagus to delineate this structure during image acquisition (*black arrow*). The black asterisk indicates the cervical vertebrae. Reproduced with permission from Journal of Herpetological Medicine and Surgery.[22] (*D*) Horizontal beam, right radiographic view of the cranial coelom of a ball python (*Python regius*) demonstrating multifocal areas of increased soft tissue density throughout the vascular lung due to mycobacteriosis. (*Courtesy of* Stephen Divers.)

Cytology and Microbiology

The ability to diagnose pathologic changes within the respiratory system of snakes is relatively straightforward if initial reliance is placed on the collection of material for cytology or histopathology and microbiology. Snakes should not be treated with broad spectrum antimicrobials unless attempts to demonstrate and characterize a bacterial disease have been undertaken.

The upper respiratory tract, including the nares, choana, larynx, and cranial trachea, can be visualized and often sampled directly without anesthesia. Small-diameter culturettes permit the collection of samples, although care is required to avoid contamination by oral commensals. Swabs can be submitted for cytologic evaluation, microbiologic staining, and culture (**Fig. 6**).

The transtracheal lavage is often preferred as the initial diagnostic tool for investigating lower respiratory tract disease and can be safely performed in most snakes (**Fig. 7**). Patients should be appropriately stabilized before short-term anesthesia, and the lavage should be undertaken after the acquisition of radiographs or CT. The larynx is identified and intubated with a sterile endotracheal tube, before inserting a sterile catheter of appropriate diameter and length through the endotracheal tube, and down the trachea, and if possible, into a lung. Sterile saline (5 mL/kg) of 0.9% sterile saline is instilled into the lung while the animal is positioned in a horizontal position.

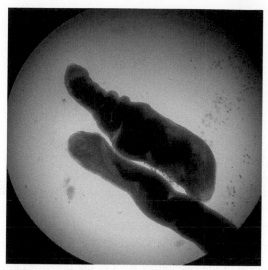

Fig. 6. Renifers (digenetic trematodes) recovered from the larynx of a free-ranging black rat snake (*Pantherophis obsoletus*) (unstained x10). (*Courtesy of* Stephen Divers.)

It helps to draw up the saline into a larger syringe to provide greater aspiration ability (ie, for a 1 kg reptile, draw up 5 mL into a 60 mL syringe). The patient is then gently inverted, rolled, or rocked for 10 to 15 seconds before attempting aspiration. If no fluid is aspirated, then a second dose of saline is infused. It is often helpful to tilt the reptile head down and continue aspiration as the catheter is withdrawn up the trachea.[10] Any residual saline is readily absorbed from the lungs. In cases of severe pneumonia, it may be possible to aspirate without the need for instilling saline, or quantities greater than the amount infused may be retrieved. The catheter should ideally be inserted to 30% to 40% SVL; however, in larger snakes a tracheal lavage may be all that is possible. The collected fluid can be used for cytology and microbiology (including bacterial and fungal cultures or PCR) (**Fig. 8**). Depending on the volume and quality of the sample obtained, material should be divided and submitted as requested by the laboratory.

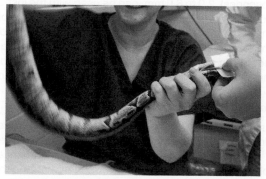

Fig. 7. Tracheal lavage in a ball python. In larger reptiles a sterile endotracheal tube should be placed into the trachea before inserting the lavage catheter. (*Courtesy of* Stephen Divers.)

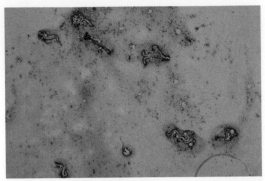

Fig. 8. Tracheal lavage from a ball python demonstrating multiple small larval nematodes (DiffQuik, x10). (*Courtesy of* Stephen Divers.)

ENDOSCOPY

Endoscopic evaluation of the respiratory tract is the preferred imaging and sample collection system in domesticated animals and humans, and the same is true for snakes. Depending on the size of the animal and the endoscopy equipment available, endoscopic examination of the nasal cavity, choana, larynx, trachea, bronchi, and lungs is often practical and provides a minimally invasive means of direct examination and biopsy for microbiology and histopathology (**Fig. 9**). Routine surgical considerations before general anesthesia and endoscopy should be undertaken. Transglottal endoscopy of the trachea, bronchi, and lungs is a noninvasive procedure that can be undertaken during short-term anesthesia in larger snakes with fine-diameter flexible or rigid endoscopes. Transcutaneous pulmonoscopy requires a more involved, albeit minimally invasive, surgical approach and longer anesthesia times.[10,11]

Transglottal Endoscopy

The use of fine-diameter rigid telescopes and flexible fiberscopes or videoscopes permits endoscopic access to, and biopsy of, the trachea in many snakes.[10,11] Semirigid or rigid endoscopes, 1.0 to 4.0 mm, can be used to evaluate the glottis and trachea as far as their diameter and length permits. In small snakes, this may include access to the cranial aspect of the lungs. For deeper access, flexible endoscopes (often urethroscopes or bronchoscopes), 2.0 to 6.0 mm, can be used with the instrument channel for biopsy forceps or cytology brushes. To avoid artifacts, endoscopic biopsies should be gently shaken from the biopsy forceps into sterile saline and then decanted into histology filters before placing into formalin.[13] Individual laboratory requirements should always be followed, but in general, biopsies for microbiology are often submitted in enrichment or transport broth, whereas ethanol is generally preferred for parasitology.

Transcutaneous Endoscopy

This approach was developed to permit practitioners who have access to established avian and exotic rigid endoscopy systems the chance to examine the lower respiratory tract of snakes.[13,14] For snakes, depending on available equipment and the size of the snake, endoscopic evaluation of the distal trachea, intrapulmonary bronchus, vascular, semisaccular, and saccular lung may be possible. In most snakes a right lateral approach with the snake in left lateral recumbency is preferred, whereas in boids (with 2 lungs) left, right, or bilateral examinations can be performed, and

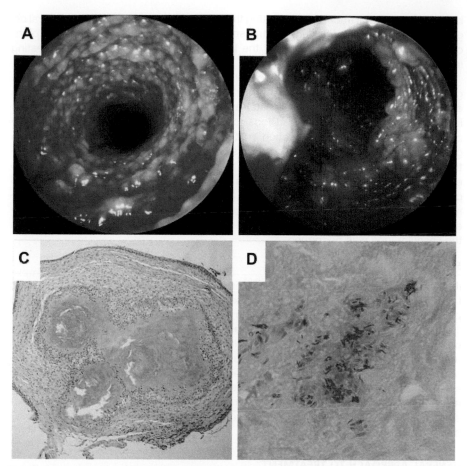

Fig. 9. (*A*) Transcutaneous pulmonoscopy of the right lung of a *Boa constrictor* using a 2.7 mm telescope. Note the severe inflammation of the faveolar parenchyma associated with acute bacterial pneumonia. (*B*) Endoscopic view of the left vascular lung of a ball python (*Python regius*) with chronic granulomatous pneumonia. (*C*) Endoscopic biopsy of the same snake demonstrating the typical histologic form of a granuloma (H&E, x10). (*D*) Gram stain of the same biopsy illustrating acid-fast bacteria consistent with *Mycobacterium sp* (Ziehl-Neelson, x1000). H&E, hematoxylin and eosin stain. (*Courtesy of* Stephen Divers.)

preference is often dictated by diagnostic imaging. With the anesthetized snake in lateral recumbency and following aseptic preparation, a small (1–2 cm) skin incision is made at the level of the semisaccular lung (or transitional zone) to avoid major hemorrhage (approximately 35%–45% SVL).[5,13,14] A ventrolateral approach can be made following a craniocaudal incision between the second and third rows of lateral scales or dorsoventrally over an intercostal space. The subcutaneous, coelomic muscle and coelomic membrane are bluntly dissected. When the wall of the lung (transparent avascular membrane) is reached, 2 fine stay sutures can be placed to elevate it to the level of the skin incision (this is often not necessary with the more lateral approach). Following perforation of the lung, the endoscope (rigid with or without the operating sheath, or, in large boids, a flexible endoscope) is introduced through the incision and directed cranially toward the vascular lung, anterior lung lobe, intrapulmonary bronchus, and distal trachea. By directing the endoscope caudally, various visceral organs can also be viewed through the transparent saccular lung wall. If there are pathologic changes, the affected part of the lungs can be sampled for further testing (cytology, culture, PCR, histology).[13,14]

Following examination via the ventrolateral approach, the lung is closed with a single, simple interrupted suture using absorbable material, with the muscle and skin closed routinely. The lateral, intercostal approach does not require closure of the lung or the muscle, just the skin.[10] Biopsies should be gently shaken from biopsy forceps into sterile saline before fixation in 10% formalin (or 2% glutaraldehyde or 2% glutaraldehyde for electron microscopy) to ensure diagnostic quality.[13] The aforementioned techniques have been performed in colubrids, pythons, and boas with good to excellent results.[14] Reevaluation of snakes months or a year or more later confirmed complete healing of the previous entry and biopsy sites.[13] The authors have not experienced any negative consequences associated with pulmonoscopy in snakes; however, greater hemorrhage would be expected if a more cranial approach through the vascular lung was performed.

Surgical Biopsy

If minimally invasive endoscopic techniques are not possible, then surgical access to the lung can be achieved by coeliotomy. There is no functional diaphragm nor negative pleural pressure to preserve. In snakes the vascular lung is typically located between 12% and 45% SVL. However, great species variation exists with regard to lung anatomy, including the presence of a tracheal lung in some elapids and viperids, left and right lungs in boids, and only a right lung in most other snakes.[5] Preoperative radiography/CT to determine the margins of the respiratory tract should be performed before surgical biopsy to ensure an accurate, targeted approach. Biopsy of the vascular cranial lung commonly results in greater hemorrhage unless appropriate hemostatic measures are taken. Biopsy of the thinner posterior lung (or air sac) is not complicated by hemorrhage.

GENERAL APPROACH TO TREATMENT

Early diagnosis and aggressive therapeutic measures, including intensive nursing, are often hallmarks for success. Patients should be maintained at the upper end of their preferred optimum temperature zone with appropriate humidity to facilitate immunologic and mucociliary functions. The use of hospital oxygen cages should be reserved for those cases in which hypoxemia is present or suspected. Fluid therapy is often required due to increased insensible losses from exacerbated respiratory rate and effort. Route of fluid administration should be consummate with urgency and degree of deficit. Anorexia is not uncommon but there is rarely an urgent need to provide nutritional support during initial case management. Assisted feedings should be delayed until dehydration has been corrected and initial diagnostics (that often require sedation or anesthesia) have been performed.

Antimicrobial Therapy

A variety of bacterial and fungal organisms can cause disease, and therefore, culture (or PCR) and sensitivity (disc diffusion or minimal inhibitory concentration [MIC]) testing is mandatory. The current culture of using advanced cephalosporins and fluoroquinolones as first-line choices is ill advised and not in keeping with published antimicrobial stewardship recommendations.[15] While awaiting microbiology results, gram-stained smears should be used to direct initial antimicrobial choices.

Antimicrobials should only be prescribed when a bacterial or fungal disease has been identified. Inappropriate use of broad-spectrum antimicrobials implies a low level of clinical expertise and predisposes to antibacterial resistance.[15]

Nebulization

Nebulization can be useful to deliver antimicrobials, especially those that may be systemically toxic, topically to the respiratory tract. Small particle size to ensure penetration deep into the respiratory tract, appropriate solution, (in sterile water or saline), and air as the carrier are important to maintain ventilation. Using oxygen as a carrier tends to suppress respiration and reduce drug delivery. Although there have been no direct studies to date, the results involving avian reptiles suggest that successful nebulization requires particle sizes of less than or equal to 3 μm delivered for 30 mins (if anesthetized and ventilated) or 2 to 4 hours (if conscious).[16,17] Once or twice daily treatments are recommended. In addition to antimicrobials (often aminoglycosides, amphotericin B), mucolytics (acetylcysteine) and benzalkonium-polyhexanide solutions (F10 Antiseptic Solution Concentrate, Health and Hygiene Ltd, South Africa) are often nebulized but should not be mixed (**Table 1**). Saline may be beneficial for mobilizing exudates. However, there is no evidence to suggest that antimicrobial nebulization is more effective than intravenous administration or that bronchodilators and mucolytics have any beneficial effects. If nebulization is pursued, a dedicated chamber should be used to facilitate creation of a thick fog for the snake, while preventing human exposure.

Intrapulmonic Treatment

Transcutaneous catheterization of the lung can provide an alternative airway in cases of tracheal obstruction or to provide a route for direct drug delivery to the lungs.[18,19] In one case of tracheal obstruction in a ball python (*Python regius*), local anesthesia was used and following a 1.5 cm surgical cut-down, the saccular lung was identified, stab incised, and a 4-mm endotracheal tube was inserted and sutured in place.[19] Although this endotracheal tube functioned as an alternative airway for 13 days before being removed and the site surgically closed, a smaller catheter could be used for drug delivery. Irritating drugs should be avoided; however, this technique can provide a route for delivering drugs that may be systemically toxic, but which are poorly absorbed across the respiratory epithelium (eg, aminoglycosides, amphotericin B). Following removal of the catheter, the site should be surgically closed.

Table 1
Suggested drugs for nebulization of reptiles[4]

Drug	Dose
Amikacin	50 mg in 10 mL saline
Tobramycin	50 mg in 10 mL saline
Ceftazidime	100 mg in 10 mL saline
Amphotericin B	10 mg in 10 mL saline
Benzalkonium/polyhexanide (F10)	54 mg/4 mg (1 mL) in 250 mL saline
Acetylcysteine	20% solution

In humans the mg quantity of drug is entirely inhaled and therefore most useful. However, reptiles are placed in a nebulization chamber such that drug concentration and duration of exposure (typically 2–4 h) are more important than the mg of drug used.

SPECIFIC RESPIRATORY TRACT DISEASES
Tracheitis and Tracheal Obstruction

Inflammation, granulomas, chondromas, lymphomas, and exudates can be associated with the trachea. If obstructive, these can lead to dyspnea, which tends to be poorly responsive to oxygen; however, dramatic improvement would be expected following creation of an alternative airway (eg, lung catheter).

Mycoplasma has been reported to cause tracheitis in a burmese python (*Python molurus bivittatus*).[20] *Salmonella arizonae* was considered the etiologic cause of tracheitis in a double-headed kingsnake (*Lampropeltis hondurensis*).[21] Nidovirus was seen in association with tracheitis in a group of ball pythons that also had bacterial pneumonia.[22,23] Tracheal chondromas and lymphoma have also been reported in several boid snakes.[20–22]

Although lethargy and respiratory compromise including dyspnea and open-mouth breathing are common, most published reports have been presented dead or were euthanatized shortly after presentation for post-mortem investigations. Ideally, endoscopic evaluation of the trachea permits evaluation and selective biopsy of specific lesions for histopathology and microbiology (culture, PCR). If unavailable, radiography, CT, and tracheal lavage may be useful, but diagnoses may be missed.

Exudates should be suctioned from the trachea, whereas firm, space occupying masses (chondromas, granulomas) typically require endoscopic debridement or tracheal resection and anastomosis.[24–26] Antimicrobial therapy is based on culture and sensitivity or MIC results, and treatment for 3 to 6 weeks is often required. Reevaluation is important to determine the effectiveness of treatment.

Endoscopic and tracheal resection have been curative for single chondromas.[21] Multiple masses/granulomas carry a less favorable prognosis. Bacterial tracheitis can often be treated. Fungal infections tend to be more granulomatous and more resistant to medical therapy. There are no reports of successful treatment of viral tracheitis, and supportive care is often all that can be provided.

Bacterial Pneumonia

Bacterial pneumonia may occur as a primary entity, secondary to stomatitis and aspiration, by hematogenous spread (eg, endocarditis) or by direct/close anatomic association (eg, hepatitis, coelomitis).[23–27] Bacterial pneumonia can be focal, multifocal, or diffuse and unilateral or, in boids, bilateral. Many infections involve commensal or environmental organisms that become pathogenic in an immunocompromised host.

Bacterial pneumonia seems common in snakes. Microbiologic results have included many bacterial species: *Mycoplasma, Aeromonas, Alcaligenes, Chlamydophila, Citrobacter, Corynebacterium, Enterobacter, Escherichia coli, Klebsiella, Morganella, Moraxella, Pasteurella, Proteus, Pseudomonas, Acinetobacter Brevibacterium, Achromobacter, Bacillus, Stenotrophomonas, Empedobacter, Salmonella,* and *Mycobacterium*.[23–32] Compared with healthy snakes with a predominance of *Providencia rettgeri* and coagulase-negative *Staphylococcus* spp, those with pneumonia exhibit moderate to heavy growth of aerobic gram-negative bacilli.[15] Anaerobic organisms (including *Bacteroides, Clostridium, Fusobacterium,* and *Peptostreptococcus species*) have been rarely reported.[33]

Cases of acute or peracute pneumonia may present as sudden death, although lethargy, anorexia, and respiratory signs, including dyspnea and open-mouth breathing, are common. Although diagnostic imaging may provide convincing evidence of lung disease, a definitive diagnosis relies on the collection of material for histopathology (or cytology) and microbiology. Therefore, endoscopic evaluation or lung lavage are typically required.

High-volume lung lavage and aspiration or coupage have been used to remove considerable quantities of exudate from the lower respiratory tract of anesthetized or sedated snakes. Systemic and local application of antimicrobials are typically required and selection should be based on microbiologic cultures or MIC results. Prolonged treatment is often required, along with correction of any predisposing husbandry or nutritional components. Reptile pharmacokinetic studies have been performed for clarithromycin and oxytetracycline, which should be used in preference to fluoroquinolones for mycoplasmosis.[34–38]

If left untreated, most cases progress to generalized sepsis and death, although chronic granulomata or abscesses can develop. Severe cases, especially involving *Mycobacterium* and *Chlamydia* sp. have a more guarded to poor prognosis.

Fungal Pneumonia

Mycotic pneumonia is occasionally diagnosed in captive reptiles, albeit rarely in snakes. Typically, fungal infections occur due to high mycotic exposure (poor environment), immunosuppression (hypothermia, hatchlings, concurrent disease), or long-term, broad-spectrum antibiotic misuse.

Several fungi have been associated with pneumonia in reptiles, including *Aspergillus, Candida, Fusarium, Mucor, Geotrichum, Penicillium, Cladosporium, Rhizopus, Chrysosporium, Paecilomyces,* and *Beauveria species*. The systemic deep mycoses occasionally diagnosed in mammals, such as blastomycosis and histoplasmosis, have not been diagnosed in reptiles to date.

Most cases are presented dead or terminal, but severe respiratory compromise would be expected. A diagnosis of fungal pneumonia is often difficult to make antemortem without biopsy. Recovery of fungal elements, hyphae, or spores or positive fungal culture from a transtracheal wash is supportive of a diagnosis but lesions may be encapsulated and nonproductive. Endoscopic evaluation and biopsy are more effective and less invasive than traditional surgical approaches. Gross pathologic changes of mycotic pneumonia include pulmonary granulomata, lung consolidation, and occasionally extension of the disease in adjacent organs.

Large encapsulated lesions require surgical removal, and even small encapsulated granulomas are often resistant to drug therapy. In acute cases and those where encapsulation is absent, antifungal medication may be effective, with both local and systemic administration combined. It is often wise to obtain antifungal MIC results and to check antifungal drug blood levels to ensure they are exceeded.

Typically the prognosis is poor when dealing with extensive disease. Single granulomas that can be surgically removed carry a fair to good prognosis, especially when combined with postoperative antifungal therapy.

Viral Pneumonia

Several viruses have been identified in association with peracute to chronic pathology of the respiratory system; however, most of the viruses identified have only been circumstantially incriminated as primary causes of disease, with few studies fulfilling Koch's postulates. Therefore, the clinician must be cautious and attempt to differentiate between *infection* and *disease*. In addition, the clinical picture is frequently complicated by secondary bacterial or fungal issues.

A variety of viruses have been detected in association with respiratory pathology. Paramyxoviruses (Ferlaviruses) are known pathogens in snakes (*Bothrops, Bitis, Crotalus, Trimeresurus, Vipera, Atheris*) where they have been associated with caseous necrotic debris, lung thickening, and edema.[39] Other species of colubrids and boids have also been affected.[40] More recently, a nidovirus has been identified as a likely etiologic agent of severe respiratory disease in pythons.[22,23] In most of the cases the association of virus with respiratory lesions is just that, an association, and a direct causal relationship has rarely been demonstrated.

Typical signs of upper and/or lower respiratory tract disease are often reported. The extent of which the clinical signs can be attributed to the virus rather than secondary infections is open to debate in many cases. Most cases of viral pneumonia are determined by PCR, histopathology, and rarely by electron microscopy, virus isolation, or genetic sequencing. However, where serologic tests exist (eg, ophidian paramyxovirus), they should be used, as paired rising titers can be useful to differentiate between active infection versus past exposure. PCR testing has revolutionized the ability to identify viruses from oral/tracheal swabs, lung lavage, or biopsy samples. However, positive results only indicate the presence of the virus and not disease. Therefore, it is important to demonstrate host pathologic response by serology, cytology, or histopathology. It may be wise to save additional biopsy or necropsy tissues at $-20°C$ in case virologic investigations are subsequently required.

There are no reports of specific antiviral therapies against paramyxoviruses or nidoviruses. There are several human drugs that have been developed, but high costs and limited commercial interests have resulted in a lack of efficacy, pharmacokinetic, safety, and clinical trials in reptiles. When dealing with an outbreak, separation of diseased animals, barrier nursing, and disinfection are critical. In many cases, immunosuppression associated with poor husbandry and nutrition may be important and should be corrected. General medical support should include fluid therapy and nutritional supplementation. Appropriate quarantine with PCR and serologic testing (when available) remain the mainstays of prevention. In collections, euthanasia of affected animals should be considered.

Viral infections may persist for protracted periods, and treatment of clinical viral disease may not resolve persistent infection. Improvements in husbandry and nutrition may be important factors in determining an individual snake's outcome.

Verminous Pneumonia

Several parasites encountered in captive reptiles have a portion of their life cycle associated with the respiratory system. Except in cases with overwhelming parasite loads, most respiratory involvement is subclinical and minor, causing primarily localized inflammation.[41] However, heavy burdens or novel host-parasite interactions can lead to significant disease, often complicated by secondary infections.

Several genera of digenetic trematodes within the Ochetosomatidae and Plagiorchiidae (renifers) family commonly inhabit the oral cavity, but adults often migrate via the glottis to the lungs and air sacs. Adults attach to the epithelial lining in the lower respiratory tract causing focal lesions that can become secondarily infected. Large trematodes (Hydrophidae) can infect the lungs of sea snakes causing mucoid exudate with hyperplasia, hemorrhage, and necrosis.[13]

Migrating nematode larvae (Ophidascaris) have caused respiratory signs and/or pulmonary lesions in pythons. Adults of the Filarioidea and Dioctophymatoidea inhabit extraintestinal sites, including the lungs. Adult lungworms (Rhabdias) reside within the lungs of snakes, where the parthenogenic females lay their eggs. The eggs are then transported up the trachea, swallowed, and passed in the feces. Migrating larvae (Strongyloides) may also be associated with pulmonary lesions. Pentastomida (segmented, wormlike) parasites undergo extensive visceral migrations before locating within the lungs (and less commonly the trachea and nasal passages). The most important genera to infect snakes are *Raillietiella, Kiricephalus, Porocephalus,* and *Armillifer*. Mammals, including humans, can act as intermediate hosts. Pentastomids can cause localized lesions, whereas molting can induce antigenic responses. The adults feed on tissue fluids within the lung and pass embryonated eggs, which pass into the oral cavity, are swallowed, and passed in the feces. Clinical disease associated with pentastomids is rare, and they are often incidental findings. However, they may cause focal irritation and, with a host antigenic response, more diffuse inflammation. Antemortem diagnosis depends on microscopic identification of the ova, which appear distended with a thinly walled capsule and may measure up to 130 mm in diameter. Larva and their hooklets may be seen within these eggs.

Although most trematode infestations are asymptomatic, heavy parasite loads may cause enough damage to predispose the animal to a secondary pneumonia. The diagnosis is made based on the identification of the typical fluke eggs on transtracheal wash. Currently, no effective and safe treatment has been advocated, although praziquantel could be considered.

Although most parasitic infections are subclinical, heavy infestations of *Rhabdias* in snakes can be associated with open mouth breathing, extended glottal tube, and severe pneumonia (including secondary bacterial pneumonia). A mucus-laden exudate may accumulate around the nares, and a proliferative pneumonia may be identified with histopathology. Antemortem diagnosis relies on the demonstration of embryonated eggs (60×35 μm) in a lung lavage.

Nematode infections may be treated with ivermectin, benzimidazoles, levamisole, or pyrantel. Pentastomids should ideally be treated by removal (often endoscopic), as anthelmintics such as ivermectin result in parasite death and massive antigenic release. Praziquantel can be considered for trematode infections. Prevention relies on acquisition of captive-bred (instead of wild caught specimens), appropriate quarantine including fecal screening, use of clean captive-bred food items, and sound hygiene.

Cases of uncomplicated verminous pneumonia often respond to medical (anthelmintic and nonsteroidal antiinflammatory drug therapy) or, in the case of pentostomids, endosurgical removal. Secondary infections, especially if severe, can significantly reduce prognosis.

Noninfectious Pneumonia

Not all inflammatory diseases are infectious by nature. Aspiration of foreign material, either iatrogenically or by chance, is certain to cause significant inflammation within the lungs. Aspiration pneumonia begins as a foreign body reaction; however, if neglected, progresses rapidly to secondary bacterial pneumonia that is poorly responsive.[42] Although it is common practice, the prophylactic use of antibiotics in patients in whom aspiration is suspected or witnessed is rarely efficacious.[43]

Diseases that compromise tidal volume may mimic primary respiratory disease, even though the respiratory tract itself is healthy. Obesity, ascites, and cranial coelomic space-occupying lesions (eg, cardiomegaly, hepatomegaly) have the potential to cause respiratory compromise. Significant respiratory disease may result in an increase in pulmonary vascular resistance. The shunting that may occur from pulmonary pathology could decrease oxygen delivery to peripheral tissues. Serious, life-threatening hypoxia and acidosis may result from overwhelming the blood's buffering systems as anaerobiosis becomes prolonged. Other conditions as innocuous as the loosening of skin around the nares immediately before ecdysis that can increase respiratory noise may be misinterpreted as disease. The "problem" is self-resolving after completion of ecdysis.

SUMMARY

The current approach to ante-mortem diagnosis of snake respiratory disease is often lacking. A better understanding of serpentine anatomy, physiology, and respiratory diseases is critical. In addition, empirical therapy, particularly the use of broad spectrum antimicrobials is commonplace but inappropriate. Snake respiratory medicine needs to elevate to similar standards found in human and domesticated animals, which focus on imaging, endoscopic evaluation, and biopsy for definitive diagnosis, accurate prognosis, and directed, specific therapy.

REFERENCES

1. Divers SJ. Diagnostic endoscopy. In: Divers SJ, Stahl SJ, editors. Mader's reptile and Amphibian medicine and surgery. 3rd edition. St Louis (MO): Elsevier; 2019. p. 604–14.
2. Comolli JR, Divers SJ. Radiography – snakes. In: Divers SJ, Stahl SJ, editors. Maders reptile and Amphibian medicine and surgery. 3rd edition. Missouri: Elsevier; 2019. p. 503–13.
3. Kischinovsky M, Divers SJ, Wendland LD, et al. Otorhinolaryngology. In: Divers SJ, Stahl SJ, editors. Maders reptile and amphibian medicine and surgery. 3rd edition. Missouri: Elsevier; 2019. p. 736–51.
4. Knotek Z, Divers SJ. Pulmonology. In: Divers SJ, Stahl SJ, editors. Maders reptile and Amphibian medicine and surgery. 3rd edition. Missouri: Elsevier; 2019. p. 786–804.
5. Wallach V. The lungs of snakes. In: Gans C, editor. Biology of the Reptilia, volume 19, morphology G, visceral organs. Society for the Study of Amphibians and Reptiles; 1998. p. 93–295.
6. Perry SF. Lungs: comparative anatomy. In: Gans C, Gaunt AS, editors. Biology of the Reptilia, volume 19. Morphology G, visceral organs, vol. 19. Ithaca (NY): Society for the Study of Amphibians and Reptiles; 1998. p. 1–92.
7. Wang T, Smits AW, Burggren WW. Pulmonary function in reptiles. In: Gans C, Gault MH, editors. Biology of the Reptilia, volume 19, morphology G, visceral organs. Ithaca: Society for the Study of Amphibians and Reptiles; 1998. p. 297–374.
8. Parsons TS. The Nose and Jacobson's Organ. In: Gans C, Parsons TS, editors. Biology of the reptilia, vol. 2. London: Academic Press; 1970. p. 99–185.
9. McCracken HE. Organ location in snakes for diagnostic and surgical evaluation. In: Fowler ME, Miller RE, editors. Zoo & wildlife medicine current therapy 4. Philadelphia: WB Saunders; 1999. p. 243–8.
10. Zehtabvar O, Tootian Z, Vajhi A, et al. Computed tomographic anatomy and topography of the lower respiratory system of the european pond turtle (Emys Orbicularis). Iranian J Vet Surg 2014;09(2):9–16.
11. Lim CK, Kirberger RM, Lane EP, et al. Computed tomography imaging of a leopard tortoise (Geochelone pardalis pardalis) with confirmed pulmonary fibrosis: a case report. Acta Vet Scand 2013;55(1):35.
12. Sharma AJ, Wyneken J. Computed tomography. In: Divers SJ, Stahl SJ, editors. Mader's reptile and Amphibian medicine and surgery. 3rd edition. St Louis (MO): Elsevier; 2019. p. 560–70.
13. Stahl SJ, Hernandez-Divers SJ, Cooper TL, et al. Evaluation of transcutaneous pulmonoscopy for examination and biopsy of the lungs of ball pythons and determination of preferred biopsy specimen handling and fixation procedures. JAVMA 2008;233(3):440–5.

14. Jekl V, Knotek Z. Endoscopic examination of snakes by access through an air sac. Vet Rec 2006;158(12):407.
15. Laundy M, Gilchrist M, Whitney L. Antimicrobial stewardship. Oxford (UK): Oxford University Press; 2016.
16. Tell LA, Stephens K, Teague SV, et al. Study of nebulization delivery of aerosolized fluorescent microspheres to the avian respiratory tract. Avian Dis 2012; 56(2):381–6.
17. Tell LA, Smiley-Jewell S, Hinds D, et al. An aerosolized fluorescent microsphere technique for evaluating particle deposition in the avian respiratory tract. Avian Dis 2006;50(2):238–44.
18. Myers DA, Wellehan JFX, Isaza R. Saccular lung cannulation in a ball python (python regius) to treat a tracheal obstruction. J Zoo Wildl Med 2009;40(1):214–6.
19. Hernandez-Divers SJ. Pulmonary candidiasis caused by Candida albicans in a Greek tortoise (Testudo graeca) and treatment with intrapulmonary amphotericin B. J Zoo Wildl Med 2001;32(3):352–9.
20. Drew ML, Phalen DN, Berridge BR, et al. Partial tracheal obstruction due to chondromas in ball pythons (Python regius). J Zoo Wildl Med 1999;30(1):151–7.
21. Diethelm G, Stauber E, Tillson M, et al. Tracheal resection and anastomosis for an intratracheal chondroma in a ball python. JAVMA 1996;209(4):786–8.
22. Summa NM, Guzman DS-M, Hawkins MG, et al. Tracheal and Colonic Resection and Anastomosis in a Boa Constrictor (Boa constrictor) with T-Cell Lymphoma. J Herp Med Surg 2015;25(3–4):87–99.
23. Schmidt V, Marschang RE, Abbas MD, et al. Detection of pathogens in Boidae and Pythonidae with and without respiratory disease. Vet Rec 2013;172(9):236.
24. Schroff S, Schmidt V, Kiefer I, et al. Ultrasonographic diagnosis of an endocarditis valvularis in a burmese python (python molurus bivittatus) with pneumonia. J Zoo Wildl Med 2010;41(4):721 4.
25. Hilf M, Wagner RA, Yu VL. A Prospective Study of Upper Airway Flora in Healthy Boid Snakes and Snakes with Pneumonia. J Zoo Wildl Med 1990;21(3):318–25.
26. Schilliger L, Tréhiou-Sechi E, Petit AMP, et al. Double Valvular Insufficiency in a Burmese Python (Python molurus bivittatus, Linnaeus, 1758) Suffering from Concomitant Bacterial Pneumonia. J Zoo Wildl Med 2010;41(4):742–4.
27. Hernandez-Divers SJ, Shearer D. Pulmonary mycobacteriosis caused by *Mycobacterium haemophilum* and *M. marinum* in a royal python. JAVMA 2002; 220(11):1661–3.
28. Penner JD, Jacobson ER, Brown DR, et al. A novel Mycoplasma sp. associated with proliferative tracheitis and pneumonia in a burmese python (Python molurus bivittatus). J Comp Pathol 1997;117(3):283–8.
29. Plenz B, Schmidt V, Grosse-Herrenthey A, et al. Characterisation of the aerobic bacterial flora of boid snakes: application of MALDI-TOF mass spectrometry. Vet Rec 2015;176(11):285.
30. Ullmann LS, das Neves Dias-Neto R, Cagnini DQ, et al. Mycobacterium genavense infection in two species of captive snakes. J Venom Anim Toxins Incl Trop Dis 2016;22(1):27.
31. Jacobson ER. Bacterial disease of reptiles. In: Jacobson ER, editor. Infectious diseases and pathology of reptiles – color atlas and text. Boca Raton (FL): CRC/Taylor and Francis Group; 2007. p. 461–526.
32. Jacobson ER, Gaskin JM, Mansell J. Chlamydial Infection in Puff Adders (Bitis arietans). J Zoo Wildl Med 1989;20(3):364–9.
33. Stewart JS. Anaerobic Bacterial Infections in Reptiles. J Zoo Wildl Med 1990; 21(2):180–4.

34. Wimsatt J, Tothill A, Offermann CF, et al. Long-term and per rectum disposition of clarithromycin in the desert tortoise (Gopherus agassizii). J Am Assoc Lab Anim Sci 2008;47(4):41–5.

35. Wimsatt J, Johnson J, Mangone BA, et al. Clarithromycin Pharmacokinetics in the Desert Tortoise (Gopherus agassizii). J Zoo Wildl Med 1999;30(1):36–43.

36. Rettenmund CL, Boyer DM, Orrico WJ, et al. Long-term oral clarithromycin administration in chelonians with subclinical Mycoplasma spp. infection. J Herp Med Surg 2017;27(1-2):58-61.

37. Harms CA, Papich MG, Stamper MA, et al. Pharmacokinetics of oxytetracycline in loggerhead sea turtles (caretta caretta) after single intravenous and intramuscular injections. J Zoo Wildl Med 2004;35(4):477–88.

38. Helmick KE, Papich MG, Vliet KA, et al. Pharmacokinetic disposition of a long-acting oxytetracycline formulation after single-dose intravenous and intramuscular administrations in the american alligator (alligator mississippiensis). J Zoo Wildl Med 2004;35(3):341–6.

39. Hyndman TH, Shilton CM, Marschang RE. Paramyxoviruses in reptiles: A review. Vet Microbiol 2013;165(3):200–13.

40. Starck JM, Neul A, Schmidt V, et al. Morphology and morphometry of the lung in corn snakes (pantherophis guttatus) infected with three different strains of ferlavirus. J Comp Pathol 2017;156(4):419–35.

41. Jacobson E. Parasites and parasitic diseases of reptiles. In: Jacobson E, editor. Infectious diseases and pathology of reptiles. Boca Raton (FL): CRC Press; 2007. p. 571–680.

42. Cameron JL, Mitchell WH, Zuidema GD. Aspiration pneumonia. Clinical outcome following documented aspiration. Arch Surg 1973;106(1):49–52.

43. Marik PE. Aspiration Pneumonitis and Aspiration Pneumonia. N Engl J Med 2001; 344(9):665–71.

Respiratory Disorders in Chelonians

Kelsea Studer, DVM, Nicola Di Girolamo, DVM, MSc(EBHC), PhD, DiplECZM (Herp), DiplACZM*

KEYWORDS

- Reptiles • Respiratory • Lungs • Trachea • Diagnostics • Tracheal flush • Turtle
- Tortoise

KEY POINTS

- Understanding of specific chelonian respiratory tract anatomy is mandatory to assess the respiratory tract.
- Radiology is a first imaging step in order to assess chelonians with respiratory disorder, but proper positioning and horizontal beam views are needed.
- Computed tomography should be currently regarded as the reference standard for imaging of lung disorders in chelonians.
- Before starting treatment, clinicians should consider using techniques that allow sampling of the lungs, such as tracheal or bronchial lavage, in order to run cytology, culture, and sensitivity testing.
- Specific infectious disease agents such as Mycoplasma spp., herpesvirus, ranavirus, and testudo intranuclear coccidia should be considered, and appropriate testing should be performed.

INTRODUCTION

Respiratory tract disease is commonly diagnosed in chelonians, which can result in significant morbidity and mortality. In a retrospective pathologic survey of diseases presented in reptiles sold through a pet store chain and submitted for postmortem examination, 10% (5/50) of the chelonians had pneumonia.[1] It is thought that respiratory tract disease in reptiles is multifactorial and may be triggered by suboptimal husbandry conditions such as inappropriate environmental temperature, humidity, or diet, resulting in immunosuppression. Infectious agents that can affect the respiratory tract of chelonians include viral, bacterial, fungal, and parasitic organisms. Noninfectious diseases, such as trauma or nutritional deficiencies, can also have influence on respiratory tract pathology. A common misconception is that respiratory signs in chelonians are always caused by respiratory tract disease. Because chelonians lack a proper diaphragm, changes in size of celomic organs, as seen for example, during

Oklahoma State University, Center for Veterinary Health Sciences, 2065 West Farm Road, Stillwater, OK 74078, USA
* Corresponding author.
E-mail address: nicoladiggi@gmail.com

Vet Clin Exot Anim 24 (2021) 341–367
https://doi.org/10.1016/j.cvex.2021.01.004
1094-9194/21/© 2021 Elsevier Inc. All rights reserved.

constipation, urinary bladder overdistension, urolithiasis, follicular stasis, and celomic effusion, among other conditions, can cause compression on the respiratory system. These conditions result in clinical signs that could be attributed to the respiratory system, such as open-mouth breathing.[2]

The initial evaluation for respiratory disease is similar to those of other domestic animals; however, several anatomic and physiologic differences exist that the clinician should be aware of. In addition, diagnostic procedures such as diagnostic imaging techniques, sample obtainment, and treatment protocols have many unique intricacies. Appropriate treatment depends on identifying underlying cause such as infectious disease as well as correcting suboptimal husbandry practices. This article outlines the unique anatomy and physiology of chelonians and discusses common clinical presentations for respiratory disease. It should be noted that further research is still required to better understand many aspects of chelonian respiratory disease such as appropriate drug dosing schemes and regimens.[3] In addition, clinicians are encouraged to perform a recent literature search before selection of treatment therapies, as novel pharmacokinetic, pharmacodynamic, and efficacy studies may have been recently published.

ANATOMY AND PHYSIOLOGY

Chelonians breath through their nares with the mouth remaining closed during normal respiration. Breathing sounds are rarely audible. Buccal pulsations can be observed but are not associated with respirations and are rather thought to be associated with olfaction.[4] Chelonians lack an epiglottis.[5] The glottis remains open during both inspiration and expiration.[4] The trachea is supported by completely closed cartilaginous rings. The larynx and anterior aspect of the trachea are supported by the hyoid apparatus and its associated ligaments. There are 2 arytenoid cartilages but the thyroid cartilage is lacking. Chelonians lack vocal cords.[5] The trachea runs along the left side of the neck and is short but flexible, allowing retraction of the head into the shell.[6]

Because of the carapace, the lungs have limited expansion abilities. As with other reptiles, chelonians lack a muscular diaphragm and instead rely on the inguinal, axial, and shoulder muscles to cause intrapulmonary pressure changes.[4,7] The postpulmonary (or horizontal) septum functions to separate the lungs from the coelomic contents.[7] All phases of respiration are active. The obliquus abdominis and serratus major muscles increase coelomic volume, thereby decreasing pressure during inspirations, whereas the transversus abdominis and pectoralis muscles increase coelomic pressure to drive expirations. These inward and outward motions compress and expand the body cavity, causing pressure changes on the lungs.[4,7] Increased respiratory effort causes increasing involvement of the head and neck.[7]

The lungs are grossly symmetric and occupy the cranial half to two-thirds of the dorsal celomic cavity (**Fig. 1**) but are reduced to a fraction of that when the head and limbs are retracted.[4,6,8] Lungs are covered by a thick pulmonary pleura and have no apparent lobation.[8,9] Terminology and anatomy of chelonians have not been standardized and some discrepancies in the literature exist. The trachea bifurcates into 2 primary bronchi, also called intrapulmonary bronchi or first-order bronchi, which travel caudal through the lung decreasing in size until terminating at the caudal border of the lung.[8,9] Secondary bronchi, also called second-order branches or chambers, arise from the primary bronchi in a lateral and medial pattern of branching.[6,9] Large cavitations referred to as niches run alongside the secondary bronchi, resulting in a corrugated appearance.[9] Secondary bronchi give rise to tertiary bronchi, or bronchioles, of decreasing diameter.[6,8] Gas exchange occurs in ediculae and faveoli.[8,9] The

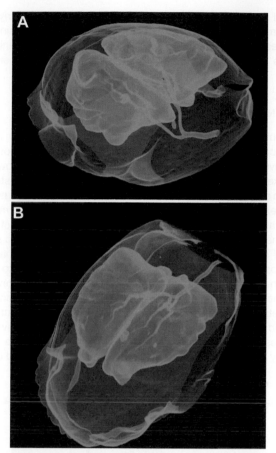

Fig. 1. Three-dimensional volume rendering of the trachea, bronchi, and lungs in a red-eared slider (*Trachemys scripta elegans*). Notice the location of the lungs, right ventral to the carapace and dorsal to the celomic structures (*A*), and the conformation of the lungs, expanded cranially and gradually reduced in volume caudally (*B*). (*Courtesy of* Nicola Di Girolamo.)

pulmonary arteries and veins follow the bronchial tree in an arborized pattern.[9] Capillaries project into the alveoli to facilitate gas exchange.[8] With the large amount of branching, niches, and alveoli or ediculae and faveoli, chelonians have larger airway to parenchyma ratio as compared with mammals.[8]

Chelonians, similar to other reptiles, have an arrhythmic breathing with variable and potentially prolonged periods of apnea.[4,7,10] Respirations are driven by numerous factors including hypoxia, hypercapnia, acid-base changes, and lung stretch receptors.[7,10] A variety of different regulatory pathways, including the vagus nerve, are involved in regulation of variables such as frequency and tidal volume.[10] Hypercapnia and hypoxia cause stimulation in respiration predominately by reducing periods of apnea.[7,10] Hypercapnia generally increases ventilation more than hypoxia. Severe hypercapnia results in nearly complete elimination of apneic periods. Frequency of respirations or tidal volume may or may not increase with these variables.[7] There is considerable amount of variation noted between species and studies.[7,10] Intrapulmonary shunts are reported in chelonians, which can result in reduced gas exchange and therefore reduced arterial P_{O_2}. Right to left shunting is seen particularly with apnea and increased parasympathetic nervous system tone. A recent study using electrocardiogram MRI reported an increased pulmonary blood flow after administration of atropine, the effects of which resulted in minimum alveolar concentration sparing effects.[11]

PHYSICAL EXAMINATION

For captive chelonians, a thorough history including diet, husbandry, and medical history before physical examination should be obtained. For the purpose of this article, those aspects involving the respiratory system are described; however, similar to other animals, examination of the musculoskeletal, neurologic, gastrointestinal, and urogenital system should also be included whenever possible. Because of their cryptic nature, physical examination of chelonians can be extremely frustrating. In small to medium chelonians, a preliminary assessment of the respiratory tract can be typically performed with manual restraint. In larger chelonians and in specific species (eg, box turtles), chemical restraint is often required. However, even in small chelonians an incorrect initial approach can significantly compromise the ability to perform a complete examination. Before restraining the animal, visual observation should be performed, which include an assessment of the body condition, mental status, head and body symmetry, posture, such as buoyancy in the case of aquatic turtles, color of the nostrils and presence of any discharge, and respiratory activity. Open-mouth breathing or excessive movements of the limbs or neck should be considered as a sign of respiratory distress (**Fig. 2**). An accurate body weight should be obtained during examination.

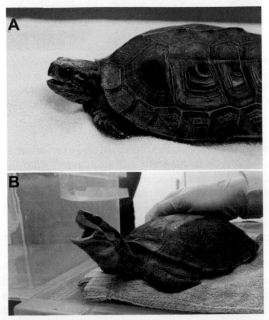

Fig. 2. Increased respiratory effort in 2 chelonians. (*A*) Open-mouth breathing in a keeled box turtle (*Cuora mouhotii*). (*B*) Open-mouth breathing with extensive neck extension in a Chinese 3-striped box turtle (*Cuora trifasciata*). (*Courtesy of* Nicola Di Girolamo.)

Nares should be assessed for patency, symmetry, discoloration, erosions, or discharge (**Fig. 3**). Chronic respiratory disease may be characterized by erosions or depigmentation of the nares (**Fig. 4**). Eyes should be evaluated for swelling or discharge. Tympanic membranes should be assessed for swellings and integrity. The assessment of the oral cavity is a crucial part of the examination of the respiratory tract and can be performed by means of a speculum or just applying gentle pressure on the side of the mandibles. The oral cavity should be inspected for the presence of plaque, excess of saliva, ulcerations, or other abnormalities. The glottis is easily visualized in most chelonians just caudal to the tongue. Mucous membrane color should be evaluated, and the oral cavity should be assessed for stringy saliva, which occurs with dehydration. Although the shell may limit auscultation, a small stethoscope may be placed in the thoracic inlet and directed dorsally on either side for auscultation (**Fig. 5A**). Some investigators have advised auscultation of the lungs with an electronic stethoscope after placement of a wet towel on the carapace (**Fig. 5B**). The heart rate can be obtained by means of a doppler. For aquatic turtles, buoyancy should also be evaluated, as atypical floating may be associated with either lung consolidation or inappropriate gas accumulation.[12] Other disorders including gas accumulation in the gastrointestinal tract or into the accessory bladders can result in positive buoyancy.[13]

HEMATOLOGY AND BLOOD CHEMISTRY

Hematology results during lung disorders may vary. There may be variations in leukocyte count, such as monocytosis, which are considered to indicate chronic underlying infection or inflammation.[14] Blood chemistry does not seem to be specific for respiratory disease; however, it could indicate other concurrent underlying systemic effects such as dehydration or inflammation.[14–16] Chronic disorders, including those affecting the respiratory tract, can result in increased or decreased packed cell volume (PCV) and increased or decreased glucose. Both these analytes are significant prognostic indicators of death in chelonians. Odds of death for chelonians with severe anemia (PCV, <10%) and moderate anemia (PCV, 11% to 20%) are 6.8 times (adjusted odds ratio [aOR], 6.8; 95% confidence interval [CI], 3.8–12.3) and 1.6 times (aOR,

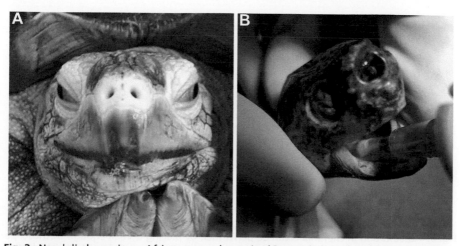

Fig. 3. Nasal discharge in an African spurred tortoise (*Centrochelys sulcata*) (*A*) and in a Hermann's tortoise (*Testudo hermanni*) (*B*). The African spurred tortoise tested negative to herpesvirus and positive to *Mycoplasma* sp. (*Courtesy of* Nicola Di Girolamo.)

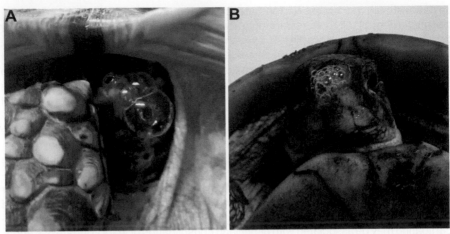

Fig. 4. Chronic changes associated with upper respiratory tract disease in chelonians. (*A*) Depigmentation of the nostrils in an African spurred tortoise (*Centrochelys sulcata*) with chronic nasal discharge that tested positive for *Mycoplasma* sp. (*B*) Severe erosion of the nostrils in a common musk turtle (*Sternotherus odoratus*). (*Courtesy of* Nicola Di Girolamo.)

1.6; 95% CI, 1.01–2.7), respectively, odds of death for chelonians with PCV within reference range. Odds of death for chelonians with severe hypoglycemia (<30 mg/dL), moderate hyperglycemia (91–150 mg/dL), and severe hyperglycemia (>181 mg/dL) are 5.3 times (aOR, 5.3; 95% CI; 2.4–11.4), 3 times (aOR, 3.0; 95% CI, 1.4–6.3), and 4.3 times (aOR, 4.3; 95% CI, 2.4–7.6), respectively, odds of death for chelonians with blood glucose concentration within reference range.[17]

Blood gases may be beneficial for evaluation of respiratory disease as in other vertebrates; however, validation is only available for individual analyzers,[18] and clear patterns correlated with disease are lacking. Arterial blood gas has considerable variation based on periods of apnea.[7] The use of venous blood gas samples in Eastern box

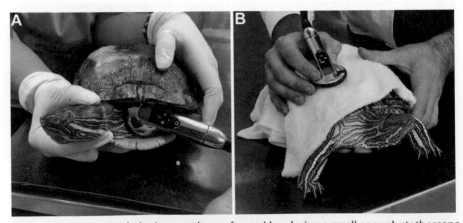

Fig. 5. Auscultation in chelonians can be performed by placing a small enough stethoscope in the cervical inlet and directed dorsally on either side (*A*) or by using an electronic stethoscope after placement of a wet towel on the carapace (*B*). Either of these techniques provide a clear assessment as in mammals. (*Courtesy of* Nicola Di Girolamo.)

turtles (*Terrapene carolina carolina*) noted variation in values depending on season, activity level, and PCV.[15] Normal values of selected blood gases for Eastern box turtles (*Terrapene carolina carolina*) and Hermann's tortoises (*Testudo hermanni*) are provided in **Table 1**.[15,18]

DIAGNOSTIC IMAGING
Radiography

Radiography is commonly the initial diagnostic imaging modality of choice for chelonians. Radiographs are quick and inexpensive as compared with computed tomography (CT) or MRI, but they are not necessarily sensitive nor specific for diagnosing lung disorders. In addition, radiographs provide limited information on the upper airways such are sinuses and nasal turbinates. Radiographic images should be obtained in multiple views to properly evaluate 3-dimensional structures in a 2-dimensional plane and maximize diagnostic accuracy. To perform radiographs, chelonians can be sedated or otherwise restrained using radiolucent materials. In most instances, appropriate positioning can be achieved safely without anesthesia and without radiation exposure to the operators. Chelonian radiographs should be obtained in 3 views, including a lateral (horizontal beam), dorsoventral (vertical beam), and a craniocaudal (horizontal beam) projection. For vertical beam radiographs, a dorsally open-faced box fitting the dimensions of the carapace helps prevent movement (**Fig 6**A, B). For horizontal beam radiographs, positioning chelonians on an elevated cylindrical surface smaller than the plastron will stimulate the animals to extend the limbs, while also preventing ambulation (**Fig. 6**C). Lateral radiographs obtained using vertical

Table 1
Reference intervals for selected blood gas values from venous blood samples of Hermann's tortoises (n = 24) and Eastern box turtles (n = 40–41) during summer measured with a portable blood gas analyzer (iSTAT, Abaxis).[15,18]

	Hermann's Tortoises (*Testudo hermanni*)			Eastern Box Turtles (*Terrapene carolina carolina*)		
	Reference Interval	90% CI	90% CI	Reference Interval	90% CI	90% CI
pH	7.14–7.51	7.10, 7.20	7.46, 7.55	7.00–7.78	6.92, 7.01	7.78, 7.88
Po_2 (mm Hg)	12.57–109.05	0, 32.59	86.72, 126.73	8–97	0, 9	97, 103
Pco_2 (mm Hg)	27.17–87.63	18.29, 37.79	76.77, 96.87	16.5–74.7	12.4, 16.6	74.4, 82.4
HCO_3 (mmol/L)				20.4–40.6	18.4, 20.4	40.5, 42.9
Lactate (mmol/L)				2.45–12.16	1.77, 2.46	12.15, 13.38
Base excess (mmol/L)				−13–14	−17, −13	14, 19

The 90% confidence intervals for the upper and lower limits of the reference intervals are provided.
Modified from: Adamovicz L et al. Venous blood gas in free-living eastern box turtles (*Terrapene Carolina Carolina*) and the effects of physiologic, demographic and environmental factors. Conserv Physiol. 2018;6(1):copy041; Di Girolamo N, Ferlizza E, Selleri P, Nardini G, Isani G. Evaluation of point-of-care analysers for blood gas and clinical chemistry in Hermann's tortoises (Testudo hermanni). J Small Anim Pract. 2018 Nov;59(11):704 to 713.

beam with animals in lateral recumbency may result in displacement of the loosely attached viscera, making diagnostic interpretation more challenging. To prevent compression of the lungs caused by celomic viscera, lateral and cranio-caudal radiographs should always be obtained with a horizontal beam. Furthermore, for maximizing expansion of the lungs, the legs, and neck of chelonians should be extended or exteriorized during horizontal beam lateral radiographs (**Fig. 7**)[19]; this may be especially clinically relevant if alterations are present at the level of the lungs, because radiographs obtained with limbs and neck extended allows a much better visualization of the area (**Fig. 8**). The dorsoventral view has limited visualization of the lungs due to superimposition with coelomic soft tissue structures; however, it can be useful to evaluate the cranio-caudal expansion of the lungs (**Fig. 9**). Lateral views provide visualization of the lungs as compared with coelomic soft tissue structures; however, the 2 lung lobes are superimposed with each other. For this reason, the craniocaudal view is essential, as it allows separate visualization of the lung fields (**Fig. 10**). Alterations of the lungs on radiographs are potentially visible also in extremely small chelonians (ie, <50 g of body weight) (**Fig. 11**).

Changes in lung opacity are difficult to be properly characterized in chelonians due to the superimposition of the carapace. Nodular, interstitial, and alveolar opacities have been described in chelonians.[20,21] It is, however, currently unclear the actual sensitivity (ie, proportion of positives that are correctly identified) and specificity (ie, proportion of negatives that are correctly identified) of radiographs for specific pulmonary diseases in chelonians. In other words, it is not known what are the chances that a chelonian with actual pulmonary disease will be correctly identified as having

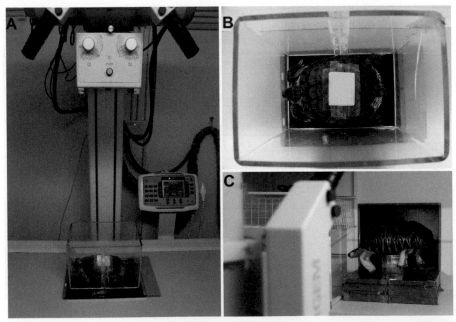

Fig. 6. Positioning of chelonians for radiographs (*A and B*). Use of a dorsally open-faced box fitting the dimensions of the carapace helps prevent movements of the animal and avoid superimposition of material on the radiographic field. (*C*) Use of an elevated cylindrical surface slightly smaller than the plastron will stimulate the animals to extend the limbs, while also preventing ambulation. (*Courtesy of* Nicola Di Girolamo.)

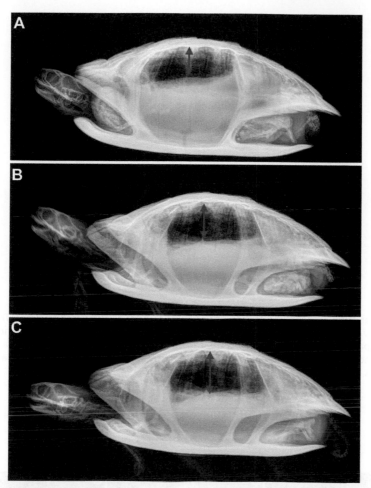

Fig. 7. Variations in expansion of the pulmonary fields depending on the extension of limbs and neck in the same red-eared slider (*Trachemys scripta elegans*) in horizontal beam lateral views. (*A*) The turtle is laying with the neck and both forelimbs and hindlimbs withdrawn in the carapace. Notice that lung expansion is minimal. (*B*) The forelimbs are extended in this radiograph, and the lung fields are slightly more expanded. (*C*) Both the forelimbs and the hindlimbs are extended in this radiograph, and the neck is more extended than on panel A, resulting in a higher expansion of the lung fields. (*Courtesy of* Nicola Di Girolamo.)

pulmonary disease based on radiographs or the opposite. It is extremely important to notice that mild to moderate changes may not be detected with radiographs and may require a more sensitive modality such as CT or MRI. Interpretation of the pulmonary tissue in chelonian radiographs may be further hindered by the compression of the coelom and deformation of the carapace. A compression of the lungs may generate artifactual changes that should not be confused with actual pathologic changes. A common reason for compression of the lungs that may result in misdiagnosis of lung pathology is the expansion of coelomic organs or coelomic fluid accumulation (**Fig. 12**). Another common reason is the change in shape of the carapace due to altered shell formation (**Fig. 13**). In both these situations, the clinician should be careful

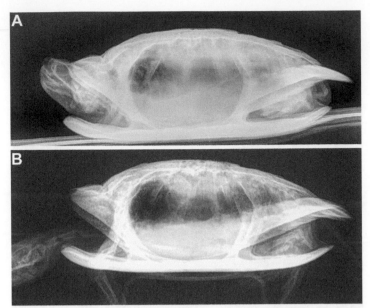

Fig. 8. Variation in the interpretation of radiographs from a yellow-bellied slider (*Trachemys scripta scripta*) with vertebral osteomyelitis. Notice that with neck and limbs withdrawn in the carapace (*A*), interpretation of the lung fields is limited. In panel (*B*), neck and limbs are extended, providing clear evidence of focal increased radiopacity in the dorsal area of the lungs. (*Courtesy of* Nicola Di Girolamo.)

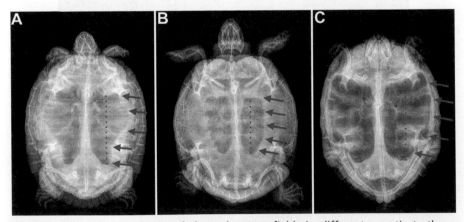

Fig. 9. Variations in expansion of the pulmonary fields in different aquatic turtles as observed in vertical beam dorsoventral radiographic views. The degree of craniocaudal and lateral expansion is considered normal in panel (*A*), decreased in panel (*B*), and increased in panel (*C*). The turtle in panel B had severe celomic effusion that contributed to compression of the lungs, whereas the turtle in panel C had prolonged anorexia and severe dehydration, resulting in overexpansion of the lungs. (*Courtesy of* Nicola Di Girolamo.)

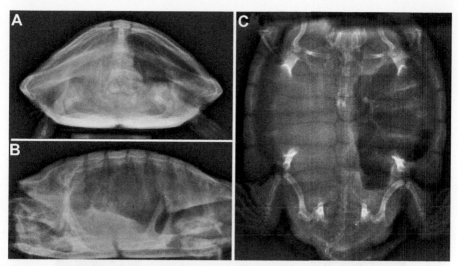

Fig. 10. Unilateral increase in radiopacity of the right lung in an adult red-eared slider (*Trachemys scripta elegans*) in craniocaudal, horizontal beam, view (*A*); lateral, horizontal beam, view (*B*); and dorsoventral, vertical beam, view (*C*). In cases similar to this one, further sampling is required to confirm pneumonia and establish the cause. Notice that both in dorsoventral and craniocaudal views the difference in lung radiopacity is evident. (*Courtesy of* Nicola Di Girolamo.)

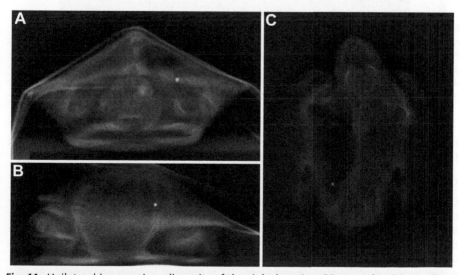

Fig. 11. Unilateral increase in radiopacity of the right lung in a 20-g, posthatchling yellow-bellied slider (*Trachemys scripta scripta*) in craniocaudal, horizontal beam, view (*A*); lateral, horizontal beam, view (*B*); and dorsoventral, vertical beam, view (*C*). The small size of a chelonian should not limit the clinician in attempting further investigations. (*Courtesy of* Nicola Di Girolamo.)

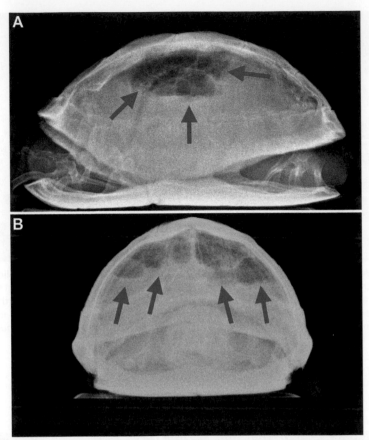

Fig. 12. Compression of the lungs in an adult female Chinese box turtle (*Cuora flavomarginata*) presenting numerous tertiary follicles and free celomic fluid as visualized in lateral, horizontal beam, view (*A*) and craniocaudal, horizontal beam, view (*B*). Because the lungs are heavily compressed, the radiopacity of the parenchyma may be artefactually increased and the symmetry in craniocaudal view may be lost, without actually representing any primary pulmonary disorder. (*Courtesy of* Nicola Di Girolamo.)

to formulate a diagnosis of primary lung disorder, because asymmetry of the lungs and focal areas with increased opacity are to be expected.

Computed Tomography

CT should be currently regarded as the reference standard for imaging of lung disorders in chelonians.[9] This modality is also of benefit when evaluating upper respiratory tissue.[22] There are several published reports of chelonians with pulmonary disorders that were not diagnosed on radiographs but were actually evident on CT.[23,24] The advantages of CT are that it is noninvasive, allows higher parenchyma detail, and avoids superimposition of the shell on the lungs. CT in medium to large chelonians can also be used for evaluation of other respiratory structures such as the sinuses. The feasibility of CT scan has been demonstrated in several publications and has been useful for diagnosing several disease processes such as pulmonary fibrosis, pneumonia, emphysema, and pulmonary abscess.[23,25]

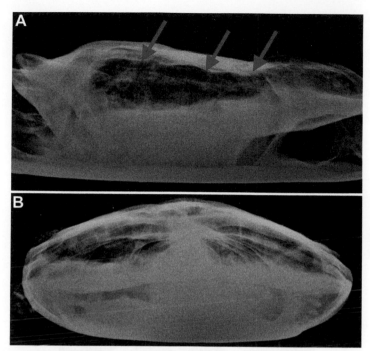

Fig. 13. Compression of the lungs in an adult female red-eared slider (*Trachemys scripta elegans*) presenting severe chronic metabolic bone disease and altered carapacial growth. (*A*) Craniocaudal, horizontal beam, view. (*B*) Lateral, horizontal beam, view. In this case, the shell was deformed and flattened resulting in dorsal compression of the lungs. Same as in **Fig. 12**, the radiopacity of the parenchyma may be artefactually increased and the symmetry in cranio-caudal view may be lost, without actually representing any primary pulmonary disorder. (*Courtesy of* Nicola Di Girolamo.)

CT in reptiles can be performed with or without sedation or anesthesia and the same applies for chelonians.[19] Most CT scanners currently available to veterinarians can scan a whole medium-sized chelonian in few seconds. If CT is performed without chemical restraint, the patient can be either restrained within a tight fighting box or propped on a block to limit patient motion. Different chelonians will react differently after being placed on a block, and clinicians should be ready to convert to sedation. Positioning in vertical recumbency is not recommended, as this significantly limits lung volume. However, if the purpose of the examination is to evaluate the pulmonary parenchyma, the head and limbs should be extended.[19] Injection of intravenous contrast is beneficial for visualization of the pulmonary vasculature, potentially allowing for diagnosis of pulmonary embolism, and makes a tremendous difference in the evaluation of soft tissue organs in the coelom. Intravenous contrast can be administered after catheter placement, the most accessible vessel being the jugular vein, or through an intravenous injection. The subcarapacial plexus should not be used for this purpose due to previously reported complications.[26]

The lungs appear in an arborization-like pattern with bronchioles extending from the main bronchus within the right and left lung (**Figs. 14–16**). Airway cavitations, referred to as niches, are found throughout the parenchyma causing an increased airway to parenchyma ratio in a honey-comb–like pattern.[9] In specific situations, serial imaging with CT scan may be helpful to monitor disease progression.

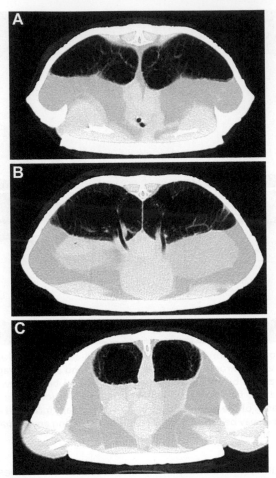

Fig. 14. Axial sections of the lungs in an adult female red-eared slider (*Trachemys scripta elegans*). (*A*) Section cranial to the heart, showing the first visualization of the lungs progressing in a cranial to caudal direction. (*B*) Section at the level of the heart, showing the access of the main bronchi in the lungs. Notice maximum expansion of the lungs. (*C*) Section at the level of the prefemoral fossa, showing a distinct reduction in the size of the lungs. (*Courtesy of* Nicola Di Girolamo.)

MRI

MRI can be used to identify respiratory tract in chelonians, the main advantage of this technique being the lack of radiation exposure to the patient. Because of the long time generally involved with MRI, sedation or anesthesia may be required.[27] It is currently unclear if MRI is advantageous as compared with CT for diagnosis of specific conditions of the lungs in chelonians.

Endoscopy

Rhinoscopy and tracheobroncoscopy are a key tool for the diagnosis of respiratory diseases in mammals. The advantage of endoscopy is that it allows sample collection for cytology, histology, culture, and molecular biology while remaining a technique

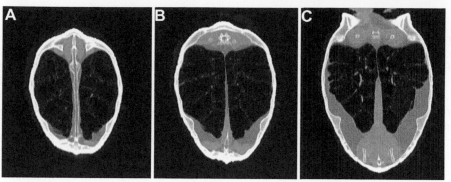

Fig. 15. Coronal sections of the lungs in the same red-eared slider (*Trachemys scripta elegans*) as in **Fig. 17**. Notice how the lungs occupy the entire carapacial space at the level of the vertebrae (*A*) and gradually decrease in size in sections closer to the plastron (*B, C*). In C, the prominent pulmonary vasculature can be visualized. (*Courtesy of* Nicola Di Girolamo.)

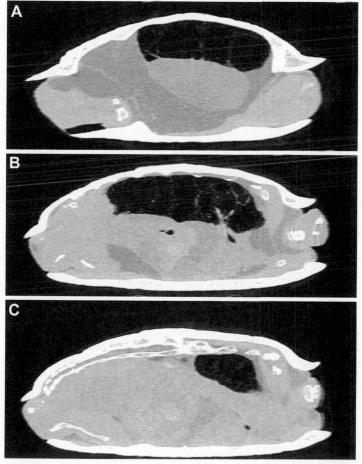

Fig. 16. Parasagittal sections of the lungs in the same red-eared slider (*Trachemys scripta elegans*) as in **Fig. 17**. Progressing from more lateral (*A*) to more median (*C*), the right lung progressively extends caudally and then reduces to a small cranial area. In (*B*), the prominent pulmonary vasculature can be visualized. (*Courtesy of* Nicola Di Girolamo.)

relatively noninvasive. In chelonians, the size of the animal and the size and type of instrument available to the clinician limit feasibility of intraluminal endoscopy. Rhinoscopy and tracheoscopy can be performed to visualize the upper respiratory tract; however, the narrow trachea and sharp deviations to primary bronchi may limit visualization of the lower airways in small- and medium-sized chelonians. For this reason, alternative approaches such as carapace osteotomy or a craniodorsal prefemoral approach have been developed.[28,29] The invasiveness of these approaches requires previous localization of lesions with either radiographs, CT, or MRI for a more targeted diagnostic procedure.

SAMPLE COLLECTION

In order to obtain a correct diagnosis, diagnostic imaging needs often to be followed by sample collection for cytology, histology, culture, and antibiotic sensitivity testing and molecular biology. Upper respiratory samples including culture and cytology may be obtained via nasal flush (**Fig. 17**), which may also have a therapeutic effect (mucous clogging the nasal passages (**Fig. 17**B) or vegetal foreign bodies (**Fig. 17**D) removal). Sampling from the lower airway tract can be conducted via tracheal wash (**Fig. 18**).[29] When respiratory tract samples are obtained, it is always advisable to perform cytology plus aerobic, anaerobic, and fungal cultures. Granulomas may require biopsy for culture and histopathology via either surgery or endoscopy.[29]

Specialized infectious disease testing, such as for *Mycoplasma*, herpesvirus, or intranuclear coccidiosis, should be considered in many cases. Tests such as serology may not appropriately reflect disease exposure due to poor humeral antibody response. When possible, culture of pathogens is the preferred diagnostic modality; however, particular agents such as *Mycoplasma* may difficult to isolate through culture alone.[30] Various polymerase chain reaction (PCR) tests are available and is advantageous, as the suspected agent does not need to be viable. PCR tests, however, rely on obtaining appropriate samples containing the actual pathogen; therefore, negative tests cannot completely rule out that the pathogen can be present in other anatomic localization.[31]

SPIROMETRY

Spirometry is a test routinely performed in humans that assess how well the lungs work by measuring how much air is inhaled and exhaled, among other values. Spirometry and pulmonary function tests have been described in 2 ill and 2 healthy olive ridley sea turtles.[12] The results of this study showed that those with positive buoyancy disorders had higher tidal volumes, lower breathing frequency patterns, and higher expiration rates. These findings showed that the metabolic cost of breathing with positive buoyancy was much greater, approximately 8 times, as compared with the clinically normal turtles.[12] Currently, the use and interpretation of spirometry in clinical chelonian practice is limited by the lack of normal reference intervals for commonly kept species.

SPECIFIC DISORDERS
Infectious Diseases

Infectious agents may result in either upper or lower respiratory tract infections. Upper respiratory infections may be characterized by ocular or nasal discharge, erosions of the nares, or oral stomatitis or plaques formation. Pneumonia may occur as a primary or secondary opportunistic infection due to underlying disease or suboptimal

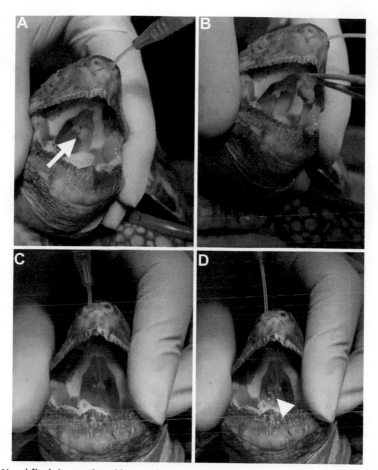

Fig. 17. Nasal flush in a sedated leopard tortoise (*Stigmochelys pardalis*). This procedure can have both diagnostics and therapeutic purposes. In this case, a large mucous clog was removed from the left nasal cavity at the level of the choanae (*arrow*) (*A, B*), whereas a vegetal foreign body was removed from the right nasal cavity (*C, D*). Some chelonians may be open-mouth breathing because of the occlusion of the nasal cavities. (*Courtesy of* Nicola Di Girolamo.)

husbandry. Because of tolerance for anaerobic conditions, many chelonians will not exhibit clinical signs until disease is severe. Although variable, clinical signs may include anorexia, lethargy, increased respiratory rate or effort, increased or abnormal respiratory sounds, abnormal stretching of the neck while breathing, or positive buoyancy in aquatic species.

Bacterial

It is commonly reported that normal bacterial flora of chelonians is predominately Gram negative and that these bacteria may become opportunistic in times of underlying stress or systemic illness.[29] Gram-negative bacteria reported include *Klebsiella, Pseudomonas, Aeromonas, Proteus, Pasteurella*, and *Salmonella*.[16,32] *Pasteurella testudines* has been isolated from healthy tortoises but may also be associated with primary infection.[16,30] Gram-positive and anaerobic infections, including

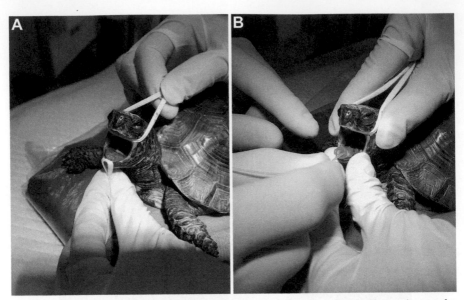

Fig. 18. Tracheal flush in a sedated keeled box turtle (*Cuora mouhotii*). The author prefers to intubate the animal first and only then pass the sampling tube (in this case a 1-mm cat urinary catheter) in the endotracheal tube. This technique may reduce contamination of the sampling tube with bacteria normally present at the level of the glottis. (*Courtesy of* Nicola Di Girolamo.)

Fusobacterium, Clostridium, and *Bacteroides,* have also been reported.[33] Intracellular bacterial infections may also be considered as a differential for atypical pneumonia, particularly granulomatous in appearance. *Chlamydia* has been isolated uncommonly as a potential source of pneumonia.[34,35] *Mycobacterium* has also been reported predominately within wild populations; however, reports in captive populations also exist.[34] Considering the potential for multiresistant bacteria currently affecting reptiles and other animals, the authors suggest to always perform culture and sensitivity testing before treating any chelonian with respiratory signs.[36]

Mycoplasma has been extensively documented to cause both upper and lower bacterial respiratory infections both in wild and captive chelonian populations.[31,37,38] The most common *Mycoplasma* documented is *Mycoplasma agassizii.* A separate species *Mycoplasma testudo* was also isolated and associated with clinical disease, but the bacteria seems to have a lower pathogenicity than M. agassizii.[38] In addition, mixed respiratory tract infections with either *M agassizii and Mycoplasma testudines, P testudines,* intranuclear coccidiosis, iridovirus, adenovirus, and herpesvirus have been also reported.[14,16,30,39,40] Transmission is suspected to be by direct contact though environmental transmission. The disease is, however, likely multifactorial, and outbreaks are often associated with environmental stress or other underlying pathology such as heavy metal intoxication.[16,30] Clinical signs are variable depending on patient and chronicity. Acute cases are reported to show clinical signs such as rhinitis; conjunctivitis; nasal or ocular discharge; and palpebral, periocular, or conjunctival edema, whereas chronic cases may show depigmentation of nares and vertical erosions ventral to the nares.[30–32,38] Damage to the respiratory and olfactory epithelial surfaces can result in inability to identify food.[30] Host inflammatory response may vary between individuals, and overexuberant host response may result in additional dysplastic changes to nasal mucosa.[16] Subclinical and asymptomatic cases can also occur.[30]

Several diagnostic options are available for *Mycoplasma* including culture, enzyme-linked immunosorbent assay (ELISA) and PCR. Bacterial culture is often unrewarding due to the slow growing and fastidious nature of *Mycoplasma*.[31,32] ELISA is based on antibody response of either serum or plasma and indicates exposure. Serology is of limited value, as it may be difficult to distinguish an active infection without using paired titers.[32] In addition, because of the extremely slow response of reptilian immune system, significant delays in response or lack of antibody response may occur. In one study, a range of 420 to 494 days until antibody response postinoculation of herpesvirus was noted.[41] PCR tests are also available and may be useful to identify acute infection, but it is very sensitive but less specific than ELISA.[32] Samples may include either nasal flush or other respiratory samples. Multiple studies have noted that nasal flush is less sensitive than actual testing of the nasal mucosal; therefore false negatives should be considered possible if nasal flush is performed.[37,42]

Mycoplasma has historically been treated with fluoroquinolones and macrolides, with recent suggestion for the use of azithromycin, clarithromycin, or danofloxacin.[43] Although treatment may resolve clinical signs, chelonians previously diagnosed with *Mycoplasma* should be considered positive life long, as latency with relapse later in life is reported.[30,32]

Viral

Herpesvirus is currently the most prevalent viral infection documented in both wild and captive chelonians. Transmission has been shown experimentally both intranasally and intramuscularly.[44] Clinical signs include anorexia, lethargy, rhinitis, conjunctivitis, stomatitis, or oral plaques. Based on these clinical signs, it is difficult to distinguish herpesvirus from *Mycoplasma* infection.[32,44] Additional lesions include tracheitis and bronchopneumonia. Nonrespiratory infections include cutaneous, neurologic, gastrointestinal, or hepatic forms. In addition, secondary bacterial infections or other coinfections are reported.[1] Similar to other herpesviral infections, clinical signs and shedding of the virus can be cyclic and have periods of latency. Development of neutralizing antibodies does not seem to prevent recurrence of clinical signs.[44]

Diagnostic testing available for herpesvirus include antibody testing using serum neutralization test or ELISA. Accuracy between these 2 tests is similar; however, ELISA may be more rapidly available.[44] Several PCR tests that can be run on tissues or swabs are also commercially available.[45–47] Similar to *Mycoplasma*, PCR is recommended during acute outbreaks in which antibodies may not be present. With monitoring and quarantine programs, a combination of antibody testing and PCR may be considered.[32,44] Histopathology may also show changes such as the presence of eosinophilic intranuclear inclusions, syncytial giant cells, and bacterial granulomas but would either require an appropriate antemortem biopsy or is obtained post-mortem.[32] Indirect and direct immunoperoxidase techniques can be also used to detect herpesviral antigen and antiherpes immunoglobulin in serum and tissues.[48]

Ranavirus, from the family Iridoviridae, is an emerging virus with the ability to infect amphibians, fish, and reptiles.[14,49] Molecular studies have found that the ranavirus infecting chelonians are of amphibian origin. Amphibians are therefore a likely reservoir for susceptible chelonians resulting in spill-over events.[14] Although not primary pulmonary in origin, ranavirus causes systemic vasculitis that can result in inflammation, necrosis, and thrombosis in multiple areas of the body including the upper respiratory tract and lungs.[49–53] Clinical signs reported are variable but may include nasal and ocular discharge, conjunctivitis, palpebral edema, and caseous plaques within the oral cavity.[14,32,49] Asymptomatic carriers may also occur.[54] Coinfections with herpesvirus and *Mycoplasma* have been documented as well.[14] Previous infection with iridovirus may not prevent reinfection but may cause reduced apparent clinical signs.[14]

Numerous diagnostic techniques for ranavirus testing have been reported. Multiple PCR tests have been developed, and the samples for PCR can be obtained by either oral swabs, cloacal swabs, or via vein puncture (whole blood samples).[14,55,56] PCR has been found to be most sensitive with blood samples in comparison with oral or cloacal swabs.[51,55] Numerous other diagnostic methods including ELISA, electron microscopy, virus neutralization, and immunohistochemistry are available.[32,53] Intracytoplasmic inclusion bodies may also be visualized with histopathology or occasionally in blood smears.[52,53,56,57]

Treatment reported for these viral infections are largely supportive in nature and include antiviral therapy, nutritional support, fluid therapy, ambient temperature management, and antimicrobials for prevention of secondary infections.[51,55] Antiviral therapy has not been evaluated in proper clinical trials in order to provide a definitive confirmation of its effectiveness and safety. Acyclovir inhibited the growth of a testudinid HV 3 (teHV3) in vitro;[58] however, its effectiveness in vivo needs yet to be established. Increased environmental temperature has shown variable response to treatment, with one study showing decreased mortality and increased median survival time in adult red-eared sliders (*Trachemys scripta elegans*) housed at 28°C versus 22°C.[51,55] In contrary, in juvenile red-eared sliders the shortest median survival time was in those housed at 27°C versus 22°C.[52]

Other viral infections, as well as coinfections, are less commonly reported but should be considered. Coinfection with adenovirus and *M agassizii* has been reported in an ornate box turtle (*Terrapene ornate ornate*).[39] In addition, in a report of 50 Sulawesi tortoises (*Indotestudo forstenii*) with systemic adenovirus, 24 were reported to have histopathologic changes of the respiratory tract, including rhinitis, pharyngitis, tracheitis, and pneumonia.[59] Paramyxovirus was isolated in a leopard tortoise (*Stigmochelys pardalis*), although it is unknown if paramyxovirus was the causative agent for the reported respiratory disease.[60] Coinfections with picornavirus or ferlavirus with *Mycoplasma* have also been reported.[61]

Fungal

Fungal pneumonia can occur secondary to underlying systemic disease, immunosuppression, or because of antibiotics overuse.[32] Several fungi including *Aspergillus*, *Candida*, *Penicillium*, *Mucor*, *Geotrichum*, *Cladosporium*, *Rhizopus*, *Beauveria*, *Sporotrichum*, *Basidiobolus* and *Paecilomyces* have been isolated in the chelonian respiratory disease.[28,62] Diagnostic imaging may show granulomatous-like lesions or increased opacity of the lungs, but it is not pathognomic. Definitive diagnosis can be made via fungal culture, cytology, or histopathology. Treatment should be focused on treating any underlying systemic disease or husbandry discrepancies along with antifungal medication.[32] Direct treatment of pulmonary candidiasis with an intrapulmonary catheter was reported in a Greek tortoise (*Testudo graeca*).[28]

Parasitic

Parasitic disease within the respiratory tract is generally not primary pulmonary in nature but rather associated with systemic or aberrant infections.[32] Disseminated intranuclear coccidiosis has been reported in several chelonian species with variable systemic lesions including chronic rhinosinusitis, oronasal fistulas, and pneumonia (**Fig. 19**).[40,63] Preferred antemortem diagnosis is via PCR of either conjunctival oral choanal or cloacal swabs.[64,65] Cytology of nasal discharge with Wright-Giemsa,

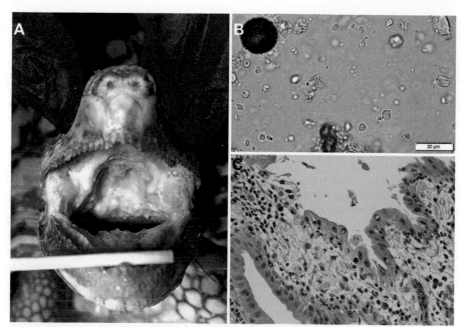

Fig. 19. Oral cavity (*A*), fecal flotation (*B*), and histology of the lungs (*C*) of a leopard tortoise (*Stigmochelys pardalis*) with disseminated testudo intranuclear coccidiosis (TINC) that affected primarily the lungs. The disease was confirmed on postmortem examination and histology of major organs. The animal tested negative for ranavirus and herpesvirus and positive for *Mycoplasma* sp. ((*A*) *Courtesy of* Nicola Di Girolamo; (*B*) *Courtesy of* Yoko Nagamori; (*C*) *Courtesy of* Oklahoma Animal Disease Diagnostic Laboratory at Oklahoma State University College of Veterinary Medicine; with permission.)

acid-fast, or periodic acid-Schiff techniques may reveal mononuclear inflammation and occasionally the presence of coccidia organisms.[40] Tissue histopathology and electron microscopy may also be used but are more likely a postmortem diagnostic.[63,64,66] Although various treatments, such as toltrazuril and ponazuril, have been described for gastrointestinal coccidiosis, the efficacy of these medications in disseminated cases is unknown. In addition, even with the elimination of coccidia, secondary tissue sclerosis may cause long-term damage.[64]

Aberrant parasitic migration such as ascarid larval migration has also been reported causing secondary bacterial pneumonia.[32] Spirorchid flukes have been reported in aquatic turtles, which, in disseminated form, can result in infection of the cardiopulmonary system. Although infection is thought to generally be incidental, occasionally egg release can cause severe multifocal granulomatous pneumonia among other systemic effects.[1,67]

Noninfectious Diseases

Chelonians in captivity commonly have multifactorial disease including underlying husbandry deficits such as inappropriate temperature, humidity, or nutrition. Hypovitaminosis A is commonly reported in captive aquatic turtles that are accustomed to higher levels of vitamin A in their natural diet. Hypovitaminosis A results in squamous metaplasia and immunosuppression. Clinical signs may be mild such as bilateral periorbital swelling but can result in more severe secondary bacterial pneumonia. Aural abscesses and caseous debris covering the corneas may also be present.[1,32]

Traumatic events such as motor vehicular trauma, predatory bite wounds, or penetrating foreign bodies, such as fishhooks, can result in trauma to the respiratory system. Acute consequences may include pulmonary contusions, trauma, or pneumocoelom (**Fig. 20**); however, more chronic complications such as secondary bacterial or fungal pneumonia may also occur.[32] In sea turtles, cold stunning can result in life-threatening hypothermia and respiratory depression.[24] Idiopathic pulmonary fibrosis has been reported in a leopard tortoise (*Geochelone pardalis pardalis*), although underlying systemic infection, such as *Mycoplasma*, could not be completely ruled out.[23] Although uncommon, intoxication may result in respiratory clinical signs such as ivermectin, which can result in respiratory paralysis.[68] Unilateral pulmonary aplasia, thought to be congenital in nature, has also been reported in common snapping turtle (*Chelydra serpentine*).[6]

Neoplasia in chelonians is uncommon; however, it should be considered particularly with mass effects or granulomatous-like disease.[20] Multicentric neoplasia including lymphoblastic lymphoma and multicentric pulmonary low-grade fibromyxoid sarcoma have been reported in sea turtles.[69,70] Underlying viral infections, such as herpesvirus, leading to viral-induced oncogenic neoplasia could be considered as well.[70]

Finally, nonrespiratory disorders are of particular importance to consider, as compression on the lungs can result in respiratory signs (see **Fig. 12**), which include differentials such as organomegaly or coelomic effusion. Female chelonians may have prolific follicular or egg development. Gastrointestinal distension may occur from foreign body ingestion, constipation, or functional ileus. Urinary bladder stones or retropulsed eggs that have entered the urinary bladder can cause bladder distension and compression on the caudal aspect of the lungs.[29] One chelonian diagnosed with flaccid urinary bladder presented with severely compressed lungs and open-

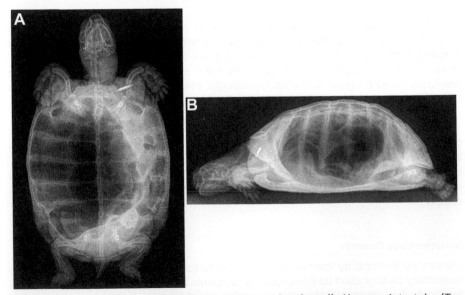

Fig. 20. Pneumocoelom of presumed traumatic cause in a juvenile Hermann's tortoise (*Testudo hermanni*) presented with significant breathing difficulty. (*A*) Dorsoventral, vertical beam, view. (*B*) Lateral, horizontal beam, view. (*Courtesy of* Nicola Di Girolamo.)

mouth breathing, which resolved after voiding of the urinary bladder.[2] Other organomegaly or coelomic effusion should also be considered.

CLINICS CARE POINTS

- Increased respiratory effort or open-mouth breathing in chelonians is not always caused by primary respiratory disorders and may also be the result of extrarespiratory disorders.

- During the physical examination of aquatic chelonians, buoyancy should be evaluated, as atypical floating may be associated with either lung consolidation or inappropriate gas accumulation.

- Nasal flushes have a diagnostic and also a therapeutic effect as mucous or foreign material clogging the nasal passages.

- For proper imaging of the lungs, it is fundamental that horizontal beam is used in lateral and craniocaudal radiographs.

- Blood gases may be beneficial for evaluation of respiratory disease as in other vertebrates; however, validation is only available for individual instruments, and clear correlation between results and disease in chelonians are currently lacking.

DISCLOSURES

The authors do not have any relationship with commercial companies that have a direct financial interest in subject matter or materials discussed in article or with companies making a competing product.

REFERENCES

1. Reavill DR, Griffin C. Common pathology and diseases seen in pet store reptiles. In: Mader DR, Divers SJ, editors. Current therapy in reptile medicine and surgery. St. Louis (MO): Elsevier; 2014. p. p13–9.
2. Di Girolamo N, Selleri P. What is your diagnosis? J Am Vet Med Assoc 2016; 249(3):271–3.
3. Caron M, Smead C, Brandão J, et al. A twenty-year trend in type of references used for reptile drug dosages in an exotic animal formulary. Exoticscon 2019;p564.
4. Gans C, Hughes GM. The mechanism of lung ventilation in the tortoise Testudo graeca Linné. J Exp Biol 1967;47(1):1–20.
5. Sacchi R, Galeotti P, Fasola M, et al. Larynx morphology and sound production in three species of testudinidae. J Morphol 2004;261(2):175–83.
6. Schachner ER, Sedlmayr JC, Schott R, et al. Pulmonary anatomy and a case of unilateral aplasia in a common snapping turtle (Chelydra serpentina): developmental perspectives on cryptodiran lungs. J Anat 2017;231(6):835–48.
7. Trevizan-Baú P, Abe AS, Klein W. Effects of environmental hypoxia and hypercarbia on ventilation and gas exchange in Testudines. PeerJ 2018;6:e5137.
8. Solomon SE, Purton M. The respiratory epithelium of the lung in the green turtle (Chelonia mydas L.). J Anat 1984;139(2):353–70.
9. Ricciardi M, Franchini D, Valastro C, et al. Multidetector computed tomographic anatomy of the lungs in the loggerhead sea turtle (Caretta caretta). Anat Rec (Hoboken) 2019;302(9):1658–65.
10. Milsom WK, Jones DR. The role of vagal afferent information and hypercapnia in control of the breathing pattern in chelonia. J Exp Biol 1980;87:53–63.

11. Greunz EM, Williams C, Ringgaard S, et al. Elimination of intracardiac shunting provides stable gas anesthesia in tortoises. Sci Rep 2018;8(1):17124.

12. Schmitt TL, Munns S, Adams L, et al. The use of spirometry to evaluate pulmonary function in olive ridley sea turtles (Lepidochelys olivacea) with positive buoyancy disorders. J Zoo Wildl Med 2013;44(3):645–53.

13. Scifo A, DeVoe RS, Goe A. Positive buoyancy secondary to gas accumulation within the accessory bladders in a florida cooter (Pseudemys floridana floridana). J Herpetol Med Surg 2020;30(1):9–13.

14. Adamovicz L, Allender MC, Archer G, et al. Investigation of multiple mortality events in eastern box turtles (Terrapene Carolina Carolina). PLoS One 2018; 13(4):e0195617.

15. Adamovicz L, Leister K, Byrd J, et al. Venous blood gas in free-living eastern box turtles (Terrapene carolina carolina) and effects of physiologic, demographic and environmental factors. Conserv Physiol 2018;6(1):coy041.

16. Jacobson ER, Gaskin JM, Brown MB, et al. Chronic upper respiratory tract disease of free-ranging desert tortoises (Xerobates agassizii). J Wildl Dis 1991; 27(2):296–316.

17. Colon VA, Di Girolamo N. Prognostic value of packed cell volume and blood glucose concentration in 954 client-owned chelonians. J Am Vet Med Assoc 2020;257(12):1265–72.

18. Di Girolamo N, Ferlizza E, Selleri P, et al. Evaluation of point-of-care analysers for blood gas and clinical chemistry in Hermann's tortoises (Testudo hermanni). J Small Anim Pract 2018;59(11):704–13.

19. Mans C, Drees R, Sladky KK, et al. Effects of body position and extension of the neck and extremities on lung volume measured via computed tomography in red-eared slider turtles (Trachemys scripta elegans). J Am Vet Med Assoc 2013; 243(8):1190–6.

20. Chrisman J, Devau M, Wilson-Robles H, et al. Oncology of reptiles: disease, diagnosis, and treatment. Vet Clin Exot Anim 2017;20:87–110.

21. Schumacher J, Toal RL. Advanced radiography and ultrasonography in reptiles. Semin Avian Exot Pet Med 2001;10(4):162–8.

22. Yamaguchi Y, Kitayama C, Shinichi T, et al. Computed tomographic analysis of internal structures within the nasal cavities of loggerhead and leatherback sea turtles. Anat Rec 2020;1–7.

23. Lim CK, Kirberger RM, Lane EP, et al. Computed tomography imaging of a leopard tortoise (Geochelone pardalis pardalis) with confirmed pulmonary fibrosis: a case report. Acta Vet Scand 2013;55(1):35.

24. Stockman J, Innis CJ, Solano M, et al. Prevalence, distribution, and progression of radiographic abnormalities in the lungs of cold-stunned Kemp's ridley sea turtles (Lepidochelys kempii): 89 cases (2002-2005). J Am Vet Med Assoc 2013; 242(5):675–81.

25. Gumpenberger M, Henninger W. The use of computed tomography in avian and reptile medicine. Semin Avian Exot Pet Med 2001;10(4):174–80.

26. Innis CJ, De Voe R, et al. A call for additional study on the safety of subcarapacial venipuncture in chelonians. Proc Assoc Reptilian Amphibian Veterinarians 2010;8–10..

27. Straub J, Jurina K. Magnetic resonance imaging in chelonians. Semin Avian Exot Pet Med 2001;10(4):181–6.

28. Hernandez-Divers SJ. Pulmonary Candidiasis caused by candida albicans in a greek tortoise (Testudo graeca) and treatment with intrapulmonary amphotericin b. J Zoo Wildl Med 2001;32(3):352–9.

29. Knotek Z, Divers SJ. Pulmonology. In: Mader DR, Divers SJ, Stahl S, editors. Reptile and amphibian medicine and surgery. 3rd edition. St. Louis (MO): Elsevier; 2019. p. 786–804.

30. Jacobson ER, Brown MB, Wendland LD, et al. Mycoplasmosis and upper respiratory tract disease of tortoises: A review and update. Vet J 2014;201(3):257–64.

31. Goessling JM, Guyer C, et al. Upper respiratory tract disease and associated diagnostic tests of mycoplasmosis in Alabama populations of Gopher tortoises, *Gopherus polyphemus*. PLoS One 2019;24(4):e0214845.

32. Bennett T. The chelonian respiratory system. Veterinary Clin North Am Exot Anim Pract 2011;14(2):225–v.

33. Stewart JS. Anaerobic bacterial infections in reptiles. J Zoo Wildl Med 1990;21(2): 180–4.

34. Soldati G, Lu ZH, Vaughan L, et al. Detection of mycobacteria and chlamydiae in granulomatous inflammation of reptiles: a retrospective study. Vet Pathol 2004; 41(4):388–97.

35. Vanrompay D, De Meurichy W, Ducatelle R, et al. Pneumonia in Moorish tortoises (*Testudo graeca*) associated with avian serovar A *Chlamydia psittaci*. Vet Rec 1994;135(12):284–5.

36. Foti M, Giacopello C, Fisichella V, et al. Multidrug-resistant *Pseudomonas aeruginosa* isolates from captive reptiles. J Exot Pet Med 2013;22(3):270–4.

37. Braun J, Schrenzel M, Witte C, et al. Molecular methods to detect Mycoplasma spp. And Testudinid herpesvirus 2 in desert tortoises (Gopherus agassizii) and implications for disease management. J Wildl Dis 2014;50(4):757–66.

38. Jacobson ER, Berry KH. *Mycoplasma testudineum* in free-ranging desert tortoises, *Gopherus agassizii*. J Wildl Dis 2012;48(4):1063–8.

39. Farkas SL, Gal J. Adenovirus and mycoplasma infection in an ornate box turtle (Terrapene ornata ornata) in Hungary. Vet Microbiol 2009;138(1–2):169–73.

40. Innis CJ, Garner MM, Johnson AJ, et al. Antemortem diagnosis and characterization of nasal intranuclear coccidiosis in Sulawesi tortoises (*Indotestudo forsteni*). J Vet Diagn Invest 2007;19(6):660–7.

41. Drake KK, Aiello CM, Bowen L, et al. Complex immune responses and molecular reactions to pathogens and disease in a desert reptile (*Gopherus agassizii*). Ecol Evol 2019;9(5):2516–34.

42. Sandmeier FC, Weitzman CL, Maloney KN, et al. Comparison of current methods for the detection of chronic mycoplasmal urtd in wild populations of the mojave desert tortoise (gopherus agassizii). J Wildl Dis 2017;53(1):91–101.

43. Gibbons PM. Advances in reptile clinical therapeutics. J Exot Pet Med 2014; 23(1):21–38.

44. Origii FC, Romero CH, Bloom DC, et al. Experimental transmission of herpesvirus in Greek tortoises (*Testudo graeca*). Vet Pathol 2004;41:50–61.

45. Kane LP, Bunick D, Abd-Eldaim M, et al. Development and validation of quantitative PCR for detection of Terrapene herpesvirus 1 utilizing free-ranging eastern box turtles (Terrapene carolina carolina). J Virol Methods 2016;232:57–61.

46. Murakami M, Matsuba C, Une Y, et al. Development of species-specific PCR techniques for the detection of tortoise herpesvirus. J Vet Diagn Invest 2001; 13(6):513–6.

47. VanDevanter DR, Warrener P, Bennett L, et al. Detection and analysis of diverse herpesviral species by consensus primer PCR. J Clin Microbiol 1996;34(7): 1666–71.

48. Origii FC, Tucker S, et al. Application of immunoperoxidase-based techniques to detect herpesvirus in tortoises. J Vet Diagn Invest 2003;15(2):133–40.

49. Johnson AJ, Pessier AP, Jacobson ER. Experimental transmission and induction of ranaviral disease in Western Ornate box turtles (Terrapene ornata ornata) and red-eared sliders (Trachemys scripta elegans). Vet Pathol 2004;44(3):285–97.

50. Huang Y, Huang X, Liu H, et al. Complete sequence determination of a novel reptile iridovirus isolated from soft-shelled turtle and evolutionary analysis of *Iridoviridae*. BMC Genomics 2009;10(224):224.

51. Allender M. Characterizing the epidemiology of ranavirus in North American chelonians: diagnosis, surveillance, pathogenesis, and treatment. Diss. University of Illinois at Urbana-Champaign, 2012. Available at: https://www.ideals.illinois.edu/handle/2142/34286. Accessed August 28, 2020.

52. Allender MC, Barthel AC, Rayl JM, et al. Experimental transmission of frog virus 3-like ranavirus in juvenile chelonians at two temperatures. J Wildl Dis 2018;54(4):716–25.

53. Westhouse RA, Jacobson ER, Harris RK, et al. Respiratory and pharyngoesophageal iridovirus infection in a gopher tortoise (*Gopherus Polyphemus*). J Wildl Dis 1996;32(4):682–6.

54. Allender MC, Bunick D, Mitchell MA. Development and validation of TaqMan quantitative PCR for detection of frog virus 3-like virus in eastern box turtles (Terrapene carolina carolina). J Virol Methods 2013;188(1–2):121–5.

55. Allender MC, Mitchell MA, Torres T, et al. Pathogenicity of frog virus 3-like virus in red-eared slider turtles (Trachemys scripta elegans) at two environmental temperatures. J Comp Pathol 2013;149(2–3):356–67.

56. Hausmann JC, Wack AN, Allender MC, et al. Experimental challenge study of FV3-like Ranavirus infection in previously FV3-like ranavirus infected eastern box turtles (*Terrapene Carolina Carolina*) to assess infection and survival. J Zoo Wildl Med 2015;46(4):732–46.

57. Allender MC, Fry MM, Irizarry AR, et al. Intracytoplasmic inclusions in circulating leukocytes from an eastern box turtle (*Terrapene Carolina Carolina*) with iridoviral infection. J Wildl Dis 2006;42(3):677–84.

58. Marschang RE, Gravendyck M, Kaleta EF. Herpesviruses in tortoises: investigations into virus isolation and the treatment of viral stomatitis in *Testudo hermanni* and *T. graeca*. Zentralbl Veterinarmed B 1997;44(7):385–94.

59. Rivera S, Wellehan JF, McManamon R, et al. Systemic adenovirus infection in Sulawesi tortoises (Indotestudo forsteni) caused by a novel siadenovirus. J Vet Diagn Invest 2009;21(4):415–26.

60. Papp T, Seybold J, Marschang RE. Paramyxovirus infection in a leopard tortoise (*Geochelone pardalis babcocki*) with respiratory disease. J Herpetological Med Surg 2010;20(2):64–8.

61. Kolesnik E, Obiegala A, Marschang RE. Detection of Mycoplasma spp., herpesviruses, topiviruses, and ferlaviruses in samples from chelonians in Europe. J Vet Diagn Invest 2017;29(6):820–32.

62. Schumacher J. Fungal diseases of reptiles. Veterinary Clin North Am Exot Anim Pract 2003;6(2):327–vi.

63. Garner MM, Gardiner CH, Wellehan JF, et al. Intranuclear coccidiosis in tortoises: nine cases. Vet Pathol 2006;43(3):311–20.

64. Gibbons PM, Steffes ZJ. Emerging infectious diseases of chelonians. Veterinary Clin North Am Exot Anim Pract 2013;16(2):303–17.

65. Alvarez WA, Gibbons PM, Rivera S, et al. Development of a quantitative PCR for rapid and sensitive diagnosis of an intranuclear coccidian parasite in Testudines (TINC), and detection in the critically endangered Arakan forest turtle (Heosemys depressa). Vet Parasitol 2013;193(1–3):66–70.

66. Hofmannová L, Kvičerová J, Bízková K, et al. Intranuclear coccidiosis in tortoises - discovery of its causative agent and transmission. Eur J Protistol 2019;67:71–6.
67. Gordon AN, Kelly WR, Cribb TH. Lesions caused by cardiovascular flukes (Digenea: Spirorchidae) in stranded green turtles (Chelonia mydas). Vet Pathol 1998; 35(1):21–30.
68. Teare JA, Bush M. Toxicity and efficacy of ivermectin in chelonians. J Am Vet Med Assoc 1983;183(11):1195–7.
69. Orós J, Torrent A, Espinosa de los Monteros A, et al. Multicentric lymphoblastic lymphoma in a loggerhead sea turtle (*Caretta caretta*). Vet Pathol 2001;38(4): 464–7.
70. Díaz-Delgado J, Gomes-Borges JC, Silveira AM, et al. Primary multicentric pulmonary low-grade fibromyxoid sarcoma and chelonid alphaherpesvirus 5 detection in a leatherback sea turtle (*Dermochelys coriacea*). J Comp Pathol 2019; 168:1–7.

Diagnostics of Infectious Respiratory Pathogens in Reptiles

Rachel E. Marschang, PD, Dr med vet, Dipl ECZM (Herpetology), FTÄ Mikrobiologie[a],*, Ekaterina Salzmann, Dr med vet[a], Michael Pees, Dr med vet, Dipl ECZM (Avian), Dipl ECZM (Herpetology)[b]

KEYWORDS

- Ferlavirus • Herpesvirus • Mycoplasma • Nidovirus • PCR • Serpentovirus
- Tracheal wash

KEY POINTS

- Respiratory disease is often caused by a combination of factors, including environmental, host-specific, and microbial factors.
- The quality of samples submitted for laboratory diagnostics for infectious agents will strongly influence the reliability of results.
- Contact your laboratory to discuss sampling and testing to optimize your protocols and get the most out of your results.
- Detection of infectious agents in reptiles should always be interpreted in conjunction with clinical signs and additional diagnostic testing.

INTRODUCTION

Respiratory diseases are common in various reptiles, and infectious agents can be a major contributing factor. Both upper- and lower-respiratory-tract diseases are commonly observed in reptiles presented to veterinarians. Although there are several agents that have been proven by transmission studies to be a primary cause of upper- and/or lower-respiratory-tract disease (**Box 1**), in many cases multiple factors will influence disease development, including host species, husbandry, environment, stress, pathogen strain, and other infections. Laboratory diagnosis of infectious agents should always be interpreted in conjunction with the animal's history and clinical findings, and treatment will always need to take these factors into account.

[a] Laboklin GmbH & Co. KG, Steubenstr. 4, Bad Kissingen 97688, Germany; [b] Department for Birds and Reptiles, University Veterinary Teaching Hospital, University of Leipzig, Clinic for Birds and Reptiles, An den Tierkliniken 17, Leipzig 04103, Germany
* Corresponding author.
E-mail address: rachel.marschang@gmail.com

Vet Clin Exot Anim 24 (2021) 369–395
https://doi.org/10.1016/j.cvex.2021.01.007
1094-9194/21/© 2021 Elsevier Inc. All rights reserved.

> **Box 1**
> **Infectious agents with known relevance as primary causes of respiratory disease in reptiles**
>
> Upper-respiratory-tract disease
> - Serpentoviruses
> - Herpesviruses
> - Mycoplasma
>
> Lower-respiratory-tract disease
> - Serpentoviruses
> - Ferlaviruses
> - Reoviruses
> - Rhabdias spp

Possible causes of respiratory disease include a wide range of viruses, bacteria, fungi, and parasites. This article provides a short overview of many of the agents that have been associated with respiratory disease in these animals. Although some, as mentioned, are primary causes of respiratory diseases, others may more often be associated with other clinical signs, and many can sometimes be found in clinically healthy individuals. The variability in the roles of specific agents in disease makes interpretation of laboratory diagnostics particularly difficult.

DIAGNOSTIC METHODS
Clinical Examination

Except for nasal discharge, clinical signs of respiratory diseases are normally delayed and only occur in advanced stages of disease, if the respiratory function is severely reduced. The late appearance of clinical signs is due to the huge spare capacity of the reptile lung, and the ability of reptiles to adjust their metabolism to anaerobic processes, thereby compensating for lack of oxygen. Therefore, respiratory sounds, increased respiratory rates, and open-mouth breathing (**Fig. 1**) should always be interpreted as a possible sign of severe and possibly life-threatening respiratory disease. Disease of the lower-respiratory tract can be associated with secretion from the

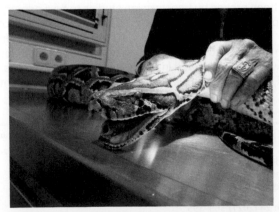

Fig. 1. Dyspnea (open-mouth breathing) in a Burmese python (*Python molurus*) with tracheitis and severe pneumonia.

trachea; however, because of the lack of a diaphragm and a poor mucociliary apparatus, secretions often remain only in the lung or lower trachea. Pharyngitis and tracheitis are regularly seen (**Fig. 2**), especially in snakes. In chelonians, mucus secretion primarily from the nares is a common finding (**Fig. 3**), and this can become purulent because of secondary infections.

Sample Collection Methods

The method and correct sampling procedure are essential for the detection of pathogens as well as the interpretation of results. On the one hand, it is important to obtain the correct material in a sufficient quantity for the detection method to work as sensitively as possible; this is relevant for all pathogens. On the other hand, especially for the detection of bacteria and fungi, it is particularly important for the interpretation of results that the localization of the samples taken is specific. For example, bacterial growth from a sample of the lower-respiratory system has a completely different meaning than from a sample of the oral cavity, and contamination of the sample must be prevented. Aside from etiologic diagnostics, laboratory diagnostics can also be used to determine an immune response or the extent of an inflammatory reaction, for example, using cytology, hematology, blood chemistry, and serology.

For etiologic diagnostics, swabs from the oral cavity, the nares, and the cloaca are commonly used and recommended, as they provide information from the main shedding orifices. Tracheal (opening) swabs, in contrast, are of limited value, as they do not specifically represent the respiratory system. Tracheal wash samples, if performed

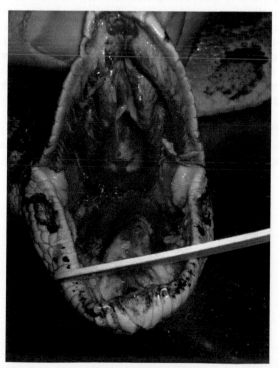

Fig. 2. Severe stomatitis and tracheitis in a Burmese python also suffering from severe pneumonia. These clinical signs are often found in the oral cavity of snakes with prolonged lower-respiratory disease. Note the foamy secretion from the tracheal opening.

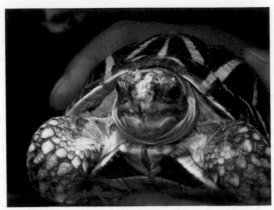

Fig. 3. Rhinitis and conjunctivitis as a sign of upper-respiratory disease in an Indian star tortoise (*Geochelone elegans*).

correctly, have been found to be more sensitive and specific for bacterial cultures as well as virus detection from respiratory tissue.[1–3] The sampling procedure is easy to perform in snakes (**Fig. 4**) but limited in tortoises and lizards. Using a sterile tube of an appropriate diameter and length, sterile saline (up to approximately 5 mL/kg) is introduced into the lower trachea. It is essential to use a mucosal disinfectant to prevent contamination of the tube during insertion into the trachea. The fluid is then instilled with the snake in an upright position, allowing the fluid to pass into the cranial part of the lung lumen. Then, the head and trachea are lowered, and as much fluid as possible is sucked back into the tube and syringe. The material can be used for cytologic as well as microbiological assessment of the lower-respiratory system (**Fig. 5**). Ideally, samples can also be obtained from the respiratory tissue itself, but this involves endoscopy and direct sampling under optical control. In these cases, biopsies can be taken and further examined.

Pathogen Detection

In clinically ill patients, pathogen detection is generally necessary in order to determine an etiologic diagnosis. Pathogen detection can encompass visualization of a

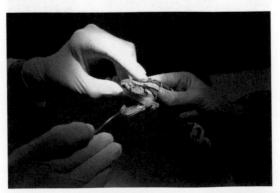

Fig. 4. Tracheal wash procedure: the sterile tube is inserted into the trachea during the respiratory cycle activity (glottis open). After application of sterile saline, the snake is held upside down and fluid is sucked back into the syringe.

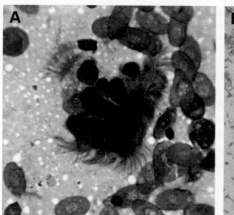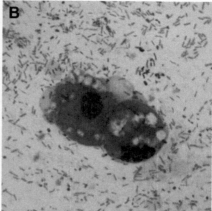

Fig. 5. Tracheal wash sample from a Burmese python with clinical signs of a lung infection (Diff-Quik-stain, original magnification ×400); normal tracheal epithelial cell (*middle*) and red and white blood cells indicating an inflammatory reaction (*A*), various bacterial rod cells, and inflammatory reaction (*B*). (*Courtesy of* Dr Volker Schmidt.)

pathogen, isolation, or detection of specific portions of the infectious agent, for example, part of the genome or specific proteins. Direct detection and visualization of pathogens in clinical samples can be used, for example, for some parasites; light microscopy, sometimes following staining, can be used for parasites, fungi, and bacteria. Isolation is frequently used for bacteria and fungi. Isolation of some viruses in cell culture has also been described but is rarely used in routine diagnostics. Polymerase chain reaction (PCR) is a commonly used technique to detect DNA or RNA of potential pathogens in clinical samples. Other methods for the detection of parts (eg, proteins) of infectious agents are much less common in reptile medicine. No matter the method used, it is important to understand the strengths and weaknesses of each and to confirm results. Not all methods are specific. Identification of pathogens seen by light microscopy or isolated or detected in a laboratory by additional testing is necessary, and any pathogens detected by PCR need to be identified, for example, using sequencing or specific probes (in the case of real-time PCRs). Detection of a specific agent does not necessarily indicate that it is a cause of disease.

Serology

The detection of an immune response to a specific pathogen is only rarely used in reptile medicine and is often not helpful in assessing a case with acute illness. Although the immune response is made up of many different parts, available laboratory testing generally detects only antibodies against specific pathogens. The reptile immune system is dependent on external influences, particularly temperature, but also species, husbandry, and pathogen. An immune response often develops more slowly than in mammals, so that antibody detection is only possible after several weeks in most cases. Serologic assays are therefore mostly used to determine infection status in quarantine or in a specific collection of animals. The pathogens for which serologic testing is commercially available are limited and depend on the country in which one resides. They can include some herpesviruses of tortoises, ferlaviruses, torchiviruses, and mycoplasma. Methods used include virus neutralization (for herpes and torchiviruses), hemagglutination inhibition (HI) (for ferlaviruses), and enzyme-linked immunosorbent assay (ELISAs; for herpesviruses and mycoplasma). Blood or plasma samples are used for the detection of antibodies.

Sample Storage and Transport

How samples are stored, whether a transport medium is used, and how soon they must be examined will depend on the test used and the pathogen of interest (**Table 1**). In general, it is best to contact your laboratory to discuss any specific recommendations. Most diagnostic laboratories will also offer supplies for sample collection and transportation. For detection of infectious agents by light microscopy (eg, for parasitology or for detection of bacteria or fungi), it is generally best to examine the samples as soon after collection as possible, and sensitivity of detection will be lower the longer the samples are stored.

SPECIFIC PATHOGENS AND THEIR DETECTION

Many agents have been associated with respiratory disease in reptiles (**Table 2**). In many cases, multiple pathogens may be involved in clinical disease. Specific testing and samples will depend on the pathogen and host species (**Table 3**).

Viruses

Serpentoviruses (nidoviruses)

Serpentoviruses are large, enveloped, single-stranded RNA (ssRNA) viruses in the order *Nidovirales* and are often referred to as nidoviruses. The nidoviruses infecting reptiles are found in the family *Tobaniviridae*, subfamily *Serpentovirinae*. These viruses have been shown to be an important cause of upper- and lower-respiratory disease in pythons.[4–7] Similar viruses have also been found in boas[7,8] and colubrids.[7] Serpentoviruses have also been described in skinks (*Tiliqua* spp) with upper-respiratory signs in Australia[9] and in association with a severe disease outbreak in Bellinger River snapping turtles (*Myuchelys georgisi*) with swollen eyelids and conjunctivitis in Australia.[10] Infected pythons may have abundant mucus in the oral cavity and reddening of the oral mucosa. Rhinitis, stomatitis, tracheitis, glossitis, and cranial esophagitis are found in early infection. Later during infection, the lung is increasingly affected, and snakes develop interstitial pneumonia. Virus is shed in oroesophageal, choanal, and cloacal swabs and has also been isolated from feces of infected snakes.[6] Later in infection, highest viral loads may be found in the lungs of infected snakes.[4] Infection has been shown to persist for extended periods of time.[7] In that study, infected snakes remained persistently infected over the 28 months of the study, and many, although not all, developed disease during that time.

Transmission of serpentoviruses in pythons has been shown to be possible via the oral cavity.[6] Because the viruses have a tropism for epithelial cells of the respiratory tract and upper esophagus, it is considered likely that they are transmitted via oral secretions and possibly fomites and aerosols. Fecal-oral transmission may also occur because virus is also shed via the cloaca.

Serpentovirus detection is most commonly done using PCR.[7,8] Serpentoviruses found in snakes have been shown to be genetically diverse,[5,7] and there is some indication that some of these viruses may be species specific. It is therefore important to discuss the method used for detection with the laboratory to ensure it is appropriate for the species. The most common samples used for virus detection are oral swabs, and this is the current recommended sample type for clinical diagnostics. There is currently no serologic test available to detect serpentovirus antibodies.

Table 1
Sample preparation and submission for detection of respiratory pathogens in reptiles

Sample Type	Test Type	Medium	Storage	Comments
Swabs	Bacterial or fungal culture	Use transport medium (eg, Amies)	Samples should be cooled but not frozen	Samples should be transported to the laboratory as quickly as possible (eg, overnight). Samples in medium (eg, Amies) cannot be used for PCR
	PCR	Can be submitted dry, in a small amount of sterile fluid (eg, saline), or in a solution designed to preserve DNA or RNA in the sample (eg, RNAlater)	Samples should be cooled. Can be frozen for testing later. If frozen, recommend adding fluid	
Tissues	Bacterial or fungal culture	No transport medium necessary. Separate tissues into separate sterile containers	Best if cooled and transported to the laboratory as quickly as possible	
	Virus isolation in cell culture	Samples for cell culture are best stored in a small amount of sterile cell culture medium	Best if cooled and transported to the laboratory as quickly as possible. Can be frozen for testing later. Freezing at −80°C (−112°F) best	
	PCR	Either without transport medium or in a solution designed to preserve DNA or RNA in the sample (eg, RNAlater)	Cooled or frozen if transport to laboratory is delayed	Tissues embedded in paraffin for histology can also be used for PCR. However, sensitivity is generally reduced. Formalin degrades nucleic acids, so tissues that have been fixed in formalin for an extended period are not appropriate for PCR testing
Serum or plasma	Serology	No medium necessary	Cooled or frozen	Blood should be centrifuged, and serum or plasma separated for transportation to the laboratory, because hemolysis can interfere with tests

Note. It is best to contact your laboratory for specific recommendations before submission.

Table 2
Infectious causes of respiratory disease in reptiles

Host Order	Host Subgroup	Pathogen Category	Pathogens[a]
Chelonians	Tortoises	Viruses	Herpesviruses
			Ranaviruses
			Torchiviruses
			Ferlaviruses
			Adenoviruses
			Reoviruses
		Bacteria	Mycoplasma
			Gram-negative bacteria
		Fungi	Multiple sporulating fungi described, for example, *Aspergillus*, *Purpureocillium* (*Paecilomyces*), *Penicillium* spp
			Yeasts
		Parasites	TINC
			Migrating ascarid larvae
	Turtles	Viruses	Ranaviruses
			Herpesviruses
			Adenoviruses
			Serpento(Nido-)viruses
		Bacteria	Gram-negative bacteria
			Mycoplasma
		Fungi	Multiple fungi described
		Parasites	TINC
			Pentastomids
	Sea turtles	Viruses	Herpesviruses
		Bacteria	Gram-negative bacteria
		Fungi	Multiple hyphal fungi described, for example, *Fusarium* spp
			Yeasts
		Parasites	Trematodes
Squamates	Pythons	Viruses	Serpento(Nido-)viruses
			Ferlaviruses
			Sunshinevirus
			Adenoviruses
			Reoviruses
			Reptarenaviruses
			Ranaviruses
		Bacteria	Gram-negative bacteria
			Mycoplasma
		Fungi	Various hyphal fungi
		Parasites	*Strongyloides*
			Pentastomids
			Migrating ascarid larvae
			Rhabdias
	Boas	Viruses	Reptarenaviruses
			Serpento(Nido-)viruses
			Ferlaviruses
			Adenoviruses
			Reoviruses
		Bacteria	Gram-negative bacteria
			Mycobacteria
		Fungi	Various species, rare

(*continued on next page*)

Table 2
(continued)

Host Order	Host Subgroup	Pathogen Category	Pathogens[a]
		Parasites	*Strongyloides*
			Pentastomids
			Rhabdias
	Other snakes	Viruses	Ferlaviruses
			Adenoviruses
			Reoviruses
			Serpento(Nido-)viruses
		Bacteria	Gram-negative bacteria
		Fungi	Various species, rare
		Parasites	*Rhabdias*
			Strongyloides
			Pentastomids
			Renifers
	Agamas	Viruses	Adenoviruses
			Ferlaviruses
		Bacteria	Gram-negative bacteria
		Fungi	Rare
		Parasites	Rare
	Other squamates	Viruses	Ferlaviruses
			Adenoviruses
			Serpento(Nido-)viruses
			Herpesviruses
		Bacteria	Gram-negative bacteria
		Fungi	*Metarhizium* spp
			Other fungi also reported
		Parasites	Pentastomids
			Migrating ascarid larvae
Crocodilians		Viruses	Herpesviruses
			Flaviviruses (West Nile virus)
		Bacteria	Mycoplasma
			Gram-negative bacteria
			Mycobacteria
			Chlamydia
		Fungi	Multiple fungi described, for example, *Metarhizium* spp, *Purpureocillium* (*Paecilomyces*) spp
		Parasites	Pentastomids
			Coccidia

Abbreviation: TINC, intranuclear coccidiosis of tortoises.

Many of the pathogens listed are frequently associated with disease not related to the respiratory tract, and many can also be found in clinically healthy individuals.

[a] Where possible, these have been ordered according to frequency with which infections associated with respiratory disease have been reported in the author's experience.

Ferlaviruses

Ferlaviruses are enveloped ssRNA viruses belonging to the family *Paramyxoviridae*. The ferlaviruses are genetically somewhat diverse, and several genotypes, A, B, C, and tortoise, have been described.[11] These viruses are known to cause severe pneumonia in viperid snakes[12] and have also been found in other snake species,[13,14]

Table 3
Laboratory diagnostic testing and clinical samples for infectious respiratory disease in reptiles

Category	Pathogen	Other Names Used for the Pathogen in Literature	Hosts	Diagnostic Tests[a]	Clinical Sample[b]	Priority Tissue Samples if Known	Serology[c]
Viruses	Serpentoviruses	Nidoviruses	Mostly pythons, also other snakes, similar viruses described in lizards and chelonians in individual cases	PCR, NGS, immunohistochemistry, in situ hybridization, virus isolation	Oral swab, tracheal wash	Oral mucosa, lung	Not described
	Ferlaviruses	Ophidian paramyxovirus	Snakes, occasionally other squamates and chelonians	PCR, virus isolation, immunohistochemistry, in situ hybridization	Tracheal wash, oral and cloacal swabs	Lung	HI, differences depending on virus strain
	Adenoviruses	Atadenoviruses, siadenoviruses, others	Squamates, chelonians, crocodilians	PCR, virus isolation, histology	Cloacal swabs, oral swabs	Liver, intestine	(Virus neutralization)
	Reoviruses		Squamates, occasionally chelonians	PCR, virus isolation	Oral and cloacal swabs	Not described	(Virus neutralization)
	Sunshinevirus		Pythons	PCR, virus isolation	Oral and cloacal swabs	Brain	Not described
	Herpesviruses	Scutaviruses (chelonians)	Mostly chelonians, occasionally squamates, crocodilians	PCR, immunohistochemistry, in situ hybridization, virus isolation, cytology, histology	Oral swabs, lesions	Lesions, tongue, liver	Virus neutralization and ELISA for some testudinid herpesviruses
	Ranaviruses	Iridoviruses	Most often in chelonians, also in squamates	PCR, virus isolation, immunohistology, in situ hybridization	Oral swabs, blood, tail clips, skin, lesions	Liver, other tissues	(ELISA)
	Reptarenaviruses	Arenaviruses, IBD	Boas and pythons	PCR, cytology, immunohistochemistry, NGS	Esophageal swabs, whole blood, liver biopsies, cloacal swabs	Brain	(ELISA, immunoblotting)
	Torchiviruses	Tortoise picornavirus, virus "x"	Tortoises	PCR, virus isolation	Oral swabs, cloacal swabs, conjunctival swabs	Tongue, kidney, intestine	Virus neutralization

						ELISA
Bacteria	Mycoplasma	Mycoplasma aggasizii, M testudineum, Mycoplasma spp	Mostly chelonians, occasionally snakes, crocodylians	PCR, culture	Nasal lavage, nasal, oral and conjunctival swabs	Nasal mucosa
	Chlamydia	Chlamydia pneumoniae, others	Various reptile species	PCR, immunohistology	Nasal lavage, oral and cloacal swabs, blood, lesions	Lesions, various tissues	Not described
	Gram negative bacteria		Various reptile species	Culture	Tracheal washes, lung biopsies	Lesions, lung	Not described
Fungi	Yeasts	For example, Cryptococcus, Candida	Various reptile species	Culture, PCR	Tracheal (pulmonal) washes, lesions	Lung, lesions	Not described
	Hyphal fungi	For example, Coccidioides, Fusarium, Metarhizium, Purpureocillium	Various reptile species	Culture, histology/cytology, PCR	Tracheal/pulmonal washes, lung biopsies, lesions	Lung, lesions	Not described
Parasites	Intranuclear coccidia of tortoises	TINC	Tortoises	PCR, light and electron microscopy	Conjunctival, oral, and cloacal swabs, feces, blood	Various tissues	Not described
	Rhabdias spp	Lungworms	Mostly snakes, other squamates	Eggs: Flotation Larvae: Direct examination, light microscopy, enrichment	Feces, tracheal wash, oropharyngeal mucous	Lung	Not described
	Other nematodes		Various reptiles	Flotation, light microscopy	Feces	Intestine	Not described
	Pentastomids	Armillifer, Raillietiella, others	Various reptiles, mostly snakes	Eggs: Flotation, light microscopy Adults: Endoscopy, other imaging methods	Feces, tracheal wash	Lung	Not described

(continued on next page)

Table 3
(continued)

Category Pathogen	Other Names Used for the Pathogen in Literature	Hosts	Diagnostic Tests[a]	Clinical Sample[b]	Priority Tissue Samples if Known	Serology[c]
Trematodes	Some referred to as renifers	Various reptiles, mostly marine turtles, other turtles, snakes	Eggs: Light microscopy (native, SAF enrichment, or sedimentation) Adults: Direct observation, light microscopy	Feces, tracheal wash	Lungs, lesions	Not described

Abbreviations: NGS, next-generation sequencing; SAF, sodium acetate-acetic acid formalin-solution; TINC, intranuclear coccidiosis of tortoises.

[a] Underlined: testing commercially available in some laboratories.

[b] **Underlined:** priority sample.

[c] Methods listed in parentheses have been described in the literature but are not currently commercially available for diagnostic testing.

various lizard species, and tortoises in several cases.[12] Infected snakes most commonly develop respiratory disease, and pathologic changes are mostly found in the lungs.[11,15] Other clinical signs that have been reported in infected animals include central nervous system (CNS) signs,[13,16] anorexia,[17] and sudden death with no preliminary signs of disease.[13,17] In some cases, ferlaviruses have been detected in reptiles with no concurrent signs of disease noted. Development of clinical disease depends on the virus strain involved in the infection and likely also on the host species.[11]

Ferlaviruses affect mostly the lungs of infected snakes, but can also be found in other tissues.[11,15] They are likely transmitted via fomites and aerosols as well as via direct contact.[18,19] Virus has been shown to be shed mostly through the mouth, but can also be found in the cloaca.[19]

Diagnosis of ferlavirus infections has been described using virus isolation, immunohistochemistry, and PCR, but PCR is currently the most commonly available method. Many different PCRs have been used to detect these viruses in clinical samples.[20] Because genetically variable viruses can be associated with disease, methods capable of detecting all known variants are generally preferable. Sensitivity can be a problem when testing clinical samples. One study found a very low sensitivity when testing tracheal wash samples compared with lung tissue in infected viperid snakes,[17] although the PCR method used will likely influence this.[20] In a study with corn snakes (*Pantherophis guttatus*) infected with genogroup A, B, and C viruses, tracheal washes were recommended as the best clinical samples independent of virus type.[19] Virus was most often detected in lungs from infected snakes, followed by intestine, pancreas, brain, and kidney (in that particular order).

Serologic testing for anti–ferlavirus antibodies can be done using HI testing. Antibody development has been shown to depend on the virus genotype involved in the infection, with the most pathogenic strain associated with the lowest seroconversion rate.[21] Results of HI depend on the virus used, and a comparative study showed that different laboratories may report very different results from the same samples, possibly because of differences in techniques and virus strains used, making interpretation of results difficult.[22] In addition, although there have been anecdotal reports of possible persistent ferlavirus infections, it is not known whether serologically positive reptiles may be carriers or not.

Herpesviruses

In reptiles, herpesviruses are most commonly found in chelonians. Most chelonian herpesviruses characterized so far are genetically somewhat diverse, but all cluster together in the genus *Scutavirus*, subfamily *Alphaherpesvirinae*.[23] There is some indication of species specificity for some of these viruses, with some types found only in individual host species or genera, whereas others (eg, *Testudinid alphaherpesvirus 3*) are able to switch hosts, at least within a family (Testudinidae in that case). Herpesviruses cause latent infections in their hosts, so that herpesvirus-infected animals remain life-long carriers.

In chelonians, herpesviruses have been associated with upper-respiratory and upper-digestive-tract disease in tortoises,[24] sea turtles,[25,26] and aquatic turtles.[27,28] In some cases, herpesviruses have also been associated with pneumonia.[25–28] In squamates, herpesviruses have sporadically been associated with upper-respiratory and upper-digestive tract lesions.[29,30] Herpesviruses associated with conjunctivitis and/or pharyngitis have recently been found in farmed crocodiles in Australia.[31] Transmission studies have confirmed the role of herpesviruses in upper-respiratory and upper-digestive tract disease in tortoises.[23]

Several methods have been described for the detection of herpesviruses in infected reptiles. Infected cells may develop intranuclear inclusions, which can aid diagnostics. Inclusions have been detected in epithelial cells from tongue swabs from acutely infected tortoises.[32] However, this method is likely to be relatively insensitive and unspecific. Virus isolation has also been described for some of the herpesviruses found in tortoises. The most common method used is PCR for the detection of viral DNA. Because there are many genetically distinct herpesviruses found in reptiles, a method capable of detecting a wide range of viruses in the family *Herpesviridae*[33] is most often used for this purpose; this allows the detection of previously undescribed herpesviruses as well as of various herpesviruses capable of infecting individual species. Numerous strain- or species-specific herpesvirus PCRs have also been described. These herpesvirus PCRs can be more sensitive but are limited in that they may only detect a single or limited number of specific viruses. The clinical sample most often used for the detection of herpesviruses associated with upper-respiratory and upper-digestive-tract disease is an oral or choanal swab. In tortoises, swabbing of the base of the tongue is generally recommended.[32]

Serologic testing is available for the detection of antibodies against some of the herpesviruses found in tortoises. Testudinid herpesvirus 1 and *Testudinid alphaherpesvirus 3* have both been isolated in cell culture, and virus neutralization tests are commercially available for antibody detection against each in Europe. The two do not serologically cross-react,[34] and it is unlikely that these tests would be able to detect antibodies against other herpesviruses. An ELISA has also been described for the detection of antibodies against *Testudinid alphaherpesvirus 3*.[35] Antibody detection appears to also depend on the host species, and some species are less likely to develop antibodies against specific viruses than others. Because herpesviruses cause life-long persistent infections, detection of antibodies against herpesviruses should always be considered an indication of infection. Serology is therefore often included in quarantine examinations in tortoises.

Adenoviruses

In reptiles, adenoviruses have most often been found in squamates, and almost all of these have been in the genus *Atadenovirus*. Adenovirus infections appear to be much rarer in chelonians, and more genetically diverse adenoviruses, including a siadenovirus, an atadenovirus, and several viruses in a proposed additional "testadenovirus" genus, have been described in these animals. In most cases, adenovirus infection in reptiles has been associated with liver and intestinal lesions. However, less commonly, upper- and/or lower-respiratory and upper digestive tract lesions have been described. These lesions have included ulcerations in the oral cavity and nasal and ocular discharge in tortoises with a systemic severe siadenovirus infection.[36] In squamates, atadenoviruses have been detected in bearded dragons with dyspnea[37] and pneumonia,[38] a common agama with an oral abscess,[39] vipers with stomatitis and esophagitis,[40] and in a death adder (*Acanthophis antarcticus*) with pneumonia.[41] In some cases, dyspnea or detection of a lesion(s) in lungs has been associated with mixed infections, with adenoviruses possibly playing a role.[14,42]

Adenovirus detection is most often done by PCR using a PCR capable of detecting viruses in all of the described genera.[43] Choice of PCR method is important, because adenoviruses of reptiles are genetically very diverse. Several PCRs have been developed to detect individual adenoviruses in specific species, for example, agamid adenovirus 1.[44] However, little is known about specific adenoviruses that may be involved in respiratory disease, making a broader diagnostic approach a better option. The clinical sample most commonly used for adenovirus detection is a cloacal swab. If these viruses are considered a possible cause of lesions in the respiratory and upper digestive tract, it may be useful to also collect an oral swab for testing. Serologic detection of antibodies against several different reptile adenoviruses has been described,[45] but is not commercially available.

Ranaviruses

Ranaviruses are large, double-stranded DNA viruses belonging to the family *Iridoviridae*. They can infect amphibians, fish, and reptiles and have a wide range of hosts, with some able to switch hosts between animal classes.[46] They have been associated with various clinical signs and systemic disease in multiple reptile species. Stomatitis, rhinitis, conjunctivitis, tracheitis, pneumonia, esophagitis, and facial and cervical swelling have been described in disease outbreaks associated with ranaviruses in both wild and captive chelonians, including a variety of species.[46] Infection can also impact other tissues. Oral lesions have also been described in ranavirus-infected squamates in individual cases.[47,48]

Diagnosis of ranavirus infections is most often by PCR. Several conventional and real-time PCRs have been described for this purpose.[49–52] When choosing a method for ranavirus detection in reptiles, it is important to note that depending on the geographic location of the animal, genetically variable viruses have been found in reptiles. Ranaviruses in reptiles in North America have generally been very closely related to the species *Frog virus 3*, whereas more diverse ranaviruses have been found in reptiles on other continents.[46] The detection method should be chosen with this in mind. The choice of clinical sample for ranavirus detection can also be difficult. Oral swabs have been used, but may lack sensitivity.[53,54] Virus has also been detected in cloacal swabs and blood of infected animals,[53,55] and there is some indication that more invasive sampling of tissues may lead to higher rates of identification of infected animals.[56] An ELISA has been described for the detection of antibodies against ranaviruses in chelonians, but is not commercially available.[57]

Reoviruses

In reptiles, reoviruses have most often been found in squamates, where they have been associated with a variety of clinical signs and pathologic conditions, including gastrointestinal, CNS, respiratory, and hepatic disease.[24] A reovirus was shown to cause interstitial pneumonia in rat snakes.[58] In chelonians, reports of reovirus infections are rare and have been associated with stomatitis.[24]

Reoviruses have most often been detected by virus isolation. They grow on various reptile cell lines at 28°C (82.4°F). A consensus nested PCR has been described that can detect the reoviruses found in reptiles so far.[59] Sampling protocols for reovirus detection are not well defined because most virus detections have been from various tissues from dead animals. Oral and cloacal swabs may be suitable. Neutralization tests have been used for the detection of antibodies against reoviruses in both captive and wild-caught reptiles,[60–62] indicating some circulation of these viruses in both settings; however, serologic testing is not currently commercially available, and there is some indication that different reoviruses from reptiles may differ genetically and serologically,[63,64] making it necessary to use appropriate viruses in any serologic test.

Sunshinevirus

Sunshineviruses are enveloped, ssRNA viruses in the order *Mononegavirales*. They are distantly related to ferlaviruses. Sunshinevirus has mostly been detected in pythons in Australia,[65] but there are a few reports of possible infection in pythons outside of Australia.[66,67] Infected snakes may remain clinically healthy, but can develop respiratory, CNS, or nonspecific disease.[65] Diagnosis of infection is generally by PCR. Virus has been detected in oral and cloacal swabs, but brain is considered the optimal sample.[65] There is currently no serologic test for the presence of antibodies against sunshinevirus.

Reptarenaviruses

Reptarenaviruses (family *Arenaviridae*) have been shown to cause inclusion body disease (IBD) in boas and pythons.[68] IBD and reptarenavirus infection are most often associated with CNS disease, but can also manifest in a variety of other clinical signs, including upper- and lower-respiratory-tract disease.[69] Disease in pythons often develops more quickly and is often associated with more severe neurologic disease, whereas boas may develop more chronic disease with a wider variety of possible clinical signs. Why animals with IBD develop respiratory disease is not known. It is possible that it is a result of infection with reptarenaviruses but could also be a result of immunosuppression and consequent secondary infections. Diagnosis can be challenging, especially in pythons, and can be based on virus detection by PCR and/or detection of inclusion bodies in cells of affected animals. Virus detection by PCR can be done using a variety of clinical samples. Oral swabs, esophageal swabs, combined oral-cloacal swabs, whole blood, and liver biopsies have been reported to be useful for this purpose.[68,70,71] In pythons, virus may be difficult to detect and require repeat testing over an extended period of time,[71] or it may only be detectable in the brain.[68] Reptarenaviruses have been shown to be genetically extremely variable[72,73]; this can be relevant for PCR diagnostics with possible false negative results depending on the virus or viruses involved and the primers used. Inclusion body detection in blood smears, liver, or esophageal tonsil biopsies appears to correlate well with virus detection in boas, but in pythons, inclusions are rarely found.[74] Detection of antibodies against reptarenaviruses by ELISA and immunoblotting has been described, but relatively few animals appear to develop detectable antibodies.[75]

Torchiviruses

Torchiviruses are also known as tortoise picornaviruses or virus "x." They have been described in numerous tortoise species, most often in spur-thighed tortoises (*Testudo graeca*).[76–78] Although torchiviruses are known to cause kidney disease and extreme softening of the carapace in juvenile tortoises,[79] they have also been associated with rhinitis, stomatitis, pharyngitis, and pneumonia as well as other changes in adult tortoises and have also been found in apparently clinically healthy animals.[77] Torchivirus detection has been carried out by virus isolation in Terrapene heart cells (TH-1) and by PCR.[54,77] These viruses are genetically variable making PCR detection more difficult. The best clinical sample for virus detection is generally an oral swab, but virus can also be detected in other samples, for example, conjunctival and cloacal swabs.[79,80] Virus shedding was found to be intermittent in some animals following experimental infection.[79] Antibodies against torchiviruses can be detected using virus neutralization assays.[78,81]

Bacteria and Fungi

General considerations

Reptiles are known to harbor a large range of aerobic bacteria and fungi as a normal part of their microbial gut flora, including both gram-positive and gram-negative bacteria and to some extent also yeast and other fungi.[3,82] This diverse microbiome makes it difficult to interpret results from samples from the oral cavity, the nares, or even the upper-respiratory tract. Interpretation always needs to consider the sampling point and the clinical condition, as well as concurrent infections. Although primary bacterial infection in the lower airways is described and may arise following oral transmission as well as via the blood system, most bacterial infections are a consequence of a primary impact, for example, a virus infection, a toxic cause, or a chronic alimentary or husbandry deficit. For ferlavirus infections, it is postulated that the possible virulence of the virus strain is connected to a lack of (local) immune reaction and therefore severe secondary bacterial infection,[62,83,84] and there is evidence that secondary bacterial infection plays a role in the severity and clinical progression of serpentovirus infections.[7]

Because bacterial and fungal infections, once they reach the lower-respiratory system, are of high relevance, and identification is essential for effective treatment, the correct sampling procedure, mostly a tracheal wash sample (see **Fig. 4**), needs to be carried out as sterilely as possible and following published standards (see above).

Aside from the correct sampling technique, recent studies also indicate that the identification of the bacterial species can be challenging and that biochemical identification kits used for standard diagnostics are not suitable in reptiles, because they focus on bacteria of relevance in human (or mammalian) medicine. More sensitive methods, such as MALDI-TOF mass spectrometry, are more suitable, although references for species identification are often still lacking in the respective databases.[85]

Despite the colonization of the intestinal as well as the upper-respiratory system with various species of bacteria, the normal, healthy lung in reptiles is sterile.[11] Diagnostic testing for lower-respiratory-tract disease must therefore aim to obtain samples from the lung surface (via endoscopy) or at least the lower trachea using a suitable washing tube. Imaging methods, such as computed tomography (CT), are also of great help in interpreting the extent of a lung tissue infection.

Mycoplasma

Mycoplasma is a common cause of upper-respiratory-tract disease, especially in chelonians. In tortoises, upper-respiratory-tract disease can be caused by *Mycoplasma agassizii*, and disease association has been proven by experimental transmission studies.[86,87] *Mycoplasma testudineum* also causes upper-respiratory-tract disease but is thought to be less pathogenic than *M agassizii*.[88] Diverse related *Mycoplasma* spp have been detected in European tortoise species[54,89] and chelonians of the family Emydidae.[90–93] Although mycoplasma in chelonians is well studied, mycoplasma infection in other reptiles has only sporadically been reported, mostly in snakes.[84,94,95] Although the numbers of such reports are increasing, the association between mycoplasma infections and clinical disease in these reptiles is still unclear.

Clinical signs associated with mycoplasma infections are chronic rhinitis and conjunctivitis with nasal and ocular discharge.[86,96,97] However, clinical signs can vary from severe to asymptomatic carriers.[87,97,98]

Detection of mycoplasma is most often done by PCR. Mycoplasma culture is complex and rarely used for routine diagnostics.[86] Various conventional[92,99,100] and quantitative PCRs[101,102] have been described. Nasal lavage has been described as the sample with the highest sensitivity, especially when the samples were cultivated in SP4 broth for 24 to 48 hours before PCR.[87] However, nasal and oral swabs have also been shown to be suitable for mycoplasma detection.[54,89,92]

ELISAs have been used for the detection of antibodies against *M agassizii* in various tortoise species[88,103] and against *M testudineum* in desert tortoises.[88] Experimental infections have shown that antibodies develop within 2 months after infection.[86,87] Cross-reactions between closely related mycoplasma species, such as *M agassizii* and *M testudineum*, are likely.[104]

Chlamydia

Chlamydia spp are occasionally isolated from reptiles and can be related to systemic and local diseases, even acting as a primary and fatal collection disease, for example, in a collection of emerald tree boas.[105] Chlamydia can cause a variety of clinical diseases associated with various tissues. Pneumonia can occur as a concurrent or even main sign.[106] Diagnosis is normally confirmed using suitable PCR protocols, and nasal flushes or tracheal wash sample fluid is recommended. Immunostaining of tissue sections from granulomas has been described to identify the antigens in the inflammatory reaction.[105]

Gram-negative bacteria

Infections of the lower-respiratory system involving gram-negative bacteria are commonly associated with concurrent inflammatory reactions in the oral cavity (stomatitis) as well as tracheitis. Therefore, it is conceivable that a severe infection in the upper-respiratory system can spread into the lower parts and then affect one or both lungs and the air sacs. The standard diagnostic procedures for bacterial species identification include aerobic culture, followed by assessment of growth characteristics on agar plates, colony morphology, staining patterns, and further identification with biochemical or more advanced methods.[85,107] A variety of gram-negative species are reported to be involved in boid snakes with bacterial pneumonia; predominantly described are Pseudomonas spp, Aeromonas spp, Stenotrophomonas spp, Klebsiella spp, Salmonella spp, and Proteus spp.[84,85,108] In most cases of inflammatory disease, more than 1 bacterial species can be isolated, indicating that infections often occur rather as a secondary problem.[85] The identification of the bacteria involved followed by antibiotic sensitivity testing is an essential step for an effective and optimized treatment, as bacterial infections of the lung generally require systemic antibiotic treatment. Underlying causes always need to be taken into consideration during the diagnostic workup. Because bacterial infection in the lung tissue can cause severe inflammatory reactions and purulent secretion, imaging techniques, such as endoscopy, CT, and MRI, are recommended as useful tools to assess the extent of the infection and even the success of antimicrobial treatment.[109]

Fungi

Fungi are found as secondary infections, opportunistic infections related to poor husbandry conditions, but also described as possible primary causes of a respiratory disease. Case reports indicate that severe fungal pneumonia can occur.[110,111] Aspergillus spp, Penicillium spp, and Candida spp are commonly diagnosed, but for more reptile-specific species, diagnosis can be challenging and requires specific diagnostics.[112] Aside from opportunistic infections, there are also reports on specific fungal species causing primary disease. These pathogens can be relatively specific to the host species. Metarhizium granulomatis has been described in chameleon species and can cause glossitis and pharyngitis, but can also spread to the internal organs.[113] Purpureocillium lilacinum has been reported as the fungal cause of a fatal pneumonia in a green tree python,[114] and further hypocrealean fungi are known to cause primary or secondary lung infections in reptiles.[115] Because of the granulomatous nature of most fungal infections, collection of biopsies is recommended whenever possible for diagnostic testing. For standard culture, specific agars (eg, Sabouraud agar) are used, and fungal growth may take up to 72 hours. The identification of the fungal species is then based on the culture morphology and growth characteristics. Further tools, such as MALDI-TOF, or specific PCR and sequencing protocols are recommended for further identification.

Parasites

Several parasite species are regularly found in reptiles with respiratory disease, including nematodes, trematodes, and single-celled parasites, such as coccidia (intranuclear coccidiosis of tortoises [TINC]). The life cycle of the parasite is of relevance, as most parasites with intermediate hosts are only to be expected in wild-caught reptiles.

Helminths and pentastomids

Parasitic worms can use the lung tissue as a passage compartment during their larval (migration) stadium (eg, *Strongyloides* spp) or as the final target for adult worms, as seen in trematodes, and of course, in lungworms (*Rhabdias* spp). Pentastomids (often referred to as worms, although they are crustacean parasites) also parasitize in the lung. Often, these infections do not cause clinical disease, but depending on the parasite load and the reptile immune system, reactions can range from mild to severe pneumonia, including secondary bacterial infections. Tracheal wash samples are most helpful for diagnosis; parasite eggs can also be found in fecal samples, after they have passed from the trachea into the intestines and the feces. Oral swab samples from excessive mucus secretion can be used for cytologic examination. Because the appearance of the eggs and oocysts and larvae varies and a wide variety can be found in different species, the authors refer to specific literature for identification. Adult lungworms can also be visualized directly by using imaging techniques, especially endoscopy.

Intranuclear coccidiosis of tortoises

TINC are associated with systemic disease and unspecific clinical signs.[116] Infections have also been associated with chronic rhinosinusitis and oronasal fistulae.[117] Infection has been reported most often in radiated tortoises (*Astrochelys radiata*), but also in multiple other testudinid species.[116–120] The exact life cycle and transmission route of TINC is still unknown, but fecal-oral transmission has been proven in an experimental study.[121]

TINC is most often diagnosed by PCR. Although several methods have been described, a quantitative PCR that is specific for TINC appears to be the most sensitive and specific method.[118] Suitable clinical samples are oral, conjunctival, or cloacal swabs, and nasal lavages. The detection of TINC from blood[120] and fecal samples[117,121] by PCR has also been described.

DISCUSSION

Diagnosis of infectious causes of respiratory disease in reptiles requires a combination of clinical examination, history, imaging techniques, and laboratory testing. Laboratory testing should focus on pathogen detection rather than detection of a host immune response. The quality of samples will strongly influence the quality of any laboratory results and should be carefully considered depending on the presentation and possible causes. Many of the pathogens associated with respiratory disease in reptiles appear to be facultative pathogens, and disease development will depend on a range of factors, including pathogen strain, host species, animal husbandry, and other potential pathogens and microorganisms present in the host. In general, diagnostic testing for respiratory pathogens is not standardized, and clinicians should discuss testing and interpretation with their laboratory. In addition, knowledge about the diversity of possible pathogens is growing. New scientific discoveries lead on the one hand to changes in testing options and the understanding of test specificity. They also lead to changes in the taxonomy and nomenclature of the infectious agents which in turn can make it difficult to understand older literature or call earlier conclusions on the prevalence of certain pathogens into question. Keeping up with these changes can be difficult but understanding them is key to optimizing diagnosis and treatment of disease in reptile patients.

CLINICS CARE POINTS

- Pathogens associated with upper-respiratory-tract disease are often detected using oral swabs and/or nasal flushes.
- Tracheal wash samples may be better for detection of pathogens associated with lower-respiratory-tract disease.
- Pathogen detection should always be interpreted in conjunction with clinical signs and additional testing.

DISCLOSURE

Two of the authors (R.E. Marschang and E. Salzmann) are employed by a commercial laboratory that offers diagnostic testing to veterinarians. This employment did not influence the writing or publication of this article.

REFERENCES

1. Schumacher J. Respiratory diseases of reptiles. Seminars in Avian and Exotic Pet Medicine 1997;6(4):209–15.
2. Hernandez-Divers S. Diagnostic techniques. In: Mader DR, editor. Reptile medicine and surgery. 2nd edition. St Louis (MO): Saunders Elsevier; 2006. p. 490–532.
3. Pees M, Schmidt V, Schlömer J, et al. Examination on the relevance of the sampling points and the aerobic microbiological culture for the diagnosis of respiratory infections in reptiles. Dtsch tierärztl Wochenschr 2007;114:387–92.
4. Stenglein MD, Jacobson ER, Wozniak EJ, et al. Ball python nidovirus: a candidate etiologic agent for severe respiratory disease in *Python regius*. MBio 2014; 5:e01484-14.
5. Dervas E, Hepojoki J, Laimbacher A, et al. Nidovirus-associated proliferative pneumonia in the green tree python (*Morelia viridis*). J Virol 2017. https://doi.org/10.1128/JVI.00718-17. pii: JVI.00718-17.
6. Hoon-Hanks LL, Layton ML, Ossiboff RJ, et al. Respiratory disease in ball pythons (*Python regius*) experimentally infected with ball python nidovirus. Virology 2018;517:77–87.
7. Hoon-Hanks LL, Ossiboff RJ, Bartolini P, et al. Longitudinal and cross-sectional sampling of serpentovirus (nidovirus) infection in captive snakes reveals high prevalence, persistent infection, and increased mortality in pythons and divergent serpentovirus infection in boas and colubrids. Front Vet Sci 2019;6:338.
8. Marschang RE, Kolesnik E. Detection of nidoviruses in live pythons and boas. Tierarztl Prax Ausg K Kleintiere Heimtiere 2017;45(1):22–6.
9. O'Dea MA, Jackson B, Jackson C, et al. Discovery and partial genomic characterisation of a novel nidovirus associated with respiratory disease in wild shingleback lizards (*Tiliqua rugosa*). PLoS One 2016;11(11):e0165209.
10. Zhang J, Finlaison DS, Frost MJ, et al. Identification of a novel nidovirus as a potential cause of large scale mortalities in the endangered Bellinger River snapping turtle (*Myuchelys georgesi*). PLoS One 2018;13(10):e0205209.

11. Pees M, Schmidt V, Papp T, et al. Three genetically distinct ferlaviruses have varying effects on infected corn snakes (*Pantherophis guttatus*). PLoS One 2019;14(6):e0217164.

12. Hyndman TH, Shilton CM, Marschang RE. Paramyxoviruses in reptiles: a review. Vet Microbiol 2013;165:200–13.

13. Papp T, Pees M, Schmidt V, et al. RT-PCR diagnosis followed by sequence characterization of paramyxoviruses in clinical samples from snakes reveals concurrent infections within populations and/or individuals. Vet Microbiol 2010;144: 466–72.

14. Abbas MD, Marschang RE, Schmidt V, et al. A unique novel reptilian paramyxovirus, four atadenovirus types and a reovirus identified in a concurrent infection of a corn snake (*Pantherophis guttatus*) collection in Germany. Vet Microbiol 2011;150:70–9.

15. Jacobson ER, Adams HP, Geisbert TW, et al. Pulmonary lesions in experimental ophidian paramyxovirus pneumonia of Aruba Island rattlesnakes, *Crotalus unicolor*. Vet Pathol 1997;34:450–9.

16. Jacobson ER, Gaskin JM, Wells S, et al. Epizootic of ophidian paramyxovirus in a zoological collection: pathological, microbiological, and serological findings. J Zoo Wildl Med 1992;23:318–27.

17. Flach EJ, Dagliesh MP, Feltrer Y, et al. Ferlavirus-related deaths in a collection of viperid snakes. J Zoo Wildl Med 2018;49:983–95.

18. Foelsch DW, Leloup P. Fatale endemische Infektion in einem Serpentarium. Tierarztl Prax 1976;4:527–36.

19. Pees M, Neul A, Müller K, et al. Virus distribution and detection in corn snakes (*Pantherophis guttatus*) after experimental infection with three different ferlavirus strains. Vet Microbiol 2016;182:213–22.

20. Kolesnik E, Hyndman TH, Müller E, et al. Comparison of three different PCR protocols for the detection of ferlaviruses. BMC Vet Res 2019;15:281.

21. Neul AK, Schrödl W, Marschang RE, et al. Immunologic responses in corn snakes (*Pantherophis guttatus*) after experimentally induced infection with ferlaviruses. Am J Vet Res 2017;78:482–94.

22. Allender MC, Mitchell MA, Dreslik MJ, et al. Measuring agreement and discord among hemagglutination inhibition assays against different ophidian paramyxovirus strains in the Eastern massasauga (*Sistrurus catenatus catenatus*). J Zoo Wildl Med 2008;39:358–61.

23. Gandar F, Wilkie GS, Gatherer D, et al. The genome of a tortoise herpesvirus (Testudinid herpesvirus 3) has a novel structure and contains a large region that is not required for replication in vitro or virulence in vivo. J Virol 2015. https://doi.org/10.1128/JVI.01794-15. pii: JVI.01794-15.

24. Marschang RE. Viruses infecting reptiles. Viruses 2011;3:2087–126.

25. Jacobson ER, Gaskin JM, Roelke M, et al. Conjunctivitis, tracheitis, and pneumonia associated with herpesvirus infection in green sea turtles. J Am Vet Med Assoc 1986;189:1020–3.

26. Stacy BA, Wellehan JFX, Foley AM, et al. Two herpesviruses associated with disease in wild Atlantic loggerhead sea turtles (*Caretta caretta*). Vet Microbiol 2008;126:63–73.

27. Ossiboff RJ, Newton AL, Seimon TA, et al. Emydid herpesvirus 1 infection in northern map turtles (*Graptemys geographica*) and painted turtles (*Chrysemys picta*). J Vet Diagn Invest 2015;27:392–5.

28. Sim RR, Norton TM, Bronson E, et al. Identification of a novel herpesvirus in a captive Eastern box turtles (*Terrapene carolina carolina*). Vet Microbiol 2015; 175:218–33.

29. Wellehan JFX, Nichols DK, Li L-L, et al. Three novel herpesviruses associated with stomatitis in Sudan plated lizards (*Gerrhosaurus major*) and a black-lined plated lizard (*Gerrhosaurus nigrolineatus*). J Zoo Wildl Med 2004;35:50–5.

30. Wellehan JFX, Johnson AJ, Latimer KS, et al. Varanid herpesvirus-1: a novel herpesvirus associated with proliferative stomatitis in green tree monitors (*Varanus prasinus*). Vet Microbiol 2005;105:83–92.

31. Hyndman TH, Shilton CM, Wellehan JFX, et al. Molecular identification of three novel herpesviruses found in Australian farmed saltwater crocodiles (*Crocodylus porosus*) and Australian captive freshwater crocodiles (*Crocodylus johnstoni*). Vet Microbiol 2015;181:183–9.

32. McArthur S, Blahak S, Kölle P, et al. Roundtable: chelonian herpesviruses. J Herpetol Med Surg 2002;2:14–31.

33. VanDevanter DR, Warrener P, Bennett L, et al. Detection and analysis of diverse herpesviral species by consensus primer PCR. J Clin Microbiol 1996;34(7): 1666–71.

34. Marschang RE, Frost JW, Gravendyck M, et al. Comparison of 16 chelonid herpesviruses by virus neutralization tests and restriction endonuclease digestion of viral DNA. J Vet Med B Infect Dis Vet Public Health 2001;48:393–9.

35. Origgi FC, Klein PA, Mathes K, et al. An enzyme linked immunosorbent assay (ELISA) for detecting herpesvirus exposure in Mediterranean tortoises. J Clin Microbiol 2001;39:3156–63.

36. Rivera S, Wellehan JFX, McManamon R, et al. Systemic adenovirus infection in Sulawesi tortoises (*Indotestudo forsteni*) caused by a novel siadenovirus. J Vet Diagn Invest 2009;21:415–26.

37. Papp T, Fledelius B, Schmidt V, et al. PCR-sequence characterization of new adenoviruses found in reptiles and the first successful isolation of a lizard adenovirus. Vet Microbiol 2009;134(3–4):233–40.

38. Crossland NA, DiGeronimo PM, Sokolova Y, et al. Pneumonia in a captive central bearded dragon with concurrent detection of helodermatid adenovirus 2 and a novel mycoplasma species. Vet Pathol 2018;55:900–4.

39. Ball I, Stöhr AC, Abbas MD, et al. Detection and partial characterization of an atadenovirus in a common agama (*Agama agama*). J Herpetol Med Surg 2012;22:12–6.

40. Raymond JT, Garner MM, Murray S, et al. Oroesophageal adenovirus-like infection in a palm viper, Bothriechis marchi, with inclusion body-like disease. J Herpetol Med Surg 2002;12:30–2.

41. Benge SL, Hyndman TH, Funk RS, et al. Identification of helodermatid adenovirus 2 in a captive central bearded dragon (*Pogona vitticeps*), wild Gila monsters (*Heloderma suspectum*), and a death adder (*Acanthophis antarcticus*). J Zoo Wildl Med 2019;50(1):238–42.

42. Catroxo MHB, Pires JR, Martins AMCRPF, et al. Detection of paramyxovirus, reovirus and adenovirus infection in king snakes (*Lampropeltis triangulum* spp.) by transmission electron microscopy and histopathology techniques. Inter J Environ Agric Res 2018;4:66–75.

43. Wellehan JFX, Johnson AJ, Harrach B, et al. Detection and analysis of six lizard adenoviruses by consensus primer PCR provides further evidence of a reptilian origin for the atadenoviruses. J Virol 2004;78:13366–9.

44. Fredholm DV, Coleman JK, Childress AL, et al. Development and validation of a novel hydrolysis probe real-time polymerase chain reaction for agamid adenovirus 1 in the central bearded dragon (*Pogona vitticeps*). J Vet Diagn Invest 2015;27:249–53.

45. Ball I, Öfner S, Funk RS, et al. Prevalence of neutralising antibodies against adenoviruses in lizards and snakes. Vet J 2014;202:176–81.

46. Duffus ALJ, Waltzek TB, Stöhr AC, et al. Distribution and host range of ranaviruses. In: Gray MJ, Chinchar VG, editors. Ranaviruses: lethal pathogens of ectothermic vertebrates. Cham, Switzerland: Springer Open; 2015. p. 9–58.

47. Hyatt AD, Williams M, Coupar BEH, et al. First identification of a ranavirus from green tree pythons (*Chondropython viridis*). J Wildl Dis 2002;38:239–52.

48. Marschang RE, Braun S, Becher P. Isolation of a ranavirus from a gecko (*Uroplatus fimbriatus*). J Zoo Wildl Med 2005;36:295–300.

49. Mao J, Hedrick RP, Chinchar VG. Molecular characterization, sequence analysis and taxonomic position of newly isolated fish iridoviruses. Virology 1997;229:212–20.

50. Allender MC, Bunick D, Mitchell MA. Development and validation of TaqMan quantitative PCR for detection of frog virus 3-like virus in eastern box turtles (*Terrapene carolina carolina*). J Virol Methods 2013;188:121–5.

51. Leung WTM, Thomas-Walters L, Garner TWJ, et al. A quantitative-PCR based method to estimate ranavirus viral load following normalisation by reference to an ultraconserved vertebrate target. J Virol Methods 2017;249:147–55.

52. Stilwell NK, Whittington RJ, Hick PM, et al. Partial validation of a TaqMan real-time quantitative PCR for the detection of ranaviruses. Dis Aquat Organ 2018;128:105–16.

53. Johnson AJ, Pessier AP, Jacobson ER. Experimental transmission and induction of ranaviral disease in western ornate box turtles (*Terrapene ornata ornata*) and red-eared sliders (*Trachemys scripta elegans*). Vet Pathol 2007;44:285–97.

54. Kolesnik E, Obiegala A, Marschang RE. Detection of *Mycoplasma* spp., herpesviruses, topiviruses, and ferlaviruses in samples from chelonians in Europe. J Vet Diagn Invest 2017;29:820–32.

55. Allender MC, Abd-Eldaim M, Schumacher J, et al. Ranavirus in free-ranging eastern box turtles (*Terrapene carolina carolina*) at rehabilitation centers in three southeastern US states. J Wildl Dis 2011;47:759–64.

56. Goodman RM, Miller DL, Ararso YT. Prevalence of ranavirus in Virginia turtles as detected by tail-clip sampling versus oral-cloacal swabbing. Northeast Nat (Steuben) 2013;20:325–32.

57. Johnson AJ, Wendland L, Norton TM, et al. Development and use of an indirect enzyme-linked immunosorbent assay for detection of iridovirus exposure in gopher tortoises (*Gopherus polyphemus*) and eastern box turtles (*Terrapene carolina carolina*). Vet Microbiol 2010;142:160–7.

58. Lamirande EW, Nichols DK, Owens JW, et al. Isolation and experimental transmission of a reovirus pathogenic in rat snakes (*Elaphe* species). Virus Res 1999;63:135–41.

59. Wellehan JF Jr, Childress AL, Marschang RE, et al. Consensus nested PCR amplification and sequencing of diverse reptilian, avian, and mammalian orthoreoviruses. Vet Microbiol 2009;133(1–2):34-42.

60. Gravendyck M, Ammermann P, Marschang RE, et al. Paramyxoviral and reoviral infections of iguanas on Honduran islands. J Wildl Dis 1998;34:33–8.

61. Marschang RE, Donahoe S, Manvell R, et al. Paramyxovirus and reovirus infections in wild-caught Mexican lizards (*Xenosaurus* and *Abronia* spp.). J Zoo Wildl Med 2002;33:317–21.

62. Pees M, Schmidt V, Marschang RE, et al. Prevalence of viral infections in captive collections of boid snakes in Germany. Vet Rec 2010;166:422–5.

63. Blahak S, Ott I, Vieler E. Comparison of 6 different reoviruses of various reptiles. Vet Res 1995;26:470–6.

64. Kugler R, Marschang RE, Ihász K, et al. Whole genome characterization of a chelonian orthoreovirus strain identifies significant genetic diversity and may classify reptile orthoreoviruses into distinct species. Virus Res 2016;215:94–8.

65. Hyndman TH, Marschang RE, Wellehan JFX, et al. Isolation and molecular identification of Sunshine virus, a novel paramyxovirus found in Australian snakes. Infect Genet Evol 2012;12:1436–46.

66. Marschang RE, Stöhr AC, Aqrawi T, et al. First detection of Sunshine virus in pythons (*Python regius*) in Europe. In: Baer CK, editor. Proceedings Association of Reptilian and Amphibian Veterinarians. Indianapolis (IN): Association of Reptile and Amphibian Veterinarians. 2013. p. 15.

67. Kongmakee P. Pathology and molecular diagnosis of paramysovirus infection in Boidae and Pythonidae in Thailand. Thailand: MSc Thesis, Chulalongkorn University; 2014.

68. Stenglein MD, Sanchez-Migallon Guzman D, Garcia VE, et al. Differential disease susceptibilities in experimentally reptarenavirus-infected boa constrictors and ball pythons. J Virol 2017;91:e00451-17.

69. Chang LW, Jacobson ER. Inclusion body disease, a worldwide infectious disease of boid snakes: a review. J Exot Pet Med 2010;19:216–25.

70. Aqrawi T, Stöhr AC, Knauf-Witzens T, et al. Identification of snake arenaviruses in live boas and pythons in a zoo in Germany. Tierarztl Prax Ausg K Kleintiere Heimtiere 2015;43:239–47.

71. Hyndman TH, Marschang RE, Bruce M, et al. Reptarenaviruses in apparently healthy snakes in an Australian zoological collection. Aust Vet J 2019;97(4): 93–102.

72. Hepojoki J, Salmenperä P, Sironen T, et al. Arenavirus coinfections are common in snakes with boid inclusion body disease. J Virol 2015;89:8657–60.

73. Stenglein MD, Jacobson ER, Chang LW, et al. Widespread recombination, reassortment, and transmission of unbalanced compound viral genotypes in natural arenavirus infections. PLoS Pathog 2015;11:e1004900.

74. Simard J, Marschang RE, Leineweber C, et al. Prevalence of inclusion body disease and associated comorbidity in captive collections of boid and pythonid snakes in Belgium. PLoS One 2020;15(3):e0229667.

75. Korzyukov Y, Hetzel U, Kipar A, et al. Generation of anti-boa immunoglobulin antibodies for serodiagnostic applications, and their use to detect anti-reptarenavirus antibodies in boa constrictor. PLoS One 2016;11(6):e0158417.

76. Farkas SL, Ihász K, Fehér E, et al. Sequencing and phylogenetic analysis identifies candidate members of a new picornavirus genus in terrestrial tortoise species. Arch Virol 2015;160(3):811–6.

77. Marschang RE, Ihász K, Kugler R, et al. Development of a consensus reverse transcription PCR assay for the specific detection of tortoise picornaviruses. J Vet Diagn Invest 2016;28(3):309–14.

78. Paries S, Funcke S, Lierz M. Investigations on the prevalence of tortoise picornavirus in captive tortoises in Germany. Tierarztl Prax Ausg K Kleintiere Heimtiere 2018;46(5):304–8.

79. Paries S, Funcke S, Kershaw O, et al. The role of Virus "X" (tortoise picornavirus) in kidney disease and shell weakness syndrome in European tortoise species determined by experimental infection. PLoS One 2019;14(2):e0210790.

80. Marschang RE. Isolation and characterization of irido-, herpes-, and reoviruses from tortoises and description of an uncharacterized cytopathogenic agent. DrMedVet Dissertation. Giessen (Germany): Justus Leibig University; 2000.

81. Marschang RE, Schneider RM. Antibodies against viruses in wild-caught spur-thighed tortoises (*Testudo graeca*) in Turkey. Vet Rec 2007;161:102–3.

82. Hilf M, Wagner R, Yu V. A prospective study of upper airway flora in healthy boid snakes and snakes with pneumonia. J Zoo Wildl Med 1990;21:318–25.

83. Marschang RE, Papp T, Frost JW. Comparison of paramyxovirus isolates from snakes, lizards and a tortoise. Virus Res 2009;144:272–9.

84. Schmidt V, Marschang RE, Abbas MD, et al. Detection of pathogens in Boidae and Pythonidae with and without respiratory disease. Vet Rec 2013;172:236.

85. Plenz B, Schmidt V, Grosse-Herrenthey A, et al. Characterisation of the aerobic bacterial flora of boid snakes: application of MALDI-TOF mass spectrometry. Vet Rec 2015;176:285.

86. Brown MB, Schumacher IM, Klein PA, et al. *Mycoplasma agassizii* causes upper respiratory tract disease in the desert tortoise. Infect Immun 1994;62:4580–6.

87. Brown MB, McLaughlin GS, Klein PA, et al. Upper respiratory tract disease in the gopher tortoise is caused by *Mycoplasma agassizii*. J Clin Microbiol 1999;37: 2262–9.

88. Jacobson ER, Brown MB, Wendland LD, et al. Mycoplasmosis and upper respiratory tract disease of tortoises: a review and update. Vet J 2014;201:257–64.

89. Lecis R, Paglietti B, Rubino S, et al. Detection and characterization of *Mycoplasma* spp. and *Salmonella* spp. in free-living European tortoises (*Testudo hermanni, Testudo graeca,* and *Testudo marginata*). J Wildl Dis 2011;47:717–24.

90. Feldman SH, Wimsatt J, Marschang RE, et al. Novel mycoplasma detected in association with upper respiratory disease syndrome in free-ranging eastern box turtles (*Terrapene carolina carolina*) in Virginia. J Wildl Dis 2006;42:279–89.

91. Silbernagel C, Clifford DL, Bettaso J, et al. Prevalence of selected pathogens in western pond turtles and sympatric introduced red-eared sliders in California, USA. Dis Aquat Organ 2013;107:37–47.

92. Ossiboff RJ, Raphael BL, Ammazzalorso AD, et al. A *Mycoplasma* species of Emydidae turtles in the northeastern USA. J Wildl Dis 2015;51:466–70.

93. Palmer JL, Blake S, Wellehan JF Jr, et al. Clinical *Mycoplasma* sp. infections in free-living three-toed box turtles (*Terrapene carolina triunguis*) in Missouri, USA. J Wildl Dis 2016;52:378–82.

94. Penner JD, Jacobson ER, Brown DR, et al. A novel *Mycoplasma* sp. associated with proliferative tracheitis and pneumonia in a burmese python (*Python molurus bivittatus*). J Comp Pathol 1997;117:283–8.

95. Marschang RE, Heckers KO, Dietz J, et al. Detection of a mycoplasma in a python (*Morelia spilota*) with stomatitis. J Herpetol Med Surg 2016;26:90–3.

96. Jacobson ER, Gaskin JM, Brown MB, et al. Chronic upper respiratory tract disease of free-ranging desert tortoises (*Xerobates agassizii*). J Wildl Dis 1991;27: 296–316.

97. Schumacher IM, Hardenbrook DB, Brown MB, et al. Relationship between clinical signs of upper respiratory tract disease and antibodies to *Mycoplasma agassizii* in desert tortoises from Nevada. J Wildl Dis 1997;33:261–6.

98. Brown DR, Schumacher IM, McLaughlin GS, et al. Application of diagnostic tests for mycoplasmal infections of desert and gopher tortoises, with management recommendations. Chelonian Conserv Biol 2002;4:497–507.

99. Brown DR, Crenshaw BC, McLaughlin GS, et al. Taxonomic analysis of the tortoise mycoplasmas *Mycoplasma agassizii* and *Mycoplasma testudinis* by 16S rRNA gene sequence comparison. Int J Syst Bacteriol 1995;45:348–50.

100. McGuire JL, Smith LL, Guyer C, et al. Surveillance for upper respiratory tract disease and Mycoplasma in free-ranging gopher tortoises (*Gopherus polyphemus*) in Georgia, USA. J Wildl Dis 2014;50:733–44.

101. DuPré SA, Tracy CR, Hunter KW. Quantitative PCR method for detection of mycoplasma spp. DNA in nasal lavage samples from the desert tortoise (*Gopherus agassizii*). J Microbiol Methods 2011;86:160–5.

102. Braun J, Schrenzel M, Witte C, et al. Molecular methods to detect *Mycoplasma* spp. and Testudinid herpesvirus 2 in desert tortoises (*Gopherus agassizii*) and implications for disease management. J Wildl Dis 2014;50:757–66.

103. Mathes KA. Untersuchungen zum Vorkommen von Mykoplasmen und Herpesviren bei freilebenden und in Gefangenschaft gehaltenen Mediterranen Landschildkröten (*Testudo hermanni, Testudo graeca graeca* und *Testudo graeca ibera*) in Frankreich und Marokko DrMedVet Dissertation. Giessen (Germany): Justus Leibig University; 2003.

104. Brown DR, Merritt JL, Jacobson ER, et al. *Mycoplasma testudineum* sp. nov., from a desert tortoise (*Gopherus agassizii*) with upper respiratory tract disease. Int J Syst Evol Microbiol 2004;54:1527–9.

105. Jacobson E, Origgi F, Heard D, et al. Immunohistochemical staining of chlamydial antigen in emerald tree boas (*Corallus caninus*). J Vet Diagn Invest 2002;14:487–94.

106. Jacobson ER. Bacterial diseases of reptiles. In: Jacobson ER, editor. Infectious diseases and pathology of reptiles. Boca Raton (FL): CRC press; 2007. p. 461–526.

107. Carroll KC, Weinstein MP. Manual and automated systems for detection and identification of microorganisms. In: Murray PR, Baron EJ, Jorgensen JH, et al, editors. Manual of clinical microbiology. 9th edition. Washington, DC: ASM Press; 2007. p. 192–217.

108. Murray MJ. Pneumonia and normal respiratory function. In: Mader DR, editor. Reptile medicine and surgery. 2nd edition. St. Louis (MO): Saunders Elsevier; 2006. p. 865–77.

109. Pees M, Kiefer I, Oechtering G, et al. Computed tomography for the diagnosis and treatment monitoring of bacterial pneumonia in Indian pythons (*Python molurus*). Vet Rec 2008;163(5):152–6.

110. Frelier PF, Sigler L, Nelson PE. Mycotic pneumonia caused by *Fusarium moniliforme* in an alligator. J Med Vet Mycol 1985;23:399–402.

111. Hernandez-Divers SJ. Pulmonary candidiasis caused by *Candida albicans* in a Greek tortoise (*Testudo graeca*) and treatment with intrapulmonary amphotericin B. J Zoo Wildl Med 2001;32:352–9.

112. Paré JA, Jacobson ER. Mycotic diseases of reptiles. In: Jacobson ER, editor. Infectious diseases and pathology of reptiles. Boca Raton (FL): CRC press; 2007. p. 527–47.

113. Schmidt V, Klasen L, Schneider J, et al. Fungal dermatitis, glossitis and disseminated visceral mycosis caused by different *Metarhizium granulomatis* genotypes in veiled chameleons (*Chamaeleo calyptratus*) and first isolation in healthy lizards. Vet Microbiol 2017;207:74–82.

114. Meyer J, Loncaric I, Richter B, et al. Fatal *Purpureocillium lilacinum* pneumonia in a green tree python. J Vet Diagn Invest 2018;30(2):305–9.

115. Schmidt V, Klasen L, Schneider J, et al. Pulmonary fungal granulomas and fibrinous pneumonia caused by different hypocrealean fungi in reptiles. Vet Microbiol 2018;225:58–63.

116. Garner MM, Gardiner CH, Wellehan JFX, et al. Intranuclear coccidiosis in tortoises: nine cases. Vet Pathol 2006;43:311–20.

117. Innis CJ, Garner MM, Johnson AJ, et al. Antemortem diagnosis and characterization of nasal intranuclear coccidiosis in Sulawesi tortoises (*Indotestudo forsteni*). J Vet Diagn Invest 2007;19:660–7.

118. Alvarez WA, Gibbons PM, Rivera S, et al. Development of a quantitative PCR for rapid and sensitive diagnosis of an intranuclear coccidian parasite in Testudines (TINC), and detection in the critically endangered Arakan forest turtle (*Heosemys depressa*). Vet Parasitol 2013;193:66–70.

119. Kolesnik E, Dietz J, Heckers KO, et al. Detection of intranuclear coccidiosis in tortoises in Europe and China. J Zoo Wildl Med 2017;48:328–34.

120. Stilwell JM, Stilwell NK, Stacy NI, et al. Extension of the known host range of intranuclear coccidiosis: infection in three captive red-footed tortoises (*Chelonoidis carbonaria*). J Zoo Wildl Med 2017;48:1165–71.

121. Hofmannová L, Kvičerová J, Bízková K, et al. Intranuclear coccidiosis in tortoises - discovery of its causative agent and transmission. Eur J Protistol 2019;67:71–6.

Respiratory Diseases of Parrots: Anatomy, Physiology, Diagnosis and Treatment

Lorenzo Crosta, DVM, PhD, GP Cert (Exotic Animal), Diplomate ECZM – EBVS©

KEYWORDS

• Birds • Parrots • Respiratory disease

KEY POINTS

- A general diagnosis of "respiratory disease" in parrots is not difficult, but a causative diagnosis and a proper treatment can be challenging.
- Knowledge of basic avian respiratory anatomy and physiology are important for the clinician.
- Different species and different portions of the respiratory tract can have different issues: knowing those differences and the most common problems is important.

ANATOMY AND PHYSIOLOGY

The high energy demands required for flight and the high aerobic rate of this activity create high demands for oxygen. For this reason, the respiratory apparatus of the bird is likely the most different from mammals.[1]

External Nares (Nostrils)

Most nares are found at the base of the beak either dorsal or lateral. They may be surrounded by a thick, soft cere as in the budgerigar or the pigeon, screened by feathers as in the crow or the grouse, or covered by a keratinized flap, the operculum, as in the chicken or the turkey. An operculum may also be present just inside the nares as in the parrot.

Nares are absent in some species of diving birds like the gannet.[2]

The University of Sydney, Faculty of Science, Sydney School of Veterinary Science, University Veterinary Teaching Hospital Camden, Avian, Reptile and Exotic Pet Hospital, 415 Werombi Road, Camden, New South Wales 2570, Australia
E-mail address: lorenzo.crosta@sydney.edu.au

Vet Clin Exot Anim 24 (2021) 397–418
https://doi.org/10.1016/j.cvex.2021.01.005
1094-9194/21/© 2021 Elsevier Inc. All rights reserved.

Nasal Cavities

The paired nasal cavities are separated by an ossified septum. Although the separation is complete in many birds like chickens, in others like the duck and the grebe there is a rostral opening between the 2 cavities.[3]

The cranial portion of the nasal cavity is lined with nonglandular mucosa. This transitions caudally, in the respiratory region, into a pseudostratified ciliated epithelium containing goblet cells. In the olfactory region the epithelium contains neurosensory cells. Its histologic structure is similar to that of mammals.[4]

Infraorbital Sinus

In most birds, the paired infraorbital sinuses are large triangular cavities located lateral to the nasal cavity and rostroventral to the eye.[3] Their walls are composed almost entirely of soft tissues. In some birds, such as insectivorous passerines, Anseriformes, and parrots, the sinuses communicate with each other, whereas in other birds like noninsectivorous passerines, they are separate.[2] In parrots, the sinuses extend into the upper beak and are connected by a transverse canal.[5]

Cervicocephalic Air Sac

As the name indicates, these air sacs can be subdivided into cephalic and cervical sections. Although contiguous with the infraorbital sinus, the cervicocephalic air sac or "diverticulum" does not communicate with other air sacs. In brief, it does not have anything to do with air ventilation. In some species, the cervicocephalic air sac may have some contact with the clavicular air sac.[2]

The cervicocephalic air sacs are most extensive in strong-flying species like parrots; less developed in pigeons, chicken, and ratites, and absent in diving birds.[6]

Trachea

The trachea extends the length of the neck between the larynx and the syrinx. The upper trachea lies on the midline, ventral to the esophagus. The lower trachea passes through the thoracic inlet on the ventral-midline and is closely related to the clavicular air sac, which envelops it within the thorax.[7,8]

The avian trachea consists of complete cartilaginous rings that interdigitate to produce a more resistant airpipe, compared with the mammalian counterpart.

Syrinx

Unlike the mammalian larynx, birds do not have vocal cords. Instead, the sound-producing avian organ is the syrinx.

Depending on the localization of the syrinx, this structure can be tracheal, bronchial, or the most common type: tracheobronchial (located at the level of the bifurcation of the trachea into the primary bronchi), as it is in Psittaciformes.[1]

In the chicken, the last 4 tracheal rings are considered to be part of the syrinx. The subsequent rings are no longer complete. Instead, they are joined at one or both ends to a median bridge known as the pessulus. Extending cranially from the pessulus is a mucosal fold, the *membrana semilunaris*.

Together, the cartilaginous components of the syrinx form the tympanum. Left and right lateral tympaniform membranes extend from the tympanum to the lateral side of the bronchial cartilages. Paired medial tympaniform membranes pass from the pessulus to the (incomplete) medial aspect of the bronchial cartilages. Elastic connective tissue pads known as labia project from the membranes into the lumen of the syrinx. During phonation, the membranes and labia function in a similar manner to the vocal folds of the mammalian larynx. Syringeal muscles are present in songbirds and absent in domestic poultry.[4]

Lungs

Birds lack a diaphragm; therefore, the thoracic and abdominal cavities are fused to form a single coelomic cavity or coelom.

The avian lungs are located cranio-dorsally within the coelom. The primary bronchi are formed by the upper division of the trachea, usually just distal to the syrinx, and they run along all the lung to open in the caudal thoracic air sac.

Four series of secondary bronchi are starting from each primary bronchus and are named based on their anatomic location: medioventral, mediodorsal, lateroventral, and laterodorsal.[1]

The left and right avian lungs occupy a dorsal position, either side of the vertebral column. They are not lobed. The ribs are deeply embedded in the dorsomedial portion of the lungs, forming distinctive impressions that separate the lung tissue into segments known as tori intercostales. Apart from small embryonic remnants, the lung has no associated pleura.[4]

Functionally the avian lungs are divided into neopulmo and paleopulmo systems. The paleopulmo system is found in all bird species and makes up at least 75% of lung tissue. The neopulmo system, which is less efficient in gas exchange, is absent in penguins, and very reduced in Anseriformes and Psittaciformes. The neopulmo system is well developed in Galliformes, Columbiformes, and Passeriformes.[1]

Bronchial System, Ventilation (air sacs), and Gas Exchange

The divisions of the bronchi are as follows:

- Two primary bronchi (bronchi primarii)
- Secondary bronchi (bronchi secundarii)
- Parabronchi (bronchi tertiarii) and air capillaries (pneumocapillares)

The secondary bronchi are interconnected by parabronchi, or third-order bronchi. These are the functional units of the avian lung. Parabronchi arising from secondary bronchi within the dorsal paleopulmo meet and anastomose with their ventral counterparts in the interior of the lung. The parabronchi are arranged in a parallel array of elongated tubules, from which they derive their alternative name of "air pipes." In most species, their diameter is approximately 0.5 mm.[4]

Individual parabronchi are separated by interparabronchial septa composed of connective tissue. Interparabronchial blood vessels pass through the septa. Due to the arrangement of the septa, the parabronchi appear hexagonal in transverse section.

Parabronchi have several distinctive features:

- They anastomose with one another
- Their walls contain chambers called atria
- They contain gas exchange units
- Their diameter is uniform within species[4]

In brief, the tertiary bronchi do the job that in mammals is done by the alveoli, but with a different mechanic arrangement.[1]

Internally, the parabronchi are lined with simple squamous epithelium. From the lumen, numerous small air chambers known as atria bulge outwardly into the so-called mantle of the parabronchus. The atria are lined with squamous to cuboidal epithelium containing lamellated osmiophilic bodies (surfactant) for reduction of surface tension. The epithelium is surrounded by muscle cells and elastic fibers. Several funnel-shaped infundibulae open from the atria and radiate into the mantle. These give rise to an anastomosing 3-dimensional network of tubular air capillaries. The diameter of the air capillaries varies with species from approximately 3 μm to 10 μm. Due to the high surface tension within these small caliber tubes, their diameter remains relatively constant. The air capillaries are intimately intermeshed with a dense network of blood capillaries, permitting gas exchange to take place across the blood–gas barrier.

The avian blood–gas barrier is considerably thinner than that of mammals. It consists of 3 elements:

- The endothelial cells of the blood capillaries
- The fused basal membranes of the blood and air capillaries
- The epithelium of the air capillaries

Relative to body weight, the surface area for gas exchange in birds is approximately 10 times greater than in mammals.[4]

Both inhalation and exhalation are active actions, which require the assistance of respiratory muscles. In the avian respiratory cycle, inspired air passes through the trachea, passes through the lungs, and enters the air sacs. Expired air exits from the air sacs, passes again through the lungs, and is expelled from the trachea. Most birds have 9 air sacs: paired cervical, cranial thoracic, caudal thoracic, and abdominal air sacs, as well as a single clavicular air sac. Air sacs play no role in gas exchange. Instead, they work like bellows, sucking in inspired air when expanding and eject air when they contract[1] (**Figs. 1** and **2**).

CLINICAL EXAMINATION OF THE RESPIRATORY TRACT

Due to its specific anatomic characteristics, particularly the air sacs, the avian respiratory system constitutes a substantial target for infection or compromise by husbandry-related diseases. At the same time, these anatomic features provide clinicians with a range of highly efficient options for diagnostic and therapeutic intervention.[4]

As it happens for any other organ/system, the first, but most important step, will be a careful and complete clinical examination of the patient. Like any prey animal, birds tend to hide their symptoms trying to avoid predation; hence, the common costume to start our clinical examination collecting the information we need before even touching the patient, but giving the bird the chance to relax and eventually show the symptoms. This concept, known as well as the "masking phenomenon" is very important to be understood: a sick bird will make a determined effort to look healthy, even in the absence of predators.[9]

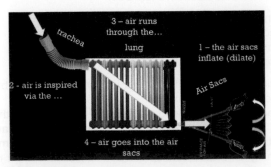

Fig. 1. Inspiratory phase of the avian respiratory system.

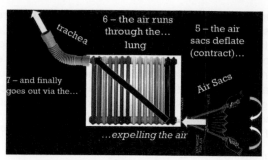

Fig. 2. Expiratory phase of the avian respiratory system.

The clinical history for respiratory diseases is a standard avian form, but it will take into consideration: the species, the breed/mutation, the type of housing, diet, presence of other birds/pets, and the daily routine of the owners, and of the bird(s).

Species is important, as some species may mimic human sounds, such a coughing. On the other hand, some species, like *Pionus* spp., may show signs resembling a respiratory distress when they are in fear, or stressed. Both those "symptoms" are false, but can lead the owner, carer, or even the veterinarian to believe there is a respiratory issue.

For what the respiratory symptoms/diseases, are concerned, much attention will be put on diet, environment, and the presence of other animals.

A dietary unbalance is well known to produce mid to long-term effect of the immune system. In this view, it is not surprising that a bad diet reflects of the health in a rather direct way. Specifically, vitamin A deficiency will lead to thinning and weakening of the respiratory epithelia, making the respiratory apparatus more accessible to pathogens of any kind.

For similar reasons, environment plays an important role for the health of the respiratory system. Wrong environment is a wide term and should be used at its broadest meaning: wrong temperatures, light cycles, neighboring animals, cage, or aviary mates can all create a "wrong environment," leading to the same problems as diet with the immune system. A wrong environment will stress the bird and chronic stress is limiting the immune response of the patient.

The presence of other animals, especially of the same, or related species, is important in case we suspect a contagious disease. It is always important to gather information about the health of other pets, cage mates, and of any other bird in the same location.

Once the aforementioned information has been gathered, the most important point, is to locate the origin of the respiratory symptoms:

- Maybe the symptoms depend on an extrarespiratory issue?
- In case of a real respiratory problem, is it an upper, or a lower respiratory tract disease?

This distinction can usually be made based on a thorough history and physical examination.[10] However, the distinction between the clinical signs is not easy, as there are symptoms that may refer to both an upper respiratory tract disease (URTD) and a lower repiratory tract disease (LRTD).

Upper airway disease does not usually present with severe respiratory distress, is usually not a life-threatening emergency, and a diagnostic plan can be formulated to determine the nature of disease.

Lower respiratory disease, including tracheal obstruction, may present with severe respiratory distress including open-mouth breathing, tail bobbing, apparent sternal movements, gurgling on inspiration or expiration, and head shaking. An acute onset of lower respiratory signs, especially with a history of recently eating (indicating possible aspiration of a foreign body), warrants immediate oxygen support and potential air sac cannula placement. Coelomic masses, ascites, or dystocia may compress the air sacs or lungs and cause signs of lower respiratory disease; placement of an air sac cannula will not help in these situations[11]

Typical signs of URTD, in parrots, would be (adapted from Ref.[10]):

Nares and nasal cavities:
- Sneezing
- Nasal discharge
- The feathers around the nostrils are stained, or soaked
- Nasal plugs, occlusion of the nares
- Abnormally shaped nares
- Swollen cere
- Scratching, or rubbing of the beak
- Head shaking
- Yawning
- Discharge, or mucous in the choanal slit
- Open beak breathing
- Epiphora, conjunctivitis
- Longitudinal groove(s) in the upper beak (chronic rhinitis)
- Possible combination of signs with sinusitis

Sinuses:
- Periorbital swelling (can be soft, fluctuating, or firm)
- Protrusion of the eye (exophthalmos)
- Sunken eye (chronic sinusitis)
- Scratching, or rubbing of the head
- Periorbital feather loss
- Possible combination of signs with rhinitis

Trachea and/or syrinx:
- Loss of vocalization
- Change of pitch or voice
- Abnormal breathing sounds, particularly on inspiration
- Head shaking
- Coughing
- Gurgling
- Dyspnea, open beak breathing
- Breathing with an extended neck.

Typical signs of LRTD would be (adapted from Ref.[12]):
- Increase respiratory movements
- Tail bobbing
- Open beak breathing
- Breathing with an extended head and neck
- Altered voice
- Respiratory noise
- Coughing (may be an imitation of human coughing)
- Reduced exercise tolerance and increase in time before normal breathing after exercise

- Weight loss (nonspecific, but common)

Clinical signs that are common to URTD and LRTD:

- Dyspnea, open beak breathing
- Breathing with an extended neck.
- Change of pitch or voice
- Respiratory noise

Considering the anatomic complexity of the avian respiratory tract, there are many possible locations of respiratory diseases in parrots. Disease processes located in different anatomic districts, will have some common and some different causes. Down here a list of the possible causes of diseases in the different parts of the respiratory system.

Causes of Rhinitis-Sinusitis

Congenital: Choanal atresia: most commonly reported in African gray parrots. Imperforate naris or nares.

Nutritional: hypovitaminosis A

Neoplasia: Nasal or sinus adenocarcinoma. Squamous cell carcinoma. Lymphoma. Fibroma, fibrosarcoma. Basal cell carcinoma. Malignant melanoma.

Immune-mediated: (allergic) rhinitis and sinusitis.

Infectious: Viral: rarely the underlying cause of rhinitis or sinusitis in companion birds: Avian influenza virus, Herpesvirus, Paramyxovirus-1, Poxvirus, Reovirus.

Primary bacterial agents (may also be considered as secondary or opportunistic agents in some cases): *Bordetella avium*, *Chlamydia psittaci*, *Enterobacter* spp, *Helicobacter* sp ("spiral bacteria") in cockatiels, *Mycoplasma* spp (budgerigars, cockatiels), *Mycobacterium* spp, *Salmonella* spp.

Secondary (opportunistic) bacterial agents: may also be considered primary agents in certain cases: *Escherichia coli*, *Haemophilus* sp, *Klebsiella* spp, *Nocardia asteroides*, *Pasteurella* spp, *Pseudomonas aeruginosa*, *Staphylococcus* spp, *Streptococcus* spp.

Fungal agents: fungal infections are often considered opportunistic and noncontagious: *Aspergillus* spp., *Candida albicans*, *Cryptococcus neoformans Mucor* sp.

Parasitic agents, *Knemidokoptes pilae* (eg, budgerigars), *Trichomonas* spp (eg, canaries).

Trauma.

Foreign bodies: food particles, wood shavings, bedding particles.

Rhinoliths: proliferative nasal granulomas, most frequently reported in African gray parrots[13] (**Fig. 3**).

Causes of Tracheitis

Tracheal stenosis following intubation: can occur up to 2 weeks after an intubation event. The exact causative event is unknown: possible physical or chemical irritation of the mucosa by the endotracheal tube itself; the constant flow of air can be responsible for focal mucosal desiccation, this may cause inflammation and promote infection locally in the trachea, which progresses in stenosis of the trachea due to excessive fibrous tissue or granuloma formation.

Foreign body (eg, millet seeds, insect part).

Infectious causes

Viral: Herpesvirus infections: Amazon laryngotracheitis in Amazon parrots and a few other psittacine species, Psittacid herpesvirus 1 (glottal lesions, mainly in green-winged macaws) (**Fig. 4**), and Psittacid herpesvirus 3 infection in Eclectus parrots

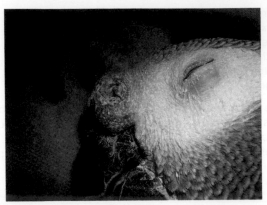

Fig. 3. A rhinolith in an African gray parrot (*Psittacus erithacus*).

and Bourke's parakeets. Poxvirus (diphtheric or wet form) in young Amazons, especially blue-fronted (*Amazona aestiva*), various parakeets, and lovebirds.

Bacterial: Various bacterial agents have been implicated in tracheitis, which may lead to tracheal stenosis either by fibrous tissue or granuloma formation: *Mycobacterium genavense*, reported in an Amazon parrot with granulomatous tracheitis.

Fungal: Aspergillus infection can be responsible for granulomas in the trachea. The syrinx seems to be a site of predilection. Commonly diagnosed in Amazon parrots, African gray parrots, and macaws (**Figs. 5** and **6**).

Parasitic: uncommon in Psittacine birds, however tracheal worms are a common finding in cranes, storks, Galliformes, and Corvidae in Europe (**Fig. 7**).

Toxic: Inhaled toxins and smoke-inhalation injuries may cause severe necrotizing tracheitis.

Trauma: Attack by a predator (uncommon in captive parrots), or a fight with a conspecific may lead to tracheal trauma and collapse.

Nutritional deficiencies: Hypovitaminosis A has been associated with epithelial changes in the trachea and notably in the syrinx. It is also a risk factor for infectious

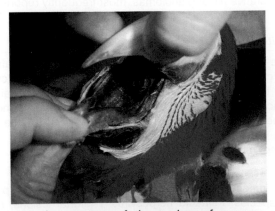

Fig. 4. A papilloma at the entrance of the trachea of a green wing macaw (*Ara chloropterus*).

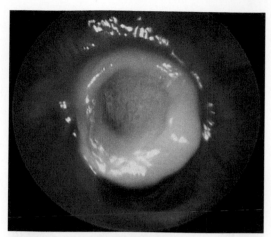

Fig. 5. A tracheal plug in a green-winged macaw (*Ara chloropterus*).

diseases of the trachea by altering the mucosal defenses and increasing air turbu-
lence. Goiter has been associated with respiratory signs in budgerigars.

Neoplasia: Uncommon. Tracheal osteochondroma has been reported in parrots.
Masses in the thoracic inlets have been associated with syringeal and bronchial
compressions.[14]

Causes of Pneumonia in Psittaciformes

Viral, including Polyomavirus, Herpesvirus, Poxvirus, Paramyxovirus (including Exotic
Newcastle Disease [END]), avian influenza (AI).

Bacterial, may be inhaled/aspirated or spread with the blood stream (sepsis); gram-
negative pathogens are commonly noted, although gram-positive organisms have
been reported as well (*Streptococcus* spp, *Staphylococcus* spp); specific etiologies
include *Nocardia*, *Chlamydia psittaci*, *Mycobacterium* (*Mycobacterium avium* or
Mycobacterium genavense), *Mycoplasma* spp (**Fig. 8**).

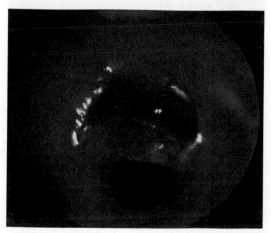

Fig. 6. Same green wing macaw of **Fig. 5**, immediately after the removal of the tracheal
plug.

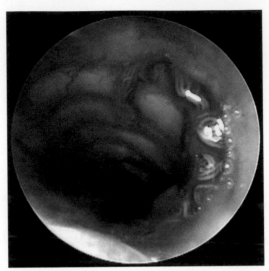

Fig. 7. Tracheal parasites (*Syngamus trachea*), in a white-necked raven (*Corvus albicollis*).

Fungal: *Aspergillus* spp, *Penicillium* spp, *Zygomycetes* (including *Mucor, Rhizopus, Absidia*), *Trichosporon* spp; *Cryptococcal* pneumonia may be associated with cryptococcal sinusitis (**Figs. 9** and **10**).

Parasitic: *Sarcocystis* spp (*Sarcocystis falcatula* most significant) especially in Old World Psittacines.

Noninfectious
Aspiration (especially hand fed birds).

Airborne toxins: most commonly related to exposure to pyrolysis products from overheating pans coated with polytetrafluoroethylene (PTFE); also includes exposure

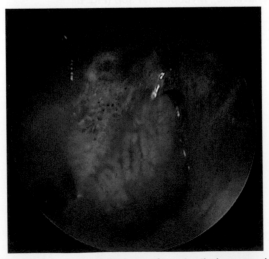

Fig. 8. Endoscopic image of the base of the lung of a red-tailed amazon (*Amazona brasiliensis*), with a chronic pneumonia.

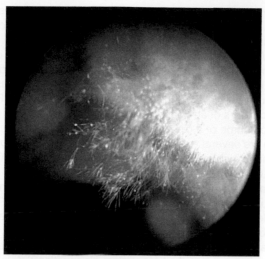

Fig. 9. Endoscopic image of celomic aspergillosis.

to aerosol sprays, paint fumes, cigarette smoke, fumes from burned food and self-cleaning ovens; most often causes acute death but birds that survive may demonstrate signs of pneumonia.[15]

DIAGNOSTICS

A generic diagnosis of respiratory disease is made with a good clinical examination, and this can also help to locate the most important issue.[4] Nevertheless, it is important to try to understand the etiology and the severity of the respiratory disease.

To achieve this, the veterinarian has several tools/techniques to use. The most commonly used are the following:

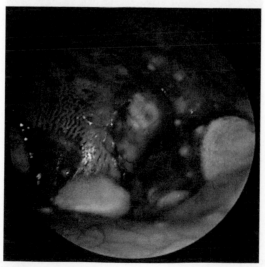

Fig. 10. Diffuse aspergillosis in a hybrid falcon.

Blood chemistry: is not particularly interesting in respiratory diseases, unless a specific organ/system is involved, or some parameters are linked to specific disease, such as Psittacosis,[16] or Aspergillosis.[17]

Hematology and protein electrophoresis: Hematology and serum chemistry in birds is considered rather indicative than diagnostic of any particular disease.[17] Protein electrophoresis (EPH) is a nonspecific diagnostic test, however, can be indicative of some diseases, such as aspergillosis.[18,19] Furthermore, even if EPH and A-G ratio are nonspecific indicators of an ongoing disease, together they are good prognostics tools for the final outcome of a disease.[20]

Serology: There are several tests, even in-house kits, available for some avian diseases, that can cause respiratory symptoms, such as Chlamydia, Aspergillus, PMV1, AI, and Herpesvirus.[16,19,21]

Polymerase chain reaction (PCR): to date an increasing number of diseases, including respiratory diseases of parrots can be diagnosed by PCR. *Mycoplasma, C psittaci*, Newcastle disease, and AI can be tested by PCR. Aspergillosis has also been diagnosed by PCR in humans and different avian species. Nevertheless, at this time, these diagnostic methods appear to have a much higher value for academic, epidemiologic, and forensic use than for clinical diagnostics[22]

Microbiology: culturing bacteria and fungi from the choanae, the trachea, of from specific lesions, as seen during and endoscopy examination is a key point of the diagnosis of respiratory disease in parrots.[23]

Cytology: samples for cytology and Gram staining are often used as a diagnostic aid in respiratory diseases of birds. Different techniques will be applied according to the prat of the respiratory system we need to sample, and/or the type of sample we want to submit.

Cytology of the Upper Respiratory System

Choanal swabs: samples should be taken from the rostral portion as the caudal portion is likely to be contaminated with oropharynx flora (**Fig. 11**).

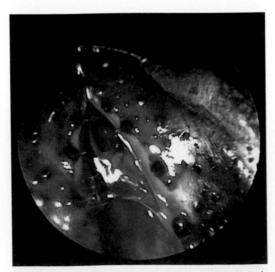

Fig. 11. Inflammatory process of the choana in an orange-winged amazon (*Amazona amazonica*).

Nasal flush: can be used to collect samples and therapeutically to clean debris and rhinoliths. A Luer lock syringe is pressed against the nares forming a seal and the fluid is infused. Drainage of the fluid should flow free from the choana into the mouth. Recommended volumes are 10 to 20 mL/kg.

Infraorbital sinus flush/aspiration: Useful for sample collection, flushing of sinuses, and medication. Advantage of minimal sample contamination. There are 2 approaches: (1) A needle is passed into the sinus at a perpendicular angle though the skin at a point midway between the imaginary line traced between the naris and the medial canthus of the eye, and (2) enter the sinus from a rostral direction by inserting the needle just caudal to the commissure of the mouth; the needle is directed ventral to the zygomatic arch ending in the sinus under the eye (**Figs. 12** and **13**).

Cytology of the lower respiratory system

Tracheal wash: with the patient anesthetized, a sterile catheter is passed through the glottis into the trachea to the point just cranial to the syrinx and 1 to 2 mL/kg of sterile saline is introduced and immediately aspirated.

Air sac lavage: 3 to 5 mL/kg of sterile saline can be injected through the body wall into the last intercostal space or through the biopsy channel of the endoscope and recovered by aspiration with a urinary catheter or similar device[24]

Histopathology: histopathology has a double value in case of respiratory diseases. For the single patient a lung, or air sac biopsy can often be important to diagnose exactly the cause of the disease process (**Fig. 14**). In case of a zoologic collection, or a breeding center, the histopathological examination of dead specimens is paramount to achieve a proper diagnosis.

Radiology: like it is for the diagnosis of respiratory diseases in any other animal species, including humans, radiographs will give a big diagnostic support in birds, as well. Although the nasal sinuses and the trachea are well visible at radiography, the lungs and the air sacs are the parts of the respiratory tract that are best explored with radiographs.

The trachea is easily spotted on radiographs, especially because it is formed of closed cartilaginous rings, which are easily recognizable; however, it is still better evaluated on the lateral view.

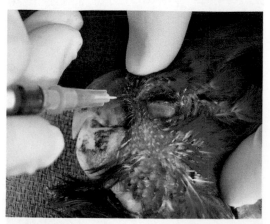

Fig. 12. Gang-gang cockatoo (*Callocephalon fimbriatum*). Insertion of a needle for sampling the nasal sinus. Two different techniques.

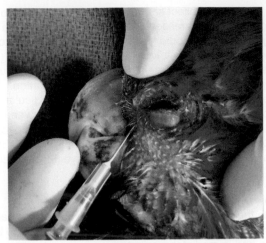

Fig. 13. Gang-gang cockatoo (*Callocephalon fimbriatum*). Insertion of a needle for sampling the nasal sinus. Two different techniques.

The lungs should be evaluated in both the left lateral (LL) and the ventrodorsal (VD) views, to fully examine any pulmonary lesions or abnormalities and reach a suspect diagnosis. Due to the structure of the distal portion of the parabronchi, in the LL views the avian lungs show a distinct honeycomb image. Any respiratory disease may alter the radiodensity of the image, making it darker, or even clearer, up to disappear (**Fig. 15**).

When radiographing the air sacs, the following must be taken into consideration:

Being virtually empty spaces, air sacs are basically identified by their borders with other organs.

Normally they are of the same opacity as the air outside the body (but consider that the soft tissues in between are altering a little the shade of gray) (**Figs. 16** and **17**).

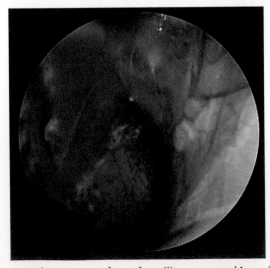

Fig. 14. Small lesions on the air sac surface of a military macaw (*Ara militaris*).

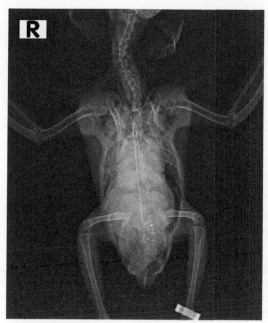

Fig. 15. Radiograph of a Hispaniolan amazon (*Amazona ventralis*). Note the lesion in the right lung.

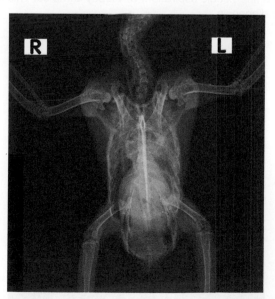

Fig. 16. Severe airsacculitis in an African gray parrot (*Psittacus erithacus*). The VD view highlights that the lesion is mostly on the left side.

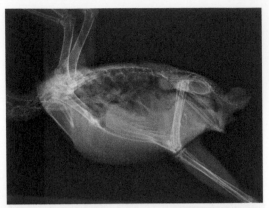

Fig. 17. Severe airsacculitis in an African gray parrot (*Psittacus erithacus*). The VD view highlights that the lesion is mostly on the left side.

In cases of an air sacculitis, the radiological appearance of the air sacs may change, both in shape and opacity, as well as for the presence of focal lesions.

It is important to remember that for a good diagnosis of air sac lesions, both a VD and an LL view must be obtained; this because some lesions may be shown only on one view, and also because the triangulation achieved comparing the 2 projections helps in locating the exact sites of the focal lesions.[25]

Computed tomography scan and MRI: examine anatomy and patency of infraorbital sinus and localize lesions in sinuses,[24] and in the lung parenchyma (**Figs. 18** and **19**).

Endoscopy: this is a direct technique to diagnose the location, extension and nature of internal (celomic) lesions of birds. Not only, the anatomic situation, makes birds ideal patients for coelioscopy. The experienced avian endoscopist can take pictures of the lesions, take fine-needle aspiration, or biopsy samples. This allows to reach a proper, causative diagnosis.

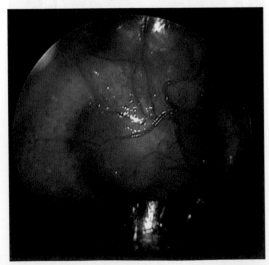

Fig. 18. Mass on unknown origin in the right lung of a Steppe eagle (*Aquila nipalensis*).

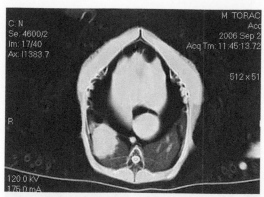

Fig. 19. Computed tomography scan of the pulmonary lesion of the bird in Fig. 16. The mass was a foreign body granuloma.

Last, but not least, the endoscope can also be used as a treatment instrument, for example, by removing a tracheal plug, or a tracheal foreign body, by directing a needle to inject a drug directly into the lesions, or even by removing entire lesions with endosurgery techniques, In few words: *"God made birds for endoscopy"*[23] (**Figs. 20–23**).

TREATMENT

Useless to say that whenever it is possible, targeting the real etiology of a disease is paramount to achieve a definitive result. Hence, bacterial diseases will be treated with antibiotics, fungal infections with antimycotics, and so on. On the other hand, the avian practitioner must be aware of the important parameters to use when selecting a treatment regimen. The questions a veterinarian working with nondomestic species must always take into consideration are as follows:

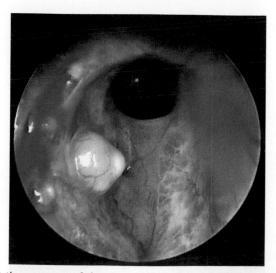

Fig. 20. Abscess at the entrance of the primary bronchus. Alexandrine parakeet (*Psittacula eupatria*).

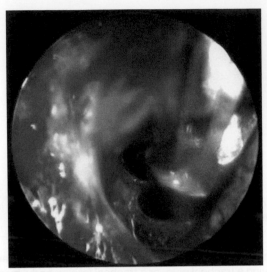

Fig. 21. Galah (*Eolophus reseicapilla*), biopsy of a small lesion in the primary bronchus.

- Will the treatment be effective against the etiologic agent?
- Will the treatment reach and be effective in the anatomic district we need to treat?
- Is the treatment safe for the animal species we are treating?

Summarizing, if a causative diagnosis is reached, if the infectious diseases will be addresses appropriately, if anti-inflammatories will be used accordingly and is a good oxygen support will be delivered to the sick parrot, the success is generally guaranteed.

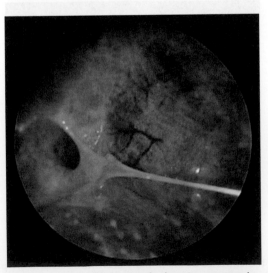

Fig. 22. Green-winged macaw (*Ara chloropterus*), chronic pneumonia and aerosacculitis.

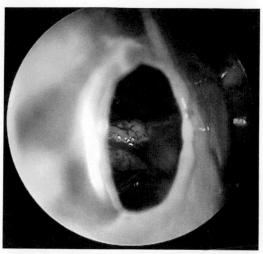

Fig. 23. Fibrinous aerosacculitis in a yellow-headed amazon (*Amazona oratrix*).

Nevertheless, the treatment of the respiratory tract can be challenging, and the different portions of this unique anatomic district tract will be treated with different approaches (**Table 1**).

Upper Airways and Nasal Sinuses

Many times, a nasal flush will help remove mucous and discharge so that the bird can breathe easier. Initial cytology and Gram stains of the fluid can help the clinician decide on treatment (antibiotics, antifungals) pending cultures and sensitivity results.

Trachea and Syrinx

Large airway obstruction requires rapid anesthetic induction with sevoflurane/isoflurane anesthesia, rapid intubation and ventilation with 100% oxygen. If there is a total upper airway obstruction, emergency air sac tube placement is performed. The bird will relax and breathe easier under inhalant anesthesia.

Lungs and Small Airway

The most effective bronchodilators are pharmaceutical agents that stimulate ß-adrenergic receptors in bronchial smooth muscle and promote smooth muscle relaxation. For this reason, they are commonly used for the treatment for bronchoconstriction causing acute respiratory distress. These ß-receptor agonists are most effective and least toxic when they are given as an aerosol that is inhaled.

The ß-receptor agonist, most commonly used in birds is terbutaline. It can be given intramuscularly in birds (0.01 mg/kg every 6–8 hours) initially and then continued by nebulization.

Nebulization is also a very good tool in the hands of the avian practitioner. A small volume of medication and a larger volume of diluent are placed into the nebulizer chamber. The veterinarian nebulizer used most commonly is an ultrasonic nebulizer that delivers particle size of 2 to 7 mm, and can be used by an owner in the home. It is not known if the particle size will reach the atria of the lung, but use of this nebulizer will deliver particles to the bronchi for treatment of bronchoconstriction.[26] In bird medicine, the approach to nebulization is to put the patient in a closed chamber (ranging

Table 1
Approach to infectious diseases of the respiratory tract

Etiology	Diagnosis	Treatment of Choice	Alternative Treatment	Comments
Chlamydia psittaci	PCR Serology CBC	Acute severe cases: Doxycycline (75–100 mg/kg IM q7d). Doxycycline (35 mg/kg PO SID for 3 wk) Milder chronic cases: Azithromycin (40 mg/kg PO q24–48h for 3 wk)	Enrofloxacin (30 mg/kg daily for 3 wk)	Besides the parenteral, or oral administration of antibiotics, most cases will benefit of a nebulization of an antibiotic dissolved in a mucolytic agent (acetylcysteine). Also, nebulization with hot steam and baking soda seem to facilitate the action of other drugs.
Bacterial pneumonia	Culture CBC	Antibiotics on sensitivity test. Widely used antibiotics: • Amoxicillin/clavulanic acid • Enrofloxacin • Marbofloxacin • Azithromycin • Ceftriaxone • Amikacin	Amikacin and gentamicin via nebulization	
Mycoplasma	PCR (if a referral laboratory is available)	Tylosin (also together with doxycycline)	Enrofloxacin Marbofloxacin	
Aspergillus spp	Culture Cytology PCR (if available) CBC Radiology Endoscopy Galactomannan assay	Voriconazole Local, intralesional (endoscopy) injection of amphotericin B Nebulization with enilconazole	Itraconazole Terbinafine	Terbinafine can be combined with itraconazole

Abbreviations: CBC, complete blood count; IM, intramuscular; PCR, polymerase chain reaction; PO, by mouth; q, every; SID, once a day.

from a professional intensive care unit to a simple cardboard box) and deliver the drug into the chamber for 15 to 20 minutes. This differs from the approach in human medicine, which is to deliver a full amount of a given drug in the shortest possible time, but would be too stressful for parrot, especially if in respiratory distress. The amount of drug and frequency of treatment depend on the single drugs, but generally is 2 to 3 times per day.

CLINICS CARE POINTS

- *Respiratory signs do not necessarily mean respiratory disease.* Birds have a peculiar respiratory mechanics and extrarespiratory problems may lead to respiratory signs, including heart diseases and behavioral patterns.

- A confirmed etiologic diagnosis is rarely achieved without laboratory test and imaging techniques.

- Nebulization is a noninvasive, nonstressful treatment technique that has great advantages in severely sick birds with respiratory signs.

- Chlamydiosis and aspergillosis can mimic each other, if diagnosis is not supported by specific techniques.

- Always consider possible environmental sources of respiratory diseases.

- The fact that some diseases are more common in a given species does not mean that that species has always, and only that diseases.

DISCLOSURE

L. Crosta declares that he has no conflict of interest.

REFERENCES

1. Crosta L. Avian Anesthesia. Proc. 11th FSAPAI CE and 18th WSAVA CE Conference, Mumbai, India, November, 21-24, 2019. p. 215–36.
2. Heard DJ. Avian respiratory anatomy and physiology. Semin Avian Exot Pet Med 1997;6(No 4):172–9.
3. King AS, McLelland J. Birds. Their structure and function. 2nd edition. Philadelphia: Bailliere Tindall; 1984.
4. König HE, Navarro M, Zengerling G, et al. Respiratory system (apparatus respiratorius). In: König HE, Korbel R, Liebich HG, editors. Avian anatomy: textbook and colour atlas. 2nd edition. Sheffield (UK): 5m Publishing; 2016. p. 118–30.
5. Baumel JJ, editor. Handbook of avian anatomy: nomina anatomica avium. 2nd edition. Cambridge (MA): Nuttall Ornithological Club; 1993.
6. Walsh MT. Clinical manifestations of cervicocephalic air sacs of psittacines. Comp Cont Ed 1984;9:783–9.
7. McLelland J. Larynx and trachea. In: King AS, McLelland J, editors. Form and function in birds, vol 4. New York: Academic; 1989. p. 69–103.
8. Morrisey JK. Diseases of the upper respiratory tract of companion birds. Semin Avian Exot Pet Med 1997;6(No 4):195–200.
9. Doneley B, Harrison GJ, Lightfoot TL. Maximising information from the physical examination. In: Harrison GJ, Lightfoot TL, editors. Clinical avian medicine, vol. 1. Palm Beach: Spix Publishing; 2006. p. 153–212.

10. Van Zeeland Y. Upper respiratory tract diseases. In: Chitty J, Monks D, editors. BSAVA manual of avian practice. A foundation manual. Gloucester (UK): BSAVA; 2018. p. 299–316.

11. Graham JE. Approach to the dyspneic avian patient. Semin Avian Exot Pet Med 2004;13:154–9.

12. Chitty J, Monks D. Lower respiratory tract diseases. In: Chitty J, Monks D, editors. BSAVA manual of avian practice. A foundation manual. Gloucester (UK): BSAVA; 2018. p. 324–33.

13. Powers LV. Rhinitis and sinusitis. In: Graham JE, editor. Blackwell's five-minute veterinary consult: avian. Incorporated: John Wiley & Sons; 2016. p. 257–9.

14. Laniesse D, Beaufrère H. Tracheitis and syringeal disease. In: Graham JE, editor. Blackwell's five-minute veterinary consult: avian. Incorporated: John Wiley & Sons; 2016. p. 281–3.

15. Strunk A. Pneumonia. In: Graham JE, editor. Blackwell's five-minute veterinary consult: avian. Incorporated: John Wiley & Sons; 2016. p. 228–30.

16. Crosta L, Melillo A, Schnitzer P. Chlamydiosis (Psittacosis). In: Speer BL, editor. Current therapy in avian medicine and surgery. St. Louis, Missouri: Elsevier; 2016. p. 82–93.

17. Martel A. Aspergillosis. In: Speer BL, editor. Current therapy in avian medicine and surgery. Elsevier; 2016. p. 63–73.

18. Cray C, Tatum LM. Applications of protein electrophoresis in avian diagnostics. J Avian Med Surg 1998;12:4–10.

19. Cray C, Watson T, Rodriguez M, et al. Application of galactomannan analysis and protein electrophoresis in the diagnosis of aspergillosis in avian species. J Zoo Wild Med 2009;40:64–70.

20. Jones MP, Orosz SE. The diagnosis of aspergillosis in birds. Semin Avian Exot Pet 2000;9:52–8.

21. Phalen DN. The use of serologic assays in avian medicine. Semin Avian Exot Pet Med 2001;10(2):77–89.

22. Fischer D, Lierz M. Diagnostic procedures and available techniques for the diagnosis of aspergillosis in birds. J Exot Pet Med 2015;24(3):283–95.

23. Crosta L. Endoscopia em Aves. In: Cubas ZS, Ramos da Silva JC, Catão-Dias JL, editors. Tratado de Medicina Veterinária de Animais Selvagens 2° edition. Brazil: Editora Roca Ltda. São Paulo; 2014. p. 1751–67.

24. Arca-Ruibal B. Disorders of the respiratory system. In: Samour J, editor. Avian medicine. 3rd edition. St. Louis, Missouri: Elsevier; 2016. p. 385–95.

25. Crosta L, Melillo A, Schnitzer P. Basic radiography. In: Chitty J, Monks D, editors. BSAVA manual of avian practice. A foundation manual. Gloucester (UK): British Small Animal Veterinary Association; 2018. p. 269–85.

26. Orosz SE, Lichtenberger M. Avian respiratory distress: etiology, diagnosis, and treatment. Vet Clin Exot Anim 2011;14:241–55.

Respiratory Diseases in Guinea Pigs, Chinchillas and Degus

María Ardiaca García, LV[a],*,
Andrés Montesinos Barceló, LV, MSc, PhD[a,b],
Cristina Bonvehí Nadeu, LV[a], Vladimír Jekl[c,d]

KEYWORDS

- Guinea pig • Chinchilla • Degu • Respiratory disease • Pneumonia

KEY POINTS

- The diagnosis and treatment of respiratory disease in pet guinea pigs, chinchillas, and degus still face serious challenges.
- The prevalence of primary and secondary respiratory pathologies seems to be high in these species.
- An effort to differentiate cardiogenic respiratory signs from primary respiratory disease is particularly important because this distinction will influence the therapeutic approach.
- First-line diagnostic techniques are radiography, computed tomography scans, cytology, and microbiological culture of samples from nasal lavage, hematology, blood gas analysis, and protein electrophoresis.
- Responsible prescription of antimicrobial drugs is vital to avoid selection of resistant micro-organisms and the potentially severe adverse effects on the digestive flora.

INTRODUCTION

The diagnosis and treatment of respiratory disease in pet guinea pigs, chinchillas, and degus still face profoundly serious challenges owing to their relatively small size, conspicuous clinical signs, insufficient scientific evidence to correlate signs and particular pathologies, and difficulty for sampling. This article is intended to summarize the available information to provide means for a systematic approach to the patients with suspected respiratory disease.

[a] Centro Veterinario Los Sauces, Calle Santa Engracia, 63, Madrid 28010, Spain; [b] Department of Animal Medicine and Surgery, Veterinary Faculty, Universidad Complutense de Madrid, Avenida Puerta de Hierro, s/n 28040 Madrid Spain; [c] Small Mammal, Department of Pharmacology and Pharmacy, Faculty of Veterinary Medicine, University of Veterinary and Pharmaceutical Sciences, Brno, Czech Republic; [d] Jekl and Hauptman Veterinary Clinic, Focused on Exotic Companion Mammal Care, Mojmírovo Náměstí 3105/6a, Brno 612 00, Czech Republic
* Corresponding author.
E-mail address: cvsauces@cvsauces.com

Vet Clin Exot Anim 24 (2021) 419–457
https://doi.org/10.1016/j.cvex.2021.02.001
1094-9194/21/© 2021 Elsevier Inc. All rights reserved.

RELEVANT ANATOMY AND PHYSIOLOGY

Guinea pigs (*Cavia porcellus*), chinchillas (*Chinchilla lanigera*), and degus (*Octodon degu*) are obligate nasal breathers. The soft palate of guinea pigs and chinchillas is fused with the base of the tongue with soft tissue folds, leaving a small hole (palatal ostium) that connects the oropharynx with the nasopharynx and larynx[1] (**Fig. 1**). The tissue around this hole is elastic, but also quite delicate and richly perfused, so it can be injured and bleed if handled roughly. The risk of hemorrhage does not seem to be exceedingly high, however, in these authors' experience. Because the larynx lies caudal to the palatal ostium, intubation in guinea pigs and chinchillas is difficult without the aid of an endoscope. For the same reason, and to prevent damage to the tube, orogastric catheterization (ie, in cases of respiratory difficulty owing to gastric bloat) should be performed under sedation in these species.[2]

The thoracic cavity of guinea pigs and chinchillas is relatively small, conic, and with the heart in cranial position. Guinea pigs generally have 14 pairs of ribs and chinchillas have 13 pairs of ribs, although some variations have been noted in both species.[2] Degus have 12 pairs of ribs.[3] The thymus in guinea pigs is located outside the thoracic cavity in the cranial cervical region in close contact with the trachea and the salivary glands.[4] The thymus progressively atrophies in the first 12 months of age, but remnant and encapsulated thymic tissue remains throughout life.[4] In the chinchilla, the thymus has an intrathoracic location and, although it experiments some histologic changes, it does not present significant atrophy through life.[5] Degus have a thymus with cervical and mediastinal components. The latter is multilobulated and amorphous, as in other rodents.[6] The cervical part is bilobed and remains active and large for the entire life of the animal, unlike the mediastinal component.[7] In these authors' experience, however, the thymus is poorly distinguished visually from intrathoracic fat on necropsy and computed tomography (CT) studies. The overall attenuation of the tissue in this area is commonly negative on precontrast studies. The lymphoid tissue presents greater enhancement in postcontrast studies and might become distinguishable from the surrounding adipose tissue on postcontrast studies on the ventral aspect of the cranial thorax (**Fig. 2**).

The pattern of lung lobulation in guinea pigs and chinchillas differs from the one in degus[8–10] (**Fig. 3**). A schematic depiction of lung lobes in different species is presented in **Fig. 4**. The pleura is thin, and interlobular or segmental differentiation by connective tissue is very scarce. For this reason, pneumonia in these species rapidly takes on a lobar character (often not allowing to distinguish between the bronchial or

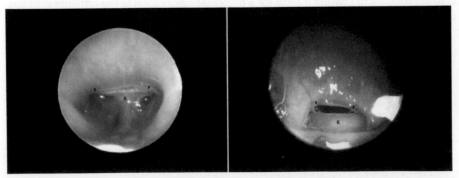

Fig. 1. Endoscopic view of the epiglottis (*E*) of a chinchilla (*left*) and a guinea pig (*right*) through the palatal ostium (*arrows*) during endoscopic intubation.

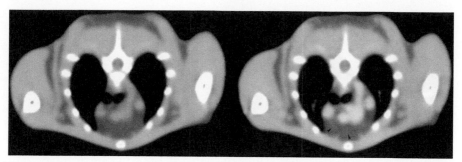

Fig. 2. Precontrast and postcontrast axial computed tomography (CT) images of the cranial thorax of an adult chinchilla. A discrete amount of intrathoracic fat is commonly found in the cranial thorax of adult chinchillas. The thymus is poorly distinguishable on the precontrast study (*left*) from the surrounding adipose tissue but becomes partially visible on postcontrast study (*right*) owing to moderate enhancement (14–30 HU) (*arrowheads*).

hematogenous origin of the infection). For the same reason, lung surgeries often require removal of the entire lobe because it is not possible to identify and isolate the bronchoalveolar segment. Rodents have several generations of bronchial arborization, but practically do not have respiratory bronchioles, and their pulmonary acini are small. The nonrespiratory bronchioles end directly in alveoli or short respiratory bronchioles.

Some authors have indicated the presence of radiodense spicular structures as a normal finding in the lungs of guinea pigs.[11] The authors of this article have never observed this radiographic finding in healthy guinea pigs. Other sources indicate

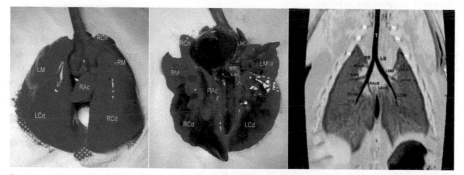

Fig. 3. Dorsal (*left*) and ventral (*middle*) views of a necropsy specimen and a multiplanar reconstruction of computed tomography (CT) images (*right*) of the normal lungs of a guinea pig showing lung lobulations and bronchial tree ramifications. Black pin point lesions owing to anthracosis are visible on the dorsal and ventral pulmonary surfaces. LAc, left accessory lobe; LAcB, left accessory secondary bronchus; LB, left primary bronchus; LCd, left caudal lobe; LCdB, left caudal secondary bronchus; LMB, left middle secondary bronchus; LMCd, caudal part of the left middle lobe; LMCdB, left middle caudal terciary bronchus; LMCn, cranial part of the left middle lobe; LMCnB, left middle cranial terciary bronchus; RAc, right accessory lobe; RAcB, right accessory secondary bronchus; RB, right primary bronchus; RCd, right caudal lobe; RCdB, right caudal secondary bronchus; RCn, right cranial lobe; RCnB, right cranial secondary bronchus; RM, right middle lobe; RMB, right middle secondary bronchus; T, trachea.

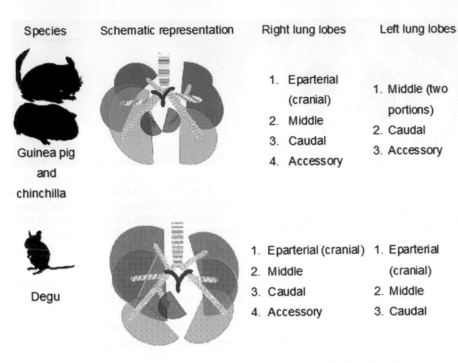

Species	Schematic representation	Right lung lobes	Left lung lobes
Guinea pig and chinchilla		1. Eparterial (cranial) 2. Middle 3. Caudal 4. Accessory	1. Middle (two portions) 2. Caudal 3. Accessory
Degu		1. Eparterial (cranial) 2. Middle 3. Caudal 4. Accessory	1. Eparterial (cranial) 2. Middle 3. Caudal

Colors legend: Orange: eparterial (cranial) lobe; Green: middle lobe; Blue: caudal lobe; Pink: accessory lobe. Red lines represent pulmonary arteries

Fig. 4. Lung lobulations in guinea pigs, chinchillas, and degus. Color legend: Orange: eparterial (cranial) lobe; Green: middle lobe; Blue: caudal lobe; Pink: accessory lobe. Red lines represent pulmonary arteries.

that in the lung tissue of apparently healthy guinea pigs, layers of bone tissue of about 7.0 to 7.5 microns (therefore, not visible on a radiograph) can be found in the interstitium and sometimes protruding into the alveoli. No inflammatory reaction is associated with this heterotopic bone tissue.[12] The reason for the high prevalence of these and other heterotopic bone lesions, such as in the ciliary body, in guinea pigs is not fully understood.[12–14]

In guinea pigs, subpleural perivascular lymphoid nodules were described in apparently healthy animals. In most cases, these are microscopic, but they might sometimes reach 0.5 mm in diameter and become visible as pinpoint whitish nodules on the lung surface. The significance of these formations is unknown.[15]

Multifocal black pinpoint discolorations in the lung surface are frequently observed during necropsy of guinea pigs (see **Fig. 3**). In these authors' experience, these lesions histologically correspond with subpleural anthracosis. It is most probably an incidental finding and is not commonly associated with fibrosis or inflammatory reaction.[16]

The respiratory and heart rates in different species are summarized in **Table 1**.

PREVALENCE OF RESPIRATORY DISORDERS, AND AGE AND SEX PREDISPOSITION

Respiratory infections, particularly pneumonia, were repeatedly cited among principal causes of mortality in farm and laboratory guinea pigs and chinchillas.[17–20] In pet

Table 1 Respiratory and cardiac rates in guinea pigs, chinchillas, and degus[1-4]		
Species	**RR (rpm)**	**HR (ppm)**
Guinea pig	40–105	230–350
Chinchilla	45–80	150–220
Degu	50–80	100–150

Note: Most of these species are easily stressed. For this reason, the reference ranges are very wide. Stress causes the respiratory and heart rates to reach the upper limit. Under anesthesia, the respiratory and heart rates usually decrease to approximately 10% below the lower limit.

animals, very scarce information is available.[13,21-25] One retrospective study on 1000 pet guinea pigs mentions that only 40 of the cases (4%) were diagnosed with respiratory disease, identifying 22 cases of pneumonia, 10 cases of rhinitis, and 8 cases of other respiratory disease (pulmonary edema, bronchitis, sinusitis, and intranasal foreign body).[13] No sex or age predisposition for respiratory disease was found in this study. Several review studies mention respiratory disease in chinchillas.[22,23,25] An unpublished study on postmortem samples from 300 pet chinchillas cites bacterial pneumonia and pleuritis, although the prevalence is not explained.[22]

The less significant stress and better environmental conditions are most probably responsible for the decreased prevalence of respiratory disease in pet guinea pigs and chinchillas compared with farm and laboratory animals. However, in these authors' experience, the respiratory disease, particularly pneumonia, in these species might have subclinical and conspicuous course, and therefore can be underdiagnosed in vivo. In our center, a histopathologic analysis of necropsy samples from guinea pigs and chinchillas showed that 65% of guinea pigs and 46% of chinchillas presented some kind of respiratory pathology at the time of death, being the interstitial pneumonia the most prevalent finding (35% of submitted samples and 65% of all respiratory pathologies).

A priori, no age or sex predisposition for respiratory pathology is consistently found in guinea pigs and chinchillas. However adult, and particularly pregnant, females might be slightly more prone to develop infectious pneumonia.[19,20] One exception is that female guinea pigs seems to be more susceptible to chlamydial infections than males.[26] Pet guinea pigs and chinchillas are more commonly exposed to respiratory pathogens when kept as a community at breeding facilities, pet shops, or shelters. Therefore, recently acquired animals, regardless the age, are probably more prone to present signs of infectious respiratory disease than those that have been living as pets for several years.

In degus, respiratory distress is commonly associated with dental disorders, which are more commonly encountered in older animals.[27] Dyspnea is associated with obstructive nasal disease caused by elodontoma formation or apical maxillary premolar and molar elongation.[28,29] Rhinitis and lung disease are relatively rare in degus; in a study of 300 pet degus, rhinitis was seen in 16 cases, of which 10 and 4 cases were associated with the presence of elodontoma and otitis media, respectively.[27] Superficial breathing (polypnea) and air gasping can be also present in cases of hyperthermia and in the final stages of any disease.

ANAMNESIS AND CLINICAL EXAMINATION

As in dog and cat medicine, when faced with a patient with respiratory symptoms, anamnesis should particularly include information about contact with other animals (conspecifics and nonconspecifics) or people experiencing signs or symptoms of zoonotic diseases and exposure to excessive cold or heat. In guinea pigs, a careful revision of the diet is important because hypovitaminosis C can be a contributing factor to immunosuppression and secondary infection of any kind.[18,25,30]

A complete clinical examination is mandatory as in any patient. In animals with suspected respiratory disease, thoracic auscultation, body temperature, respiratory and cardiac rates, and pulse oximetry are important parts of the clinical examination. An oxygen saturation of less than 92% is associated with the onset of respiratory distress. Nostrils must be checked for permeability and the presence of exudates. Most animals will consciously clean their nose, but exudates might be visible on the internal surface of the hands and forearms. A careful examination of the eyes and ears is also important because respiratory disease is frequently concomitant with ocular and otic manifestations, such as conjunctivitis, dacryocystitis, or otitis media.[31] The differential diagnosis in guinea pigs and chinchillas presenting with severe nasal discharge includes choking, esophageal obstruction, gastric torsion, omental torsion, hepatic disease, or diaphragmatic hernia that can cause regurgitation of saliva and digestive contents through the nose[32–34] (**Fig. 5**). Underlying dental disease is probably also an important contributing factor to the respiratory disease via spread of the infection, elongation of dental roots, deformity of alveolar bone, or secondary dysphagia, especially in degus[28,29] (**Fig. 6**). Any other causes of nasal airway occlusion can be a cause of respiratory distress (**Figs. 7** and **8**).

Thoracic auscultation must be performed using preferably a neonatal stethoscope. The thorax of these animals is minute, and the smallest chest piece is necessary to obtain the best possible quality of information from the auscultation. Even the neonatal chest pieces can be too large compared with the size of the thorax to be able to auscultate separately different lung and heart structures (**Fig. 9**).

The heart rate of most small mammals is much higher than that of humans, dogs, or cats, so it is advisable to have a pulse oximeter that registers up to 500 bpm. Pulse oximetry measurements can be obtained placing the probe on the hand, foot, forearm, thigh, or tail (in chinchillas). Due to the small body parts size, the readings might be impaired owing to the excessive continuous pressure of the clamp probe on the skin that impedes normal blood flow into the limb. This factor is particularly true in patients with peripheral perfusion impairment affecting the hands, feet, and tail. A small

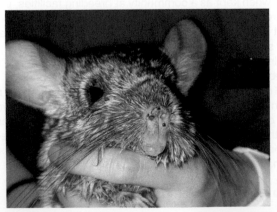

Fig. 5. Profuse nasal discharge in a chinchilla owing to dysphagia and regurgitation secondary to diaphragmatic hernia.

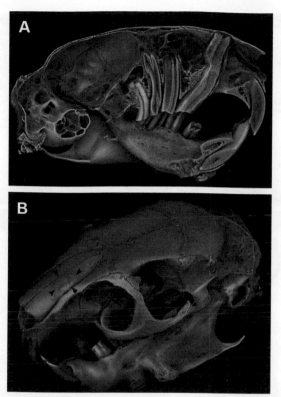

Fig. 6. Sagittal plane computed tomography (CT) images of the left maxillary dental arcade of a degu reconstructed as a 3-dimensional model, mediolateral view (*A*), and surface reconstruction (*B*). Apical elongation of all premolars and molars is obvious. Note that the apical elongation and reserve crown of the fourth premolar has erupted into the nasal cavity (*A*) with its apex bulging the nasal bone (*B*). Note the irregular structure suggesting dysplastic changes of tooth structures.

roll of gauze or other object can be placed between the parts of a clamp probe to decrease its closing pressure. Also, a periodic temporary removal of the probe and a gentle massage on the area can be helpful in these cases. Peripheral blood flow will be also decreased if the environmental temperature is low. In rodents with highly pigmented limbs skin (degus, chinchillas, and some guinea pigs) a contact probe can be placed on the shaved body surface or inside the oral cavity of an unconscious or anesthetized patient (**Fig. 10**).

A high prevalence of heart disease in guinea pigs and chinchillas is repeatedly mentioned in the literature.[13,23,25,30,35] It is particularly important to make an effort to differentiate cardiogenic lung edema as the cause of respiratory signs because this finding will affect the therapeutic approach.

COMPLEMENTARY DIAGNOSTIC TECHNIQUES

The complementary diagnostic techniques that are useful in patients with respiratory signs include diagnostic imaging and hematological, microbiological, and histopathologic analyses.

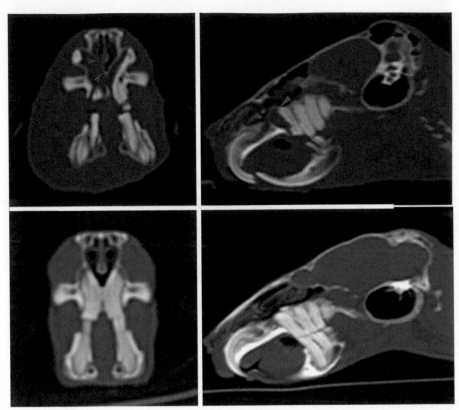

Fig. 7. Multiplanar reconstruction of computed tomography (CT) images of a chinchilla with advanced dental disease (*top row*). The elongation of the upper incisors and acquired alveolar abnormality is causing narrowing of the nasal airway (red arrowheads). In the bottom row, CT images of the same anatomic region in a chinchilla with normal occlusion are displayed for comparison.

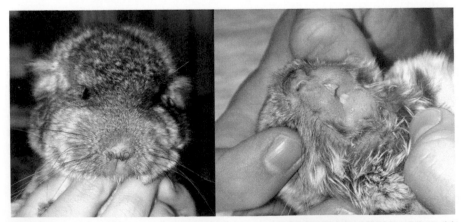

Fig. 8. Severe angioedema in a young chinchilla with acute respiratory distress presumably owing to an allergic reaction. The respiratory distress was attributed to partial occlusion of the nostrils.

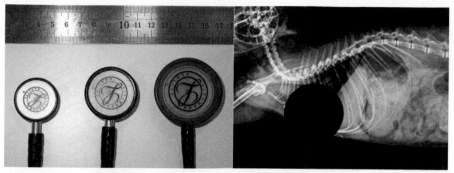

Fig. 9. Comparative size of neonatal, pediatric, and adult chest pieces of a stethoscope (*left*) and the size of the neonatal piece compared with the size of the thorax of an adult chinchilla (real size radiograph reproduction) (*right*). The smallest available chest piece should be used to obtain maximum information from the auscultation.

Diagnostic Imaging

Radiography

Radiography is a first-line diagnostic technique for evaluation of the lungs, because it is widely accessible, relatively inexpensive, and noninvasive. However, the small size of guinea pigs, chinchillas, and degus makes radiologic diagnosis difficult. The classic radiographic patterns of the lung parenchyma are not always easy to identify in patients weighing less than 1 kg. In addition to the small body size, the decrease ratio of thoracic versus abdominal volume causes superimposition of lung tissue with other intrathoracic and even abdominal organs, further hampering the evaluation. In many cases, the lesions are not clearly seen on radiographs, making radiography a specific, but relatively nonsensitive method of lung evaluation in these species (**Figs. 12 and 13**).

In contrast, when visible alterations are present, the rapid progression of some pathologic processes can create extensive alterations of the lung parenchyma in a short time. The quality of the radiography equipment, the correct positioning, and the knowledge of the anatomy of the species are of vital importance. Ventrodorsal (VD) and/or dorsoventral and right lateral and left lateral projections should be taken ideally. Some

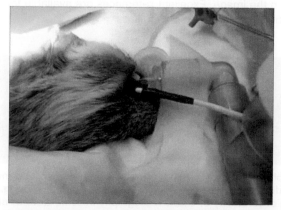

Fig. 10. Esophageal pulse oximeter probe used in the mouth of an anesthetized guinea pig.

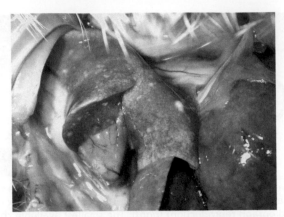

Fig. 11. Necropsy image of a miliary pneumonia in a chinchilla.

authors prefer the dorsoventral view because it causes less respiratory distress and makes the heart take a central position within the thorax with lesser overlap of heart and lungs fields. The natural collapse of the inferior lung when in lateral recumbency makes it necessary to take right and left lateral projections to better evaluate the parenchyma of both lungs. Forelimbs should be extended ventrally and slightly forward, but not fully forward, to avoid superimposing of the scapulae with the thoracic cavity. This radiographic positioning is not sensible for the detection of upper respiratory tract disease, unless an abnormality of bony structures or secondary calcification are present. However, it is advisable to include the head and neck, and not only the thorax, for all animals showing respiratory signs to avoid missing these lesions. Extreme caution and oxygen supplementation are mandatory in dyspneic animals during radiographic positioning, because it might aggravate the respiratory compromise. Sometimes, dorsoventral projection can be used instead of the classic VD image to avoid stress in patients with severely compromised ventilation.

The radiologic evaluation must begin with the verification that both the positioning of the patient and the exposure are correct. The accumulated experience with these species is still insufficient in terms of the correlation that exists between radiographic abnormalities and pulmonary pathologies. However, it is possible to recognize radiologic patterns like those that exist in dogs and cats to make at least a list of differential diagnoses based on the image. Excellent references are available for interpretation of the radiographs of guinea pigs and chinchillas.[36,37]

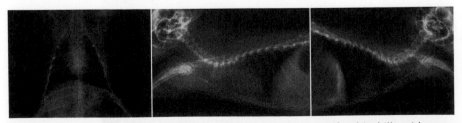

Fig. 12. Radiographs in VD and right and left lateral projections of a chinchilla with severe acute respiratory distress. Necropsy confirmed miliary pneumonia (see **Fig. 8**). These images illustrate the lack of sensitivity of classic radiography in some cases of pneumonia in this species.

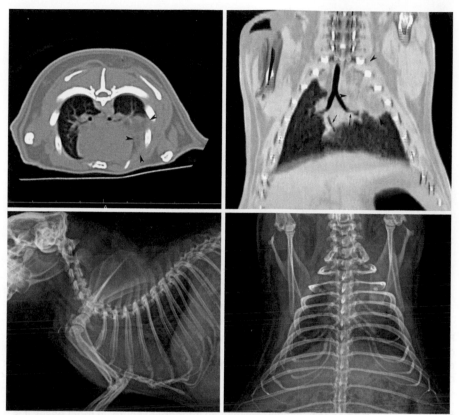

Fig. 13. Multiplanar reconstructions in axial and coronal view of a computed tomography (CT) scan (*top row*) of a guinea pig showing left middle and right accessory lobes consolidation (*arrowheads*) with air bronchograms (*arrows*). In this case CT shows advantage in both sensitivity and specificity and is more informative than plain radiographs (*bottom row*).

Increased radiodensity or opacities

Some of the alterations more frequently found are opacities or increases in radiodensity. These opacities can be due to alterations in the lung, in the pleura or in the chest wall. To differentiate between these three causes, when interpreting an increase in opacity, we must pay attention to 4 characteristics:

1. Position: if the opacity appears within the thoracic cavity in VD and lateral views, it is due to pulmonary or pleural alterations. The cardiac and diaphragmatic silhouettes must be clearly identifiable.
2. Air bronchogram: in pathologies of the lung parenchyma, the air-filled bronchi stand out on the radiodense background as radiolucent linear structures. The absence of the air bronchogram indicates that the bronchus is filled with exudates, aspirated material, or obliterated by a neoplasm (**Figs. 14–18**).
3. Silhouette sign: cardiac, diaphragmatic, great vessels, and mediastinal structures should contrast neatly against the lung parenchyma. An increased radiodensity of the lung parenchyma or presence of pleural effusion often cause blurring of these silhouettes (see **Figs. 14, 16** and **17**).

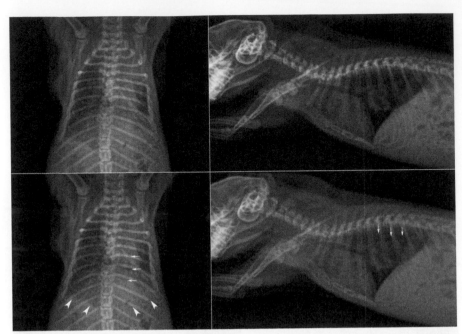

Fig. 14. Radiographic signs of pneumonia in a young guinea pig. Note the increased radio-density in the left caudal lobe with the air bronchogram (*arrows*) and blurring of the caudal edge of the lung and cardiac and diaphragmatic silhouettes on the left hemithorax compared with the other side (arrowheads).

4. Fissure sign: if an opacity exactly delimits an interlobar fissure, in most cases it is a sign of pleural effusion, but it can also appear owing to peripheral pulmonary atelectasis. This sign is also usually best seen in the VD view.

The alveolar fill pattern occurs when the alveoli are filled with exudates or aspirated liquids (mucus, serosity, blood, pus, water, etc). It can be focal or diffuse and will

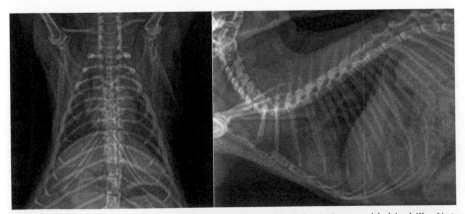

Fig. 15. Lung congestion and mild cardiogenic lung edema in a 12-year-old chinchilla. Note the diffuse hyperdensity of the lung fields with clear air bronchogram on the right hemithorax visible on the VD projection and vascular pattern recognizable on the left lateral projection.

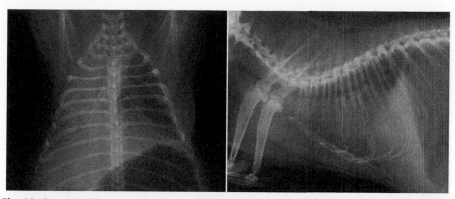

Fig. 16. Suppurative pneumonia in a guinea pig affecting right lung. Note the increased radiodensity with diffuse alveolar fill pattern pattern, the blurring of the cardiac and diaphragmatic silhouettes, and lack of air bronchogram suggesting that bronchae are filled with exudates.

generally present a nodular appearance with diffuse borders and can be associated with air bronchograms or alveologrammes. Common causes of this pattern are pneumonia and pneumonitis, aspiration, pulmonary edema, contusions, hemorrhages, and lymphomas (see **Figs. 13–18**).

The alveolar condensation with air bronchograms is typical of exudative pneumonia caused by bacterial infections (see **Figs. 16** and **17**). The absence of the air bronchogram usually indicates that the main bronchus is full of exudates or other type of material, as occurs in bronchopneumonia, aspiration pneumonia, or thromboembolism (see **Fig. 16**). The bronchioloalveolar pattern appears in early stage bronchopneumonia affecting the tributary alveoli of specific bronchioles. This pattern is seen very rarely in small animals owing to the rapid spread of the pathologic processes to the rest of the parenchyma.

The interstitial pattern is typical of viral, *Mycoplasma spp.* and *Chlamydia spp.* infections, and endotoxemic shock, but it can also be observed in other pathologies. This pattern is rarely recognizable in small mammals.

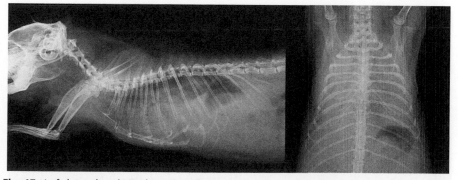

Fig. 17. Left lateral and VD thoracic radiographs of a young guinea pig with severe suppurative bronchopneumonia and pleural effusion. Note the increased radiodensity with alveolar fill pattern pattern, air bronchograms, and complete smudging of the cardiac and diaphragmatic silhouettes.

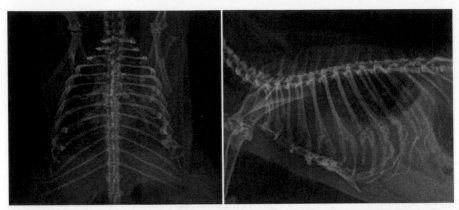

Fig. 18. Pleural effusion, increased parenchyma opacity, air bronchograms, and peripheral caudal lobe atelectasis in a guinea pig suffering with lymphoma and chronic cardiac insufficiency.

Pulmonary atelectasis is usually seen at the edges of the pulmonary lobes and is frequently seen in animals with chronic heart failure. Complete atelectasis of the pulmonary lobes can occur in cases of bronchial obstruction or compression owing to neoplasms or pneumothorax (see **Figs. 13** and **16**). Iatrogenic atelectasis associated with overinflation of the contralateral lung is seen in cases of accidental bronchial intubation owing to exceedingly long endotracheal tube.

Decreased radiopacity or hyperlucency
Hyperlucency in the thoracic cavity can be due to abnormal lung distension (ie, bullous lung emphysema) or pneumothorax. Bullous emphysema is normally associated with obstruction of the bronchae owing to aspiration, chronic inflammatory disease, or neoplasia (**Fig. 19**). It can be also seen in association with nasal obstructive disease.

Radiographic artifacts
It is important not to confuse changes in radiodensity generated by pericardial fat pads, fat in obese animals, skin folds, or other pathologies such as calcifications of

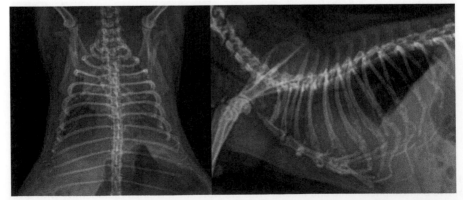

Fig. 19. Bullous lung emphysema in the caudal lobes in a guinea pig with bronchogenic adenoma.

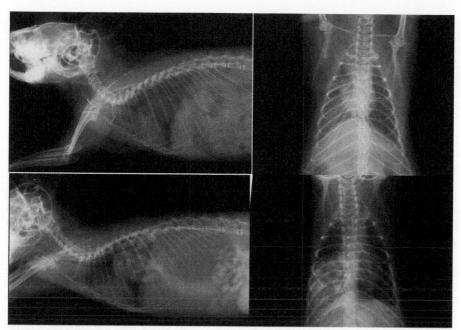

Fig. 20. Radiographs in VD (right) and right lateral (left) projections before (*top row*) and after (*bottom row*) administration of oral contrast media of a chinchilla with a diaphragmatic hernia with acute respiratory distress. Note the increased artifactual density of the lung fields owing to the herniated intestine.

the great vessels or diaphragmatic hernias that are occasionally seen in these rodents (especially chinchillas) with signs of pulmonary pathology[32,33,38] (**Fig. 20**).

Common causes of artifactual hyperlucency of the lung fields are cachexia, a loss of muscle mass. Air in the esophagus owing to aerophagia is common in cases of respiratory distress.

Computed tomography scan

CT scanning is rapidly gaining presence in veterinary medicine and allows a more detailed and advanced exploration of the nasal sinuses and thoracic cavity. Still noticeably more expensive than conventional radiology, it also requires general anesthesia to keep the patient immobilized and represents a higher dose of radiation.[39,40] Owing to the practical difficulty of intubation in these species, CT image acquisition is most commonly performed without intubation. Without intubation it is not possible to safely induce temporary apnea and therefore the motion artifact owing to cardiac and respiratory movements is often apparent. The use of modern equipment with 64-slice CT scanner or higher allows to decrease this artifact because the images acquisition is more rapid. Owing to higher cardiac rate in these species, a rapid postcontrast acquisition is also important. Authors found better results with 2 postcontrast series at 10 to 20 seconds and 30 to 50 seconds.

A CT scan is clearly more sensitive than classic radiography in the diagnosis of both upper airway diseases, such as rhinitis, sinusitis, or obstructive syndrome, and low respiratory tract diseases (see **Figs. 2**, **6**, **7** and **13**).

Peripheral lobe atelectasis, commonly seen in dogs and rabbits under anesthesia when pure oxygen is used as delivery gas, is not a common finding in guinea pigs and chinchillas in these authors' experience. Therefore, any hyperattenuating areas in peripheral lung parenchyma should be interpreted as pathologic in these species.

Other imaging techniques

Ultrasound examination is useful in the diagnosis of lung consolidation, intrathoracic abscesses or neoplasia, pneumothorax, fluid in the pleural cavity, and diaphragmatic hernias; and in diagnostic and therapeutic ultrasound-guided thoracentesis.

Echocardiography can be indicated in cases when cardiac insufficiency is suspected as the cause of dyspnea. Cardiac tamponade owing to pericardial effusion is particularly common in guinea pigs and ultrasound-guided pericardiocentesis is indicated in these cases.

Endoscopy allows evaluation of oropharynx and nasopharynx, larynx, and trachea. The nostrils of most guinea pigs and chinchillas are, however, too small to allow rhinoscopy. Endoscopy is an important ancillary technique for intubation of guinea pigs and chinchillas.[8] To date, there are no scientific descriptions of thoracoscopy with diagnostic or therapeutic purposes in these species.

MRI is another technique without the disadvantage of ionizing radiation, that in human medicine might surpass CT scanning in the diagnosis of some parenchymatous, pleural and mediastinal pathologies and is useful in cases of contraindication for contrast media used during CT studies.[41] Because it is an expensive technique that only proves useful in some particular cases, and because it has an important disadvantage because it requires much longer anesthesia times with the consequent risk for the patient, the use of MRI for diagnosis of respiratory disease is still very scarce in veterinary medicine. Moreover, most of the MRI machines available for veterinary practitioners have low-resolution images, which provide less detail than needed for the optimal evaluation of such a small thorax.

Blood analysis

Hematology, protein electrophoresis, and blood gas analysis are particularly useful when evaluating patients with respiratory disease. Hematology and protein electrophoresis allow to detect and monitor the immune response to inflammatory and infectious disease.

Arterial blood gas analysis is difficult to perform safely in small patients. Instead venous blood gas analysis can be used with limited extrapolation.[42,43] In human medicine, there is still controversy whether venous blood gas might be a good initial evaluation for patients with respiratory distress admitted for emergency care. Apparently, it correlates well for pH values. Hypercapnia (elevated P_{CO_2}) could be a sensitive but not specific indicator for respiratory acid–base disturbances. Blood oxygenation cannot be assessed in venous blood.[44,45] In these authors' experience, higher P_{CO_2} values are more common in guinea pigs when compared with other species.[42] Hypoventilation owing to restraint and stress might contribute to this fact. Guinea pigs and chinchillas will exhibit hyperlactatemia when presenting tissue hypoxia, but changes in lactatemia are difficult to interpret in these species because they have variable L-lactate levels in plasma and values of up to 15.4 mmol/L can be found in healthy animals[42] (**Table 2**). Leukocytosis of more than 25,000 white blood cells (WBC)/μL in guinea pigs is practically pathognomonic of cavian leukemia. In these author's experience, guinea pigs with chronic respiratory insufficiency will sometimes exhibit a marked increase in the hematocrit (up to 80%). Medullar biopsies and plasmatic erythropoietin measurements made us attribute this polycythemia to chronic hypoxemia in cases of chronic pneumonia, lung fibrosis, lymphoma, or chronic cardiogenic respiratory insufficiency. This

Table 2
Venous blood gas and electrolytes analysis in healthy guinea pigs (n = 64)[42] using VetScan i-STAT 1 (Abaxis©, Union City, CA USA)

	Min	Max	Reference Point	95% Reference Interval (Robust Method)
Hematocrit (%)	33	55		35–51
Hemoglobin (g/dL)	11.2	18.7		11.9–17.2
pH	7.117	7.535	7.352	7.182–7.522
HCO_3 (mmol/L)	15	34	27	19.7–35.2
TCO_2 (mmol/L)	16	36	29	20.8–37.1
BEecf (mmol/L)	−14	11	2	−8 - 11
P_{CO_2} (mm Hg)	34.7	72.6	48.5	29.9–68
Na (mmol/L)	128	149		130–148
Cl (mmol/L)	90	112		92–110
K (mmol/L)	4	6.2		3.9–6.0
Anion gap (mmol/L)	9	25	15	9–21
Calculated plasma tonicity (mOsm/L)	264	305	288	271–306
Calculated plasma osmolarity (mOsm/L)	268	315	292	274–311
Glucose				
(mg/dL)	111	504		111–408 and 98–173[a]
(mmol/L)	6.2	23.7		6.2–22.6 and 5.4–9.6[a]
Blood urea nitrogen (mmol/L)	6	27		4.6–22.3
Lactate (mmol/L)	1.1	15.4		1.4–14.7

Abbreviation: BEecf, base excess in the extracellular fluid.
[a] Glucose values of more than 300 mg/dL were found in 5 guinea pigs. These values were probably owing to stress hyperglycemia. The rest of the guinea pigs (n = 59) had glucose levels under 200 mg/dL; a second reference interval was calculated eliminating the 5 hyperglycemic animals considering them as outliers.

assumption is further supported with the fact that it will progressively remit when the underlying respiratory failure is addressed (**Fig. 21**).

Common venipuncture sampling sites in guinea pigs and chinchillas are saphenous and jugular veins and vena cava cranealis (the confluence site of the subclavian and jugular veins). When using the vena cava cranealis, care must be taken not to advance the needle too far inside the thoracic cavity, because the heart base and other great vessels are close to the thoracic inlet with some subsequent risk of hemothorax. Mild sedation is advisable in animals with respiratory distress to decrease the stress associated with restraint for venipuncture.

Microbiological tests
Microbiological culture, polymerase chain reaction, and cytology can be obtained from samples taken by nasal swabbing, nasal lavage, pleural effusion or from tissues during postmortem examinations. A tracheobronchial wash is not a routine procedure owing to small size and difficulties intubating these species.

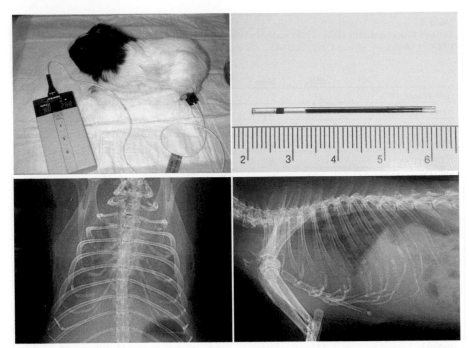

Fig. 21. Guinea pigs with chronic respiratory insufficiency will sometimes exhibit an extreme increase in hematocrit (up to 80%). The authors attribute this polycythemia to chronic hypoxemia in cases of chronic pneumonia, lung fibrosis, lymphoma or chronic cardiogenic respiratory insufficiency.

Cytology and histopathology

Of all the diagnostic tests, we can highlight cytology as the most useful, practical, and economical first-line in-house test that renders rapid results. Specimens can be obtained via nasal lavage. Swabbing is not recommended because it is more aggressive on nasal mucosa, can worsen the respiratory distress, and will render samples contaminated with blood. A routine Romanowsky stain (eg, Diff Quick) and Gram stain usually provide initial guidance on the possible etiology. Special stains reveal the presence of intracellular micro-organisms (Gimenez stain for *Mycoplasma sp*. or *Chlamydia sp*.; Ziehl-Neelsen stain for mycobacteria).

Biopsies or necropsy samples can be submitted for histopathologic analysis (see **Fig. 11**). Postmortem studies are especially important when treating communities.

TREATMENT

Little controlled scientific evidence is available regarding the treatment of respiratory disease in rodents. Data available from laboratory animals often refer to dose conditions and regimes unsuitable or not proven to be safe in pet animals. Even in human medicine, controversy is often present regarding the efficacy of certain therapeutic agents used in patients with respiratory disease. Therefore, every therapeutic intervention must be considered carefully and monitored to evaluate its benefits for each particular patient.

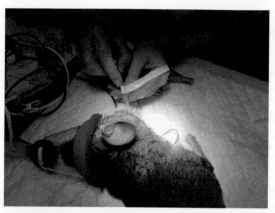

Fig. 22. A 27G intravenous catheter is placed in the right cephalic vein of an anesthetized chinchilla. Oxygen is delivered via face mask.

Oxygen Supplementation

Oxygen supplementation is important in hypoxemic animals (SatO$_2$ of <92%), but is contraindicated in animals with normal oxygen saturation. For emergency procedures up to 100% pure oxygen can be delivered via face mask, placement of an oxygen tube near the nose (flow by), or by tracheal intubation (**Figs. 22** and **23**). For a longer period of oxygen supplementation, patients are accommodated in an oxygen cage and it is recommended not surpass 40% of oxygen in the environment and deliver the gas with water vapor (oxygen bubbled through water) to avoid oxidative damage and drying of the epithelia. The inspired oxygen fraction (Fio$_2$) obtained with different methods is shown in **Table 3**.

Anxiolytics

Respiratory distress is extremely stressful to any animal. The anxiety can further decrease the effectiveness of ventilation. On the other hand, and clinical manipulation

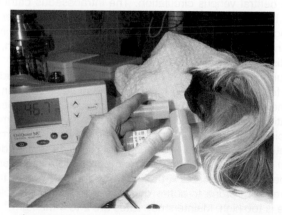

Fig. 23. Oxygen supplementation is an important therapeutic tool in hypoxemic animals. Flow by method of oxygen delivery can provide up to 55% of oxygen enrichment to the room air.

Table 3
Inspired oxygen fraction with different supplementation delivery methods using pure oxygen as a source

Method	Fio_2
Room air	0.21
Flow by (2 L/min)	0.35–0.55
Tight face mask (2 L/min)	0.8–0.9
Oxygen chamber (2–6 L/min)	0.21–0.9
Endotracheal tube	0.9–1

of the animals with respiratory distress can contribute to stress and aggravate the respiratory insufficiency. For this reason, a mild sedation is often beneficial to these patients (**Table 4**).

Fluid Therapy

Animals with severe respiratory disease are frequently dehydrated and hyporexic and need fluid therapy as a part of the treatment plan.

Commonly used emergency venous accesses in rodents include cephalic, femoral, saphenous, lateral abdominal and tail veins using needles of 25G to 30G caliber. A 24G or 27G intravenous catheter can be placed in the cephalic, lateral saphenous, dorsal metatarsal or marginal foot veins in many chinchillas, degus, and guinea pigs (see **Fig. 22**). However, saphenous veins are frequently used for blood sample collection and sometimes become disabled for catheter placement after previous venipuncture. Most adult degus and chinchillas will admit a 27G catheter in the coccygeal veins on either side of the base of the tail. In chinchillas, ear veins can be also used for intravenous access using 25G to 26G catheters.

When it is not possible to have a venous access, an intraosseous catheterization of the proximal femur or proximal tibia is possible instead by means of a 25G spinal needle in these species. The correct placement of the intraosseous catheter can be verified by radiography. The intraosseous route is analogous to the intravenous one, because the medullary cavity contains noncollapsing venous sinuses that connect directly with the central venous circulation. The intraosseous catheterization might be quite painful; it is, therefore, recommended to place the catheter under sedation and after applying local anesthesia such as infiltration of lidocaine (2 mg/kg). An intraosseous catheterization also carries a certain risk of fat embolization, iatrogenic fracture, osteomyelitis, and growth plate injury.

The optimal fluid replacement rates in rodents have not been studied, but smaller mammals seem to exhibit decreased tolerance and diuresis accommodation to high infusion rates when compared with bigger animals, such as most dogs.[46] Therefore, a more conservative approach is advisable. Shocked rodents will admit an initial bolus of warm crystalloids of up to 30 mL/kg of body weight over 20 to 30 minutes, followed by a constant rate infusion of 4 to 10 mL/kg/h to replace the fluid deficit over 12 to 24 hours. Weight and diuresis monitoring are important to avoid overhydration. Special care must be taken in animals with signs of congestive heart failure or oliguria because they are more prone to suffer overhydration and hypervolemia if the fluid replacement rate is too high. Maintenance rates are 2 to 4 mL/kg/h.[47–49] Higher rates can foment hypervolemia, edema formation, local irritation, and phlebitis. The late adds to the fact that the stiffness of the Teflon (TEF, EFTA) catheters, commonly used in clinical settings, can cause a background inflammation in catheterized vessels

Table 4
Drugs commonly used to treat respiratory disease in guinea pigs, chinchillas and degus

Drug	Dosage	Route	Frequency
Antimicrobials			
Piperacillin/tazobactam	50 mg/kg	SQ, IV	q8 h
Ceftazidime	50 mg/kg	SQ, IV	q8 h
Amikacin	15 mg/kg	SQ, IV	q24 h
Trimethoprim/ sulfamethoxazole	30–40 mg/kg	PO, SQ	q12 h
Marbofloxacin	5 mg/kg	PO, SQ	q24 h
Pradofloxacin	5 mg/kg	PO	q24 h
Doxycycline	5–10 mg/kg	PO	q24 h
Azithromycin	15–30 mg/kg	PO	q24 h
Itraconazole	5 mg/kg	PO	q24 h
Fluconazole	10 mg/kg	PO	q24 h
Nonsteroidal anti-inflammatory drugs			
Meloxicam	0.5 mg/kg	SQ, IV	q12 h
	0.8–1.5 mg/kg	PO	q8–12 h
Metamizole (dipyrone)	65–85 mg/kg	PO, SQ, IV	q8–12 h
Corticosteroids			
Dexamethasone	0.5–1 mg/kg	IV, SQ	q24 h for 1–4 d
Methylprednisolone	20–40 mg/kg	IV	q12 h for 1–4 d
Diuretics			
Furosemide	4–6 mg/kg followed by 1–2 mg/kg	PO, SQ, IM, IV	q8–12 h
Bronchodilators			
Salbutamol	0.1–0.3 mg/mL	Nebulization	q6–12 h
	0.05 mg/kg	SQ, IM, IV	
Terbutaline	0.05–0.1 mg/kg	PO, IV	q8–12 h
Mucolytics			
N-acetylcysteine	100–200 mg/kg	IV	q8–12 h
Bromhexine	5–10 mg/kg	SQ, IM, IV	q8–12 h
Ambroxol	50–100 mg/kg	PO	q8–12 h
Antihistaminics			
Diphenhydramine	2–4 mg/kg	PO, SQ	q8–12 h
Hydroxyzine	2 mg/kg	PO	q8–12 h
Anxiolytics			
Midazolam	0.5–1 mg/kg	IM, SQ, IV	q8–12 h

Some of the drugs (especially the antimicrobials) are not registered for the use in small mammal herbivores. Their administration is off-label and the practitioner needs to have the knowledge of possible adverse effects of the particular drug.
Abbreviations: IM, intramuscular; IV, intravenous; PO, by mouth; SQ, subcutaneous.

that promotes the risk of phlebitis and thrombosis. Catheters made of polyurethane, which softens with body temperature, are preferable.[50]

Warm crystalloid solutions such as 0.9% NaCl and Ringer's lactate are most used in the absence of blood gas and electrolyte analyses. Clinicians must be aware that NaCl solution is not buffered and should not be used during the maintenance phase of fluid therapy because it carries some risk of hyperchloremic acidosis. More recently, isotonic solutions with malate and acetate instead of lactate have become commercially available (Isofundin, Sterofundin ISO or Ringerfundin, Braun Vet Care) and might be preferable over lactate solutions. If a blood gas analysis is possible, the choice of fluids depends on the results and follows the general rules used in other species. Glucose can be added to these isotonic solutions to create 2.5% or 5.0% glucose concentration in cases of hypoglycemia or for the maintenance of hyporexic patients unless a contraindication is present (ie, diabetes).

The goal of the fluid therapy is restoring peripheral perfusion and hydration status. Overhydration and hypervolemia are potential risks, especially in rodents with lung disease. The signs of hydration status and tissue perfusion (heart rate, pulse, skin, and mucous membranes appearance, Capillary refill time (CRT), SatO$_2$) must be monitored. Clinical and analytical signs (hematocrit, blood gas, and electrolytes) and patient's weight gain are important when monitoring the restoration of hydration. Another important, but sometimes overlooked, factor in rodents during fluid therapy is the monitoring of the urine output. Acute renal failure with oliguria or anuria is a common complication in rodents that suffered severe dehydration or a shock state. At least whether the urine output is present or absent and approximate quantitative and qualitative (especially urine relative density) assessment must be registered. Weight gain must be also monitored because it provides a good approximation of the restoration of the hydration status, because dehydration is normally evaluated in relation to the body weight. If overhydration is overlooked, more severe signs will appear, including edema formation in the dependent areas of the body, respiratory distress, and deteriorated mental status. Close supervision of the catheter site is advisable to detect early signs of extravasation and phlebitis.

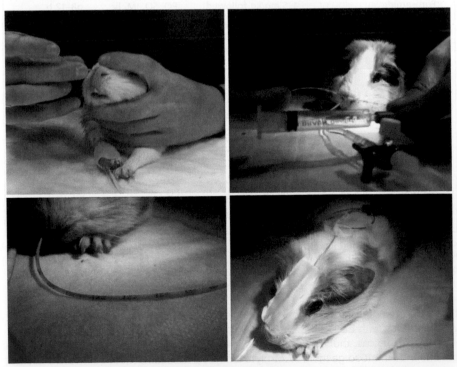

Fig. 24. Nasogastric tube (1 mm Ø) placement in a guinea pig under mild sedation.

Enteral fluid therapy can be highly effective in stable patients with a functional digestive tract. Oral fluids also promote hydration of the gastrointestinal contents, which is particularly important in herbivorous species. Monitoring the emptying of the stomach by palpation is important during any enteral therapy and before the administration any therapy. Maintenance water needs in rodents are about 50 mL/kg/d, but might be higher in animals with increased water loss (hyperthermia, dyspnea, etc). These species will admit up to 20 mL/kg of fluids at a time. Many guinea pigs and chinchillas can be forced fed and hydrated using syringe feeding. This practice is contraindicated in dyspneic animals, because it may carry a higher risk of aspiration, but can be useful in patients with a normal respiratory pattern. These animals will normally accept isotonic oral hydration solutions better than water.

Most guinea pigs and some big chinchillas will admit a soft sterile nasogastric tube of 1 mm in diameter that facilitates enteral fluid therapy and very fine ground nutritional formulas; this practice decreases the risk of aspiration (**Fig. 24**). An important limiting factor for the use of a nasogastric tube is the fact that, being guinea pigs and chinchillas and degus obligate nasal breathers, it can contribute to the risk of rhinitis.[51] Signs of rhinitis, such as exudates, must be monitored and nasogastric tubes should not be left in place for more than 3 days.

Antimicrobial Drugs

Antibiotic prescription should be based on evidence of bacterial infection caused by susceptible organisms and a previous culture whenever possible. The responsible prescription of antibiotic drugs is paramount owing to the increasing concern for antimicrobial drug-resistant micro-organisms and for the potentially severe adverse effects of antibiotic treatment on digestive flora of herbivorous animals. However, because consistently confirming or eliminating a bacterial etiology in respiratory disease in these animals is extremely difficult, an empirical antibiotic treatment is frequently established despite the risk of potentially severe adverse effects (see **Table 4**).

Ultimately, the decision for establishing or delaying antibiotic treatment is based on clinical observations and the clinician's experience. These authors consider the following factors and clinical signs in favor of antimicrobial treatment: young age or recent purchase (bacterial pneumonia is more common in young and recently acquired animals), fever, cytology of exudates or effusions suggestive of bacterial or fungal infection, mild to moderate leukocytosis (WBC counts of >25,000 WBC/μL in guinea pigs are practically pathognomonic of leukemia) and beta-globulinemia or gamma-globulinemia, and positive microbiological cultures. Antibiotic sensitivity testing should be optimally performed in all cases of respiratory infections.

Treatment for a minimum of 14 days is necessary to clear susceptible respiratory infections. It is important to make the owner understand the importance of good practices of administration of the antimicrobial drugs and teach them about the hazards of stopping treatment prematurely.

In some herbivores, complications owing to prolonged treatment with antibiotics are relatively frequent. These complications are generally mild enteritis diarrhea owing to yeast overgrowth, which usually respond to antifungals, such as nystatin, and do not require interruption of the antibiotic treatment. However, potentially fatal typhlocolitis can occur secondary to any antibiotic.

Corticosteroids

In human medicine, the use of corticosteroids in patients with acute lung disease is still controversial, but some studies suggest that it is associated with decreased morbidity and mortality in cases of pneumonia.[52–54] The benefit of corticosteroids in patients suffering from pneumonia has not been established in guinea pigs, chinchillas, or degus and probably will not be so for many years because it involves considerable resources to gather sufficient scientific evidence to draw reliable conclusions. However, there is some scientific evidence that their use can be helpful in these animals in cases of infectious pneumonia and septic shock.[55–57] In these authors' opinion, it seems to be effective to control early acute inflammatory response in cases of pneumonia, improving the respiratory function and well-being of the patients.

The main potential side effect is hyperglycemia. As bronchodilators, corticosteroids are contraindicated in cases of cardiogenic lung edema.[58] They should not be used concurrently with nonsteroidal anti-inflammatory drug medication (see **Table 4**).

Nonsteroidal Anti-inflammatory Drugs

Nonsteroidal anti-inflammatory drugs are indicated as antipyretic, anti-inflammatory, or for pain management. Their effects in pain management can be particularly beneficial in pleuritis (see **Table 4**).

Bronchodilators

The use of parenteral, enteral, or nebulized bronchodilators (salbutamol, terbutaline) can help patients with bronchospasm, which is usually accompanied by marked inspiratory and/or expiratory effort with wheezing on auscultation.[55,59,60] Pneumonia and cardiogenic lung edema do not constitute an indication for the use of bronchodilators because they have no usefulness in the absence of bronchoconstriction. Bronchodilators should be used with caution because they are associated with an increased risk of cardiovascular disease and worsening of effects of several conditions, such as ischemic heart disease, vascular congestion, cardiogenic lung edema, arrhythmias, and hypokalemia.[61] A therapeutic trial with bronchodilators must be closely supervised by veterinarians or nurses. The trial is preferably performed with inhaled bronchodilators to decrease the severity and duration of possible side effects. Normally, a visible response to the treatment in form of lesser respiratory difficulty and improved auscultation should be observed within minutes after their administration. If such a response is not observed, bronchodilators should be discontinued (see **Table 4**).

Mucolytics

Nebulized N-acetylcysteine may have a protective effect on lung tissue in guinea pigs with reactions to irritants, but its use is controversial in allergic reactions.[62,63] Other mucolytics such as bromhexine or its derivative ambroxol have similarly controversial results. Although they seem to have a clear secretagogal action and changes in the chemical properties of the mucous secretion, their therapeutic usefulness after onset of the respiratory signs and potential adverse effects are not clearly established.[64–66] Similar to bronchodilators, they should be used under close supervision (see **Table 4**).

Antihistaminics

Allergic respiratory disease has not been described and is possibly underdiagnosed in pet rodents because of the difficulty in confirming the diagnosis in clinical settings. Scientific evidence suggests that guinea pigs can develop histamine-induced rhinitis, sinusitis, and bronchospasm and that the respiratory epithelium of young guinea pigs is more sensible to histamine than in older animals.[67–72] Diagnostic and therapeutic approach to allergic respiratory disease in pet rodents still need further development (see **Table 4**).

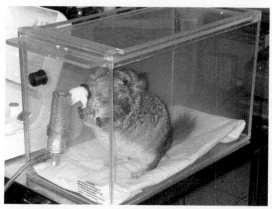

Fig. 25. Chinchilla with acute respiratory distress in a nebulization chamber.

Diuretics

Diuretic therapy can be useful in cases of cardiogenic lung edema and pleural effusions. These authors use furosemide at initial dose of 4 to 6 mg/kg intravenously or subcutaneously, followed by 1 to 2 mg/kg 2 or 3 times per day, adjusting to the minimal effective dose for each patient. The main contraindications are dehydration and severe pericardial effusion (cardiac tamponade) (see **Table 4**).

Nebulization

Nebulization with physiologic saline alone can be beneficial to moisten the exudates and promote their elimination. High environmental humidity is known to reduce sneezing in allergic rhinitis in guinea pigs.[68] Chamber nebulization can be used to deliver certain drugs, such as corticosteroids, antihistaminic or bronchodilators, topically to the respiratory epithelium (**Fig. 25**).

Nasal Lavage

Instillation of saline or hypersaline fluids can be beneficial to help eliminate the exudates and clear the airway. These authors use 0.2 to 1.0 mL/kg of fluids carefully instilled in the nostrils of animals with signs of rhinitis or sinusitis.

Primary Respiratory Tract Disorders

Congenital or hereditary disorders

Congenital or hereditary abnormalities of the respiratory system of guinea pigs, chinchillas, and degus seem to be seldom diagnosed in clinical practice. One case of a cleft palate in a chinchilla associated with absent nasal turbinates and purulent rhinosinusitis and otitis externa, media, and interna was described.[73] Cleft palate was diagnosed by authors in a 2-day old degu and a 3-day-old guinea pig. Congenital interventricular septal defects associated with respiratory signs of congestive heart failure were described in chinchillas and a degu.[35,74]

Congenital chlamydial infection is possible in guinea pigs born from an infected female.[26] This disease is usually manifested as congenital conjunctivitis.

Respiratory disease secondary to dental disease

An underlying dental disease with alveolar alterations of the incisors, premolars, or molars can cause secondary rhinitis, dacryocystitis, and upper respiratory tract

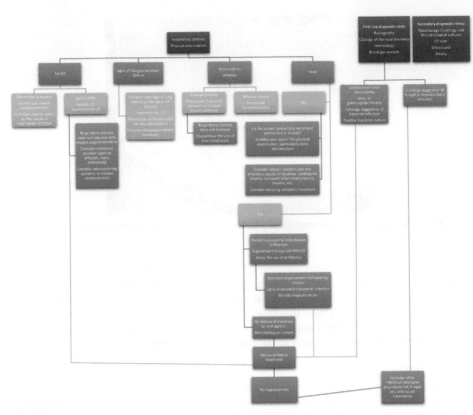

Fig. 26. Diagnostic and therapeutic approach algorithm for respiratory distress in guinea pigs and chinchillas.

disease. Particularly in degus, the elongation of the maxillary premolars and molars commonly leads to nasal cavity penetration with subsequent nasal passage obstruction and secondary bacterial infections.[29] Also in chinchillas, the elongation of the molar apices and secondary damage to the alveolar bone can lead to penetration of the nasal cavity and secondary bacterial infections.[13,20,28] Teeth migration and formation of pseudo-odontomas or elodontomas were described in degus, chinchillas, and guinea pigs.[20,28,75]

For this reason, exploration of the oral cavity, teeth, and skull (by radiography/CT scan included) is particularly important.

Owing to the difficulties we face in the diagnosis and treatment of respiratory disease in these species, diagnostic and therapeutic algorithms are still under development. The authors suggest a simplified algorithm that summarizes the information presented in this article (**Fig. 26**).

INFECTIOUS DISEASES
Bacterial Infections

The main challenge of the diagnosis of respiratory infections is that guinea pigs, chinchillas, and degus can harbor in their respiratory system several species of bacteria as asymptomatic carriers. Therefore, their presence alone is not necessarily indicative of causality and their potential to cause disease is not understood fully.[30] A positive microbial culture obtained from normally sterile sites such as the pleural cavity is more supportive of the diagnosis of infectious disease than those obtained from the nasal cavity. Having said that, infections constitute probably the most commonly diagnosed etiology of respiratory diseases in guinea pigs and chinchillas.[76]

There are some systematic reviews of spontaneous pathologies of laboratory and farm guinea pigs and chinchillas.[17,19] In 1 study, based on cultures obtained from necropsy specimens, *Pasteurella multocida*, *Bordetella bronchiseptica*, *Staphylococcus aureus*, *Pseudomonas aeruginosa*, *Streptococcus sp.*, *Klebsiella pneumoniae*, and *Listeria monocytogenes* were the most commonly isolated agents and 48% of the affected individuals presented mixed infections. Concurrent infections in other organs (pleuritis, myocarditis, and metritis) were also observed. One adult with pasteurellosis also had the presence of calicivirus in the lungs, although the association is not clear. Pneumonia caused by *Pasteurella sp.* proved to potentially present high mortality (71%) within 14 days.[19] These finding are consistent with the authors' experience with in vivo obtained microbiological cultures from nasal lavage and postmortem studies. In guinea pigs, the course of pasteurellosis includes pulmonary consolidation, pleuritis, fibrinopurulent serositis, and conjunctivitis.[10] In these authors' experience, infections with *B bronchiseptica*, *Enterobacteriaceae*, *Pseudomonadales*, and *Streptococcus sp.* are most commonly diagnosed in pet guinea pigs.

In pet chinchillas, one study isolates from conjunctival mucosa of healthy animals rendered a high prevalence (94%) of gram-positive bacteria (*Streptococcus sp*, *S aureus*, and coagulase negative *Staphylococcus sp*). In contrast, in cases of suppurative conjunctivitis, gram-negative bacteria were found frequently (62%) with *P aeruginosa* being the most common isolate (50%), followed by *Staphylococcus sp.* (27%). *P aeruginosa* was confirmed in all chinchillas with concurrent upper respiratory sings.[23] However, *Pseudomonas sp.* are also isolated commonly in asymptomatic chinchillas according to other authors and only occasionally can cause severe disease with pneumonia, otitis, conjunctivitis, septicemia, and sudden death.[77–79] Infections caused by *Pseudomonas sp.* are rare, but can be seen occasionally in guinea pigs in association with pulmonary consolidation, severe multifocal necrotizing bronchopneumonia, pulmonary botryomycosis, conjunctivitis, and otitis media.[78,79]

Among the *Enterobacteriaceae*, *Klebsiella sp*, *Enterobacter sp.*, and *Salmonella sp.* can rarely cause mild disease, such as rhinitis, otitis, or conjunctivitis, in guinea pigs and chinchillas.[80]

B bronchiseptica has historically been the most common micro-organism associated with respiratory infections in guinea pigs, possibly owing to its ease of culture.[18] The affected animals can develop immunity and clear the infection, but a small percentage remain as asymptomatic carriers. Young animals or animals kept in poor conditions are more susceptible. Bordetellosis usually presents with an accumulation of mucopurulent exudates in the nasal cavity, trachea, and tympanic bullae, which can lead to pneumonia or hematogenous systemic infection. Infected animals may show nasal and ocular discharge, signs of peripheral unilateral or bilateral vestibular syndrome, abnormal respiratory sounds, and dyspnea, as well as nonspecific signs such as fever, anorexia, or lethargy.

Both *Bordetella sp* and *Pasteurella sp* have a similar cytologic appearance of gram-negative coccobacillary rods from specimens obtained from the nasal cavity, conjunctiva, or pleural effusions.[18] The presence of a great amount of bacteria associated with inflammatory reaction is additionally supportive of the diagnosis of infection by microbial culture from nasal lavage.

Streptococcus sp. are pyogenic bacteria associated with different clinical signs. Most guinea pigs can act as asymptomatic carriers and the most common clinical presentation is abscesses formed in the cervical region (cervical lymphadenitis) in otherwise apparently healthy animals. Many guinea pigs will have inapparent upper respiratory tract infections. However, suppurative otitis, rhinitis, conjunctivitis, dyspnea, cyanosis, hematuria, hemoglobinuria, mastitis, and unexpected deaths are also possible. The cytology of the exudates, nasal lavage, or necropsy samples will reveal clusters or chains of gram-positive cocci.[26] In chinchillas, streptococcal infections are most commonly associated with otitis media and ocular disorders.[23,81] *Streptococcus equii* is considered an emergent disease in chinchilla in North America.[21,23,82] One case of streptococcal infections secondary to cleft palate in a chinchilla was described.[73]

As are humans, guinea pigs are highly susceptible to staphylococcal infections that commonly lead to acute septic shock that might present with respiratory signs.[26]

Guinea pigs are highly susceptible to *Legionella pneumophila*. The transmission rout, as in humans, depends on the environmental sources of water, such as showerheads and evaporative coolers that create an aerosolized form of the bacteria from which people and guinea pigs can become infected. As do humans, guinea pigs exhibit fever, weight loss, and respiratory difficulty approximately 1 week after infection. If left untreated, the disease presents high mortality rates owing to splenic necrosis and a severe pneumonia.[26]

In degus, infectious disease of the respiratory tract are rare and are mostly secondary to the apical maxillary premolar and molar elongation or elodontoma formations. The most commonly isolated bacteria are *S aureus* and *Streptococcus pneumoniae*. As the causative agent of bronchopneumonia, *K pneumoniae* was also described.[83]

Chlamydia and Mycoplasma sp.

Descriptions of spontaneous respiratory infections caused by *Mycoplasma sp.* are rare in guinea pigs and chinchillas. Guinea pigs can host and act as asymptomatic carriers for several species of *Mycoplasma sp.* Although these organisms were sometimes isolated from the respiratory tract, their pathogenic potential is still unknown. *Mycoplasma pulmonis* can cause respiratory disease in young guinea pigs.[84] One non–peer-reviewed report suggests that a *Mycoplasma sp.* can be related to respiratory disease (interstitial pneumonia).[85] *Mycoplasma caviae* and *Mycoplasma cavipharyngis* in particular seem to have low pathogenic potential in this species.[84,86,87]

Chlamydophila caviae infection typically causes a self-limiting conjunctivitis, but can progress to rhinitis and lower respiratory tract disease and secondary bacterial infections.[18]

Cilia-Associated Respiratory Bacillus

In guinea pigs, experimental infections with rat or mouse cilia-associated respiratory bacillus elicited antibody production but did not lead to histologic changes, suggesting that the guinea pigs are susceptible to the infection as well. However, it does not seem to be of clinical relevance in this species.[88,89]

The transmission of bacterial respiratory diseases occurs mainly by direct contact, aerosol, or fomites, and there may be interspecies transmission. *Chlamydiae* can also be transmitted via the venereal route.

Mycobacteria

Both guinea pigs and chinchilla are susceptible to mycobacterial infections.

Disseminated tuberculous and nontuberculous mycobacteriosis were reported in pet chinchillas.[90,91] A chinchilla infected with *Mycobacterium genavense* showed signs of progressive weight loss, radiographic findings consistent with bullous emphysema and severe pneumonia, and granulomatous lesions in the lungs and liver.[90] Microscopically marked intra-alveolar accumulation of foamy macrophages and giant cells associated with severe interstitial fibrosis and lymphocytic infiltration; alveolar spaces filled with fibrin, heterophils, and edema fluid; multifocal rupture of the alveolar walls; and the formation of emphysematous bullae were also observed in the lungs.[90] In the other report, a chinchilla suffering from infection with *Mycobacterium avium sbsp hominissuis* presented severe multifocal granulomatous inflammation of the lung, uterus, mediastinal and mesenteric lymph nodes, intestine, pancreas, and kidneys. Mycobacteria were also present in the vaginal discharge.[91]

Guinea pigs are used as a model of human tuberculosis in laboratory research, but no description of mycobacterial infections are available in pet guinea pigs.[92,93] The micro-organisms actively replicate in the lungs causing granulomatous inflammation with central necrosis and occasional cavitation.[92]

Fungal Infections

Respiratory infections of fungal etiology are possible, but rarer in our experience. In the literature, cases of aspergillosis, zygomycosis, and nasal candidiasis are reported in different species. Fungal rhinitis can be suspected in chronic cases refractory to antibiotic treatment or in cases of exacerbation of symptoms after treatment with antibiotics and/or corticosteroids. Cryptococcosis has recently been identified in different species as an emerging disease in the Mediterranean basin. Guinea pigs are susceptible to spontaneous disseminated cryptococcosis.[94,95] In 1 report, the affected animal showed anorexia, weight loss, generalized lymphadenomegaly, and neurologic signs. On necropsy, multifocal white lesions of approximately 0.5 mm were observed in the lungs and spleen and histopathology confirmed cryptococcal pneumonia.[94] The findings were consistent with those of experimental cryptococcosis in guinea pigs.[96]

Guinea pigs are known to host *Pneumocystis sp.* fungus, but seem to be rather resilient to experimental infections.[97] Some authors also mention spontaneous *Coccidioides sp* infection in chinchillas.[98]

No descriptions of treatment for spontaneous fungal respiratory infections are available in guinea pigs and chinchillas but, based on the information presented from other species, treatment with antifungals such as fluconazole or itraconazole for several months is probably indicated.

Viral Infections

Guinea pigs and chinchillas are susceptible to a variety of viral respiratory infections.[17,31,56,99–103] However, only influenza virus is relevant in pet rodents commonly seen in clinical practice.

Both guinea pigs and chinchillas are susceptible to human flu (influenza).[100,104–107] The transmission mechanisms and pathogenesis are very similar to influenza in ferrets, except that in guinea pigs contagion occurs more by direct contact and to a lesser extent by aerosol. The greatest peculiarity of guinea pigs with respect to influenza is the almost complete absence of clinical signs despite severe histopathologic changes in the tissues of the respiratory system. Influenza infection causes rhinitis and usually end in severe bronchointerstitial pneumonia. Infected guinea pigs may show a mucous nasal discharge by the fourth day after infection or nonspecific signs of discomfort such as ruffled fur.

Guinea pigs are susceptible to Severe Acute Respiratory Syndrome (SARS) Coronavirus infection, but seem to be not susceptible to Middle East Respiratory Syndrome (MERS). Guinea pigs show apparently low susceptibility to infection by Severe Acute Respiratory Syndrome Coronavirus-2 (SARS-CoV-2). There are no scientific data regarding the susceptibility of the chinchillas nor degus to these pathogens. There are not data supporting that these pets participate in the epidemiology of SARS, MERS, or coronavirus disease-2019 (Covid-19).[108–112]

The treatment of viral rhinitis and sinusitis focuses primarily on supportive treatment and prevention of secondary infections.

Zoonosis Considerations

Both anthroponosis and zoonosis are possible regarding respiratory pathogens of guinea pigs and chinchillas. Some of the infectious agents of respiratory diseases, such as Influenza virus, *Bordetella spp.*, *Corynebacterium spp.*, *Francisella tularensis*, *Pasteurella spp.*, *Pseudomonas spp.*, and *S pneumoniae*, *C caviae* have zoonotic potential.

Apart from humans, guinea pigs and chinchillas might act as asymptomatic carriers of pathogens for other species of animals.

Neoplasia

Among the primary respiratory neoplasia, bronchogenic papillary adenoma is common in aged guinea pigs according to some sources. Bronchogenic and alveologenic adenocarcinomas have been also documented.[25] These tumors can mimic pneumonia signs, CT studies are the most recommended technique to differentiate inflammatory pneumonia versus neoplastic disease.

Cavian leukemia is a B-cell neoplasm and, although it is a neoplasm of the lymphopoietic system, it can course with dyspnea and cyanosis. The cause is still unclear, although a viral etiology is suspected. Besides unspecific signs such as apathy, lethargy, and rough hair, enlarged peripheral and internal lymph nodes, hepatosplenomegaly, and dyspnea can occur. Affected animals typically display high leukocyte counts (25,000–250,000 WBC/µL).[76] Nonleukemic lymphoma also can affect respiratory organs and cause pleural effusion.

A single case of nasal adenocarcinoma was reported in a guinea pig that was presented with bilateral ocular purulent discharge owing to secondary *Staphylococcus sciuri* infection.[113] Metastatic mammary adenocarcinoma was reported in a chinchilla.[114]

Also not strictly a neoplastic disease, elodontomas were also associated with respiratory signs.[28,75]

Hypovitaminosis C

Guinea pigs are unable to synthetize ascorbic acid and therefore are susceptible to hypovitaminosis C if the diet is not balanced. Hypovitaminosis C is known to increase the susceptibility to infectious upper respiratory disease and conjunctivitis, particularly streptococcal diseases and enteropathies.[18,25,30] One study in 18 pet guinea pigs in Madrid, Spain, found that plasmatic vitamin C levels measured by high-performance liquid chromatography ranged from 2.8 to 17.3 µmol/L (0.05–0.30 mg/dL).[115] These levels are lower than those referenced in laboratory animals alerting on the possibility of subclinical hypovitaminosis C.[30] However, the plasmatic levels in laboratory animals could be artificially high owing to nutritional supplementation. The normal levels of plasmatic vitamin C and the true incidence of subclinical hypovitaminosis C in pet guinea pigs and its influence on their health status is still undetermined.

Iatrogenic causes of respiratory disease

Nasogastric tubes are known to cause irritation of the nasal cavity in rabbits. The risk seems to increase with the diameter of the probe used and the length of time it takes.[51] The nasal openings of guinea pigs and chinchillas are small and nasogastric tube placement is only possible in the biggest animals that normally will only admit 1-mm diameter tubes. Nasogastric tubes are useful in dyspneic animals because they decrease the risk of aspiration during assisted feeding. Normally, the placement of the tube should not increase the respiratory difficulty but, owing to the risk of nasal irritation, the authors do not recommend maintaining the tube for more than 48 to 72 hours.

Aspiration pneumonia

The primary risk factors for aspiration pneumonia are force feeding, dental disease, and general anesthesia. Aspiration pneumonia secondary to dental disease occurs owing to deficient chewing, hypersalivation, the accumulation of debris in the oral cavity, and dysphagia owing to pain or physical impediment of normal movements of the oropharyngeal structures.

In anesthetized herbivores, aspiration pneumonia also poses a risk owing to hypersalivation, debris, and regurgitation in animals that carry a nasogastric tube. Rather than using parasympathetic drugs such as atropine or glycopyrrolate, these authors prefer to give 3 to 5 mL of isotonic solution before the anesthesia and check the oral cavity with cotton swabs that must come completely clean before the anesthetic induction is started. Many herbivores, especially guinea pigs, will show coprophagy when left in a clean environment, this is the reason why they should not be left in the cage in between the mouth cleaning and anesthetic induction.

Ante mortem diagnosis of aspiration pneumonia is based on clinical signs, history of dental disease, recent force feeding, or an anesthetic episode. The initial focus is located in a bronchus and from there spreads to the adjacent parenchyma; however, a characteristic increase in segmental radiodensity or the bronchopneumonic pattern is rarely appreciated int small herbivores because the disease spreads rapidly to the rest of the lung parenchyma. A lack of air bronchogram and atelectasis might be detected radiographically.

Lipoid pneumonia

Lipoid pneumonia is caused by accumulation of lipids in the pulmonary alveoli. It is classified according to the origin of lipids as endogenous or exogenous lipoid pneumonia. Exogenous lipoid pneumonia occurs secondary to the aspiration or inhalation of exogenous lipids. The causes of endogenous lipoid pneumonia are still poorly understood, even in human medicine.[116] Lipoid pneumonia appears as a secondary reaction owing to any process causing the release of fat and cholesterol that occurs when tissue is damaged and it has been associated with lipid metabolism disorders, emphysema, and lung neoplasms. The lipids induce a variable degree of inflammatory reaction that ends up destroying the interalveolar septa and the interstitium and causing pulmonary fibrosis in chronic cases. The characteristic microscopic finding in affected lungs is abundant infiltration by macrophages laden with fat droplets.

An antemortem diagnosis can be difficult because the clinical signs and radiographic findings are consistent with many other lung diseases. Observing lipid-laden macrophages in bronchoalveolar lavages or fine needle aspiration samples could be a revealing sign in refractory pneumonias. The treatment of lipoid pneumonia in humans is based on anti-inflammatory therapy with corticosteroids.

The authors have diagnosed only 1 case of low-grade endogenous lipoid pneumonia in a 1.8-year-old female chinchilla that had concurrent uterine sarcoma and endotoxemic shock. This finding was considered incidental and not related to the death of the patient.

Nonrespiratory and extrathoracic dyspnea

There are numerous pathologic situations of nonrespiratory origin that can trigger respiratory distress.

The respiratory system is closely related to the cardiovascular system. For this reason, and as mentioned elsewhere in this article, numerous diseases of cardiac origin present with respiratory symptoms such as dyspnea, tachypnea, or cough.

Some metabolic processes such as acidosis can cause dyspnea. Metabolic acidosis is common in small herbivorous mammals and usually accompanied by compensatory hyperventilation in the early stages of the disease. Acidotic animals often show slower and deeper breathing than normal. In contrast, situations of tissue hypoxia, as occurs in cases of severe anemias, can lead to compensatory tachypnea. Coumarin and avocado toxicities can also cause dyspnea should be taken in consideration when the differential diagnoses is done.[117,118]

Abdominal masses, foreign bodies in the esophagus, diaphragmatic hernias, omental torsion, or gastric dilation are some of the pathologies that can affect the effective volume of the thoracic cavity, decrease the pulmonary capacity, and cause respiratory distress. Finally, any painful process can indirectly generate respiratory signs.

CLINICS CARE POINTS

- Complete clinical examination in animals with suspected respiratory disease must include thoracic auscultation, body temperature, respiratory and cardiac rates, and pulse oximetry.

- Oxygen supplementation and anxiolytics should be considered on arrival for any animal with respiratory distress.

- High prevalence of heart disease in guinea pigs and chinchillas is repeatedly mentioned in the literature. An effort to detect cardiogenic lung edema is important as it can mimic the signs of respiratory disease in guinea pigs and chinchillas and influence the therapeutic approach and prognosis.

- Cytological and microbiological analysis of samples obtained via nasal lavage is an important diagnostic technique.

- CT scan is more sensitive in the diagnosis of respiratory tract disorders in these species compared to classic radiography.

- Due to the practical difficulty of intubation in these species, apnea induction is not safe. Therefore rapid image acquisition using 64-slice-CT or higher is important to reduce the motion artifact. Due to higher cardiac rate in these species a rapid postcontrast acquisition is also important. Authors found better results with two post contrast series at 10-20 seconds and 30-50 seconds.

- Non-invasvie arterial blood gas analysis is not easily achieved in rodents. Venous blood gas is used instead and can be a sensitive but not specific indicator for respiratory acid-base disturbances.

- Nasogastric tubes are useful in dyspneic animals as they reduce the risk of aspiration during assisted feeding. Normally the placement of the tube should not increase the respiratory difficulty but due to the risk of nasal irritation, the authors do not recommend maintaining the tube for more than 48-72 hours.

• Hypovitaminosis C in guinea pigs and dental disease in any herbivores can be underlying causes of secondary respiratory disease.

DISCLOSURE

The authors have nothing to disclose.

REFERENCES

1. Timm KI, Jahn SE, Sedgwick CJ. The palatal ostium of the guinea pig. Lab Anim Sci 1987;37(6):801–2.
2. Hargaden M, Singer L. Anatomy, physiology, and behavior. In: Suckow MA, Stevens KA, Wilson RP, editors. The laboratory rabbit, Guinea pig, hamster, and other rodents. San Diego (CA): Elsevier Inc; 2012. p. 575–602. https://doi.org/10.1016/B978-0-12-380920-9.00020-1.
3. Beddard FE. The Cambridge Natural History. Vol X. Mammalia. Reprint Ed. (Harmer S, Shipley A, eds.). Weinheim, Germany; 1958.
4. Hale LP, Clark AG, Li J, et al. Age-related thymic atrophy in the guinea pig. Dev Comp Immunol 2001;25(5–6):509–18.
5. Cartee RE. Anatomic location and age-related changes in the chinchilla thymus. Am J Vet Res 1979;40(4):537–40. Available at: https://pubmed.ncbi.nlm.nih.gov/517827/. Accessed August 31, 2020.
6. Pearse G. Normal structure, function and histology of the thymus. Toxicol Pathol 2006;34(5):504–14.
7. Woods CA, Boraker DK. Octodon degus. Mammalian Species 1975;67:1.
8. Johnson DH. Endoscopic intubation of exotic companion mammals. Veterinary Clin North Am Exot Anim Pract 2010;13(2):273–89.
9. Malatesha G, Singh NK, Bharija A, et al. Comparison of arterial and venous pH, bicarbonate, PCO2 and PO2 in initial emergency department assessment. Emerg Med J 2007;24(8):569–71.
10. Schreider JP, Hutchens JO. Morphology of the guinea pig respiratory tract. Anat Rec 1980;196(3):313–21.
11. Kaufmann AF. Bony spicules in guinea pig lung. Lab Anim Care 1970;20(5):1002–3. Available at: https://pubmed.ncbi.nlm.nih.gov/4249262/. Accessed September 1, 2020.
12. Borst GHA, Zwart P, Mullink HWMA, et al. Bone structures in avian and mammalian lungs. Vet Pathol 1976;13(2):98–103.
13. Minarikova A, Hauptman K, Jeklova E, et al. Diseases in pet guinea pigs: a retrospective study in 1000 animals. Vet Rec 2015;177(8):200.
14. Donnelly TM, Brown C, Donnelly TM. Heterotopic bone in the eyes of a guinea pig: osseous choristoma of the ciliary body. Lab Anim (Ny) 2002;31(7):23–235.
15. Thompson SW, Hunt RD, Fox MA, et al. Perivascular nodules of lymphoid cells in the lungs of normal guinea pigs. Am J Pathol 1962;40(5):507–17. Available at: https://www.ncbi.nlm.nih.gov/pmc/articles/PMC1949553/. Accessed October 15, 2020.
16. Findlay L. The origin of pulmonary anthracosis: an experimental study. Br Med J 1911;2(2654):1278–81. Available at: https://www.jstor.org/stable/25294966. Accessed September 20, 2020.

17. Rigby C. Natural infections of guinea-pigs. Lab Anim 1976;10(2):119–42.
18. Shomer NH, Holcombe H, Harkness JE. Chapter 6 - biology and diseases of guinea pigs. In: Fox JG, Anderson LC, Loew FM, Quimby FW, editors. laboratory animal medicine. 3rd edition. San Diego (CA): Elsevier Inc; 2015. p. 247–83. https://doi.org/10.1016/B978-0-12-409527-4.00006-7.
19. Martino PE, Bautista EL, Gimeno EJ, et al. Fourteen-year status report of fatal illnesses in captive chinchilla (Chinchilla lanigera). J Appl Anim Res 2017; 45(1):310–4.
20. Lucena RB, Giaretta PR, Tessele B, et al. Doenças de chinchilas (Chinchilla lanigera). Pesqui Vet Bras 2012;32(6):529–35.
21. Mitchell CM, Johnson LK, Crim MJ, et al. Diagnosis, surveillance and management of Streptococcus equi subspecies zooepidemicus infections in chinchillas (Chinchilla lanigera). Comp Med 2020;70(4):370–5.
22. Mans C, Donnelly TM. Update on diseases of chinchillas. Veterinary Clin North Am Exot Anim Pract 2013;16(2):383–406.
23. Martel A, Donnelly T, Mans C. Update on diseases in chinchillas: 2013–2019. Veterinary Clin North Am Exot Anim Pract 2020;23(2):321–35.
24. Pignon C, Sanchez-Migallon Guzman D, Sinclair K, et al. Evaluation of heart murmurs in chinchillas (Chinchilla lanigera): 59 cases (1996-2009). J Am Vet Med Assoc 2012;241(10):1344–7.
25. Jenkins JR. Diseases of geriatric guinea pigs and chinchillas. Veterinary Clin North Am Exot Anim Pract 2010;13(1):85–93.
26. Padilla-Carlin DJ, McMurray DN, Hickey AJ. The guinea pig as a model of infectious diseases. Comp Med 2008;58(4):324–40.
27. Jekl V, Hauptman K, Knotek Z. Diseases in pet degus: a retrospective study in 300 animals. J Small Anim Pract 2011;52(2):107–12.
28. Jekl V, Hauptman K, Skoric M, et al. Elodontoma in a Degu (Octodon degus). J Exot Pet Med 2008;17(3):216–20.
29. Jekl V, Zikmund T, Hauptman K. Dyspnea in a Degu (Octodon degu) associated with maxillary cheek teeth elongation. J Exot Pet Med 2016;25(2):128–32.
30. Harkness JE, Murray KA, Wagner JE. Biology and diseases of guinea pigs. In: Fox JG, Anderson LC, Loew FM, Quimby FW, editors. Laboratory animal medicine. San Diego (CA): Elsevier; 2002. p. 203–46. https://doi.org/10.1016/b978-012263951-7/50009-0.
31. Gitiban N, Jurcisek JA, Harris RH, et al. Chinchilla and murine models of upper respiratory tract infections with respiratory syncytial virus. J Virol 2005;79(10): 6035–42.
32. Montesinos A, Ardiaca M, Bonvehi C. Hiatal hernia in two chinchillas (Chinchilla lanigera). In: Proceedings of the South European Veterinary Conference (SEVC). AVEPA. Barcelona, Spain; 2015:215-216.
33. Aymen J, Langlois I, Lanthier I. Diaphragmatic hernia in a pet chinchilla (Chinchilla lanigera). Can Vet J 2017;58(6):597–600. Available at: https://pubmed.ncbi.nlm.nih.gov/28588332/. Accessed October 17, 2020.
34. Aymen J, Langlois I, Lanthier I. Case report rapport de cas: diaphragmatic hernia in a pet chinchilla (Chinchilla lanigera). Can Vet J 2018;59(5):521–4.
35. Linde A, Summerfield NJ, Johnston M, et al. Echocardiography in the Chinchilla. J Vet Intern Med 2004;18(5):772–4.
36. Silverman S, Tell L. Radiology of rodents, rabbits, and ferrets. Elsevier Saunders; Saint Louis, MO, USA 2005. doi:10.1016/b0-7216-9789-5/x5001-7.
37. Krautwald-Junghanns M-E, Pees M, Reese S, Tully TN. Diagnostic Imaging of Exotic Pets: Birds, Small Mammals, Reptiles. (Krautwald-Junghanns M-E,

Pees M, Reese S, Tully TN, eds.). Hannover, Germany: Schlütersche Verlagsgesellschaft mbH & Co; 2010

38. Dall JA. Diaphragmatic hernia in a chinchilla. Vet Rec 1967;81(23):599.

39. Müllhaupt D, Wenger S, Kircher P, et al. Computed tomography of the thorax in rabbits: a prospective study in ten clinically healthy New Zealand White rabbits. Acta Vet Scand 2017;59. https://doi.org/10.1186/S13028-017-0340-X.

40. Masseau I, Reinero CR. Thoracic computed tomographic interpretation for clinicians to aid in the diagnosis of dogs and cats with respiratory disease. Vet J 2019;253. https://doi.org/10.1016/j.tvjl.2019.105388.

41. Biederer J, Mirsadraee S, Beer M, et al. MRI of the lung (3/3)-current applications and future perspectives. Insights Imaging 2012;3(4):373–86.

42. Ardiaca Garcia M, Montesinos Barcelo A, Bonvehi Nadeu C, et al. Point-of-care blood gas analysis abnormalities in pet guinea pigs (Cavia porcellus). In: Proceedings 2nd International Conference on Avian, Herpetological and Exotic Mammal Medicine. Paris. 2015. 2015:439.

43. Tausch KA. Untersuchungen über den Einsatz des i-STAT®-Blutanalysegerätes zur Blutgasanalyse und Bestimmung weiterer labordiagnostischer Parameter bei Kaninchen und Meerschweinchen. 2011. Available at: http://edoc.ub.uni-muenchen.de/12700/1/Tausch_Karin_Anne.pdf. Accessed September 8, 2020.

44. Byrne AL, Bennett M, Chatterji R, et al. Peripheral venous and arterial blood gas analysis in adults: are they comparable? A systematic review and meta-analysis. Respirology 2014;19:168–75.

45. Chhabra SK. Agreement and differences between venous and arterial gas analysis. Ann Thorac Med 2011;6(3):154.

46. Lichtenberger M. Shock and cardiopulmonary-cerebral resuscitation in small mammals and birds. Veterinary Clin North Am Exot Anim Pract 2007;10(2): 275–91.

47. Villela NR, dos Santos AOMT, de Miranda ML, et al. Fluid resuscitation therapy in endotoxemic hamsters improves survival and attenuates capillary perfusion deficits and inflammatory responses by a mechanism related to nitric oxide. J Transl Med 2014;12(1):232.

48. Hedrich H. In: Hedrich H, editor. The laboratory mouse. 2nd edition. Academic Press Elsevier; 2012. https://doi.org/10.1016/B978-0-12-382008-2.00001-5.

49. Marx JO, Jensen JA, Seelye S, et al. The effects of acute blood loss for diagnostic bloodwork and fluid replacement in clinically ill mice. Comp Med 2015; 65(3):202–16.

50. Turner PV, Pekow C, Vasbinder MA, et al. Administration of substances to laboratory animals: equipment considerations, vehicle selection, and solute preparation. J Am Assoc Lab Anim Sci 2011;50(5):614–27.

51. Çetin ÇB, Kara CO, Çolakoğlu N, et al. Experimental sinusitis in nasally catheterised rabbits. Rhinology 2002;40(3):154–8. Available at: https://www.researchgate.net/publication/11099276_Experimental_sinusitis_in_nasally_catheterised_rabbits. Accessed September 1, 2020.

52. Mokra D, Mikolka P, Kosutova P, et al. Corticosteroids in acute lung injury: the dilemma continues. Int J Mol Sci 2019;20(19). https://doi.org/10.3390/ijms20194765.

53. Torres A, Sibila O, Ferrer M, et al. Effect of corticosteroids on treatment failure among hospitalized patients with severe community-acquired pneumonia and high inflammatory response: a randomized clinical trial. JAMA 2015;313(7): 677–86.

54. Stern A, Skalsky K, Avni T, et al. Corticosteroids for pneumonia. Cochrane Database Syst Rev 2017;2017(12). https://doi.org/10.1002/14651858.CD007720.pub3.

55. Turner DL, Ferrari N, Ford WR, et al. Bronchoprotection in conscious guinea pigs by budesonide and the NO-donating analogue, TPI 1020, alone and combined with tiotropium or formoterol. Br J Pharmacol 2012;167(3):515–26.

56. Yamada K, Elliott WM, Hayashi S, et al. Latent adenoviral infection modifies the steroid response in allergic lung inflammation. J Allergy Clin Immunol 2000; 106(5):844–51.

57. Kamiyama K, Matsuda N, Yamamoto S, et al. Modulation of glucocorticoid receptor expression, inflammation, and cell apoptosis in septic guinea pig lungs using methylprednisolone. Am J Physiol Lung Cell Mol Physiol 2008;295(6). https://doi.org/10.1152/ajplung.00459.2007.

58. Spotorno AE, Zuleta CA, Valladares JP, et al. Chinchilla laniger. Mamm Species 2004;758(758):1–9.

59. Gan LL, Wang MW, Cheng MS, et al. Trachea relaxing effects and β2-selectivity of SPFF, a newly developed bronchodilating agent, in guinea pigs and rabbits. Biol Pharm Bull 2003;26(3):323–8.

60. Tanner L, Single AB. Animal models reflecting chronic obstructive pulmonary disease and related respiratory disorders: translating pre-clinical data into clinical relevance. J Innate Immun 2020;12(3):203–25.

61. Macie C, Wooldrage K, Manfreda J, et al. Cardiovascular morbidity and the use of inhaled bronchodilators. Int J Chron Obstruct Pulmon Dis 2008;3(1):163–9.

62. Dorsch W, Auch E, Powerlowicz P. Adverse effects of acetylcysteine on human and guinea pig bronchial asthma in vivo and on human fibroblasts and leukocytes in vitro. Int Arch Allergy Appl Immunol 1987;82(1):33–9.

63. Strapková A, Nosál'ová G, Fraňová S. Mucolytics and antioxidant activity. Life Sciences 1999;65(18-19):1923–5. https://doi.org/10.1016/S0024-3205(99)00448-8.

64. Janatuinen M, Korhonen LK. The effect of a substituted benzylamine (Bisolvon®) on mucosubstance production. Naunyn Schmiedebergs Arch Pharmakol 1969;265(2):112–7.

65. Disse BG, Ziegler HW. Pharmacodynamic mechanism and therapeutic activity of ambroxol in animal experiments. Respiration 1987;51(SUPPL. 1):15–22.

66. Becher G, Winsel K, Barleben A. Failure of ambroxol to influence the allergen induced bronchial constriction in sensitized guinea pigs. Biomed Biochim Acta 1989;48(8):589–92.

67. Duncan PG, Douglas JS. Age-related changes in guinea pig respiratory tissues: considerations for assessment of bronchodilators. Eur J Pharmacol 1985; 108(1):39–48.

68. Bahekar PC, Shah JH, Ayer UB, et al. Validation of guinea pig model of allergic rhinitis by oral and topical drugs. Int Immunopharmacol 2008;8(11):1540–51.

69. Al Suleimani M, Ying D, Walker MJA. A comprehensive model of allergic rhinitis in guinea pigs. J Pharmacol Toxicol Methods 2007;55(2):127–34.

70. Chen ZY, Zhou SH, Zhou QF, et al. Inflammation and airway remodeling of the lung in guinea pigs with allergic rhinitis. Exp Ther Med 2017;14(4):3485–90.

71. Myers AC, Kajekar R, Undem BJ. Allergic inflammation-induced neuropeptide production in rapidly adapting afferent nerves in guinea pig airways. Am J Physiol Lung Cell Mol Physiol 2002;282(4 26–4). https://doi.org/10.1152/ajplung.00353.2001.

72. Justesen DR, Braun EW, Garrison RG, et al. Pharmacological differentiation of allergic and classically conditioned asthma in the guinea pig. Science 1970; 170(3960):864–6.

73. Ozawa S, Mans C, Miller JL, et al. Cleft palate in a chinchilla (Chinchilla lanigera). J Exot Pet Med 2019;28:93–7.

74. Sanchez JN, Summa NME, Visser LC, et al. Ventricular septal defect and congestive heart failure in a common degu (Octodon degus). J Exot Pet Med 2019;31:32–5.

75. Capello V, Lennox A, Ghisleni G. Elodontoma in two guinea pigs. J Vet Dent 2015;32(2):111–9.

76. Roberts-Steel S, Oxley JA, Carroll A, et al. Frequency of owner-reported bacterial infections in pet guinea pigs. Animals 2019;9(9). https://doi.org/10.3390/ani9090649.

77. Wideman WL. Pseudomonas aeruginosa otitis media and interna in a chinchilla ranch. Can Vet J 2006;47(8):799–800. Available at: https://pubmed.ncbi.nlm.nih.gov/16933561/. Accessed October 16, 2020.

78. Hirakawa Y, Sasaki H, Kawamoto E, et al. Prevalence and analysis of Pseudomonas aeruginosa in chinchillas. BMC Vet Res 2010;6:52.

79. Doerning BJ, Brammer DW, Rush HG. Pseudomonas aeruginosa infection in a Chinchilla lanigera. Lab Anim 1993;27(2):131–3.

80. Bartoszcze M, Matras J, Palec S, et al. Klebsiella pneumoniae infection in chinchillas. Vet Rec 1990;127(5):119.

81. Yang R, Sabharwal V, Shlykova N, et al. Treatment of Streptococcus pneumoniae otitis media in a chinchilla model by transtympanic delivery of antibiotics. JCI insight 2018;3(19). https://doi.org/10.1172/jci.insight.123415.

82. Berg CC, Doss GA, Mans C. Streptococcus equi subspecies zooepidemicus infection in a pet chinchilla (Chinchilla lanigera). J Exot Pet Med 2019;31:36–8.

83. Murphy J, Crowell T, Hewes C, et al. Spontaneous lesions in the degu. In: Montali R, Migaki G, editors. The comparative pathology of zoo animals. Washington, D.C.: Smithsonian Institution Press; 1980. p. 437–44.

84. Brunner H, James WD, Horswood RL, et al. Experimental mycoplasma pneumoniae infection of young guinea pigs. J Infect Dis 1973;127(3):315–8.

85. Blazey B. Mycoplasma Pneumonia in G... Chem und Veterinäruntersuchungsamt Stuttgart. 2017. Available at: https://www.ua-bw.de/pub/beitrag.asp?subid=1&Thema_ID=8&ID=2582&lang=EN&Pdf=No. Accessed September 20, 2020.

86. Hiranuma S, Hudlicky T. Mycoplasma caviae, a new species. Tetrahedron Lett 1982;23(34):3431–4.

87. Hill AC. Mycoplasma cavipharyngis, a new species isolated from the nasopharynx of guinea-pigs. J Gen Microbiol 1984;130(12):3183–8.

88. Shoji-Darkye Y, Itoh T, Kagiyama N. Pathogenesis of CAR bacillus in rabbits, guinea pigs, Syrian hamsters, and mice. Lab Anim Sci 1991;41(6):567–71. Available at: https://europepmc.org/article/med/1667199. Accessed September 20, 2020.

89. Matsushita S, Joshima H, Matsumoto T, et al. Transmission experiments of cilia-associated respiratory bacillus in mice, rabbits and guineapigs. Lab Anim 1989; 23(2):96–102.

90. Huynh M, Pingret JL, Nicolier A. Disseminated Mycobacterium genavense infection in a chinchilla (Chinchilla lanigera). J Comp Pathol 2014;151(1):122–5.

91. Barthel Y, Drews S, Fehr M, et al. Concurrent infection with Mycobacterium avium subsp. hominissuis and Giardia duodenalis in a chinchilla (Chinchilla lanigera f. dom.). Berl Munch Tierarztl Wochenschr 2016;129(5–6):242–6.

92. Clark S, Hall Y, Williams A. Animal models of tuberculosis: guinea pigs. Cold Spring Harb Perspect Med 2015;5(5). https://doi.org/10.1101/cshperspect.a018572.

93. Kashino SS, Napolitano DR, Skobe Z, et al. Guinea pig model of Mycobacterium tuberculosis latent/dormant infection. Microbes Infect 2008;10(14–15):1469–76.

94. Brandes K, Stierstorfer B, Werckenthin C, et al. Spontaneous disseminated cryptococcosis in a guinea pig. Tierarztl Prax Ausg K Klientiere Heimtiere 2003;31(6):377–82.

95. Betty MJ. Spontaneous cryptococcal meningitis in a group of guinea pigs caused by a hyphae-producing strain. J Comp Pathol 1977;87(3):377–82.

96. Liang L, He C, Lei M, et al. Pathology of guinea pigs experimentally infected with a novel reovirus and coronavirus isolated from SARS patients. DNA Cell Biol 2005;24(8):485–90.

97. Cho SR, Park YG, Moon HN, et al. Karyotypes of Pneumocystis carinii derived from several mammals. Korean J Parasitol 1999;37(4):271–5.

98. Rezusta A, Gil J, Rubio M. Micosis Importadas. 2013. Available at: https://www.seimc.org/contenidos/ccs/revisionestematicas/micologia/Micoimpor.pdf%0Ahttps://seimc.org/contenidos/ccs/revisionestematicas/micologia/Micoimpor.pdf%0Ahttps://www.seimc.org/contenidos/ccs/revisionestematicas/micologia/Micoimpor.pdf. Accessed October 16, 2020.

99. McGillivary G, Mason KM, Jurcisek JA, et al. Respiratory syncytial virus-induced dysregulation of expression of a mucosal B-defensin augments colonization of the upper airway by non-typeable Haemophilus influenzae. Cell Microbiol 2009;11(9):1399–408.

100. Pica N, Chou Y-Y, Bouvier NM, et al. Transmission of Influenza B Viruses in the Guinea Pig. J Virol 2012;86(8):4279–87.

101. Naumann S, Kunstýř I, Langer I, et al. Lethal pneumonia in guineapigs associated with a virus. Lab Anim 1981;15(3):235–42.

102. Lazzari AM, Vargas AC de, Dutra V, et al. Agentes infecciosos isolados de Chinchilla laniger. Cienc Rural 2001;31(2):337–40.

103. Kaup FJ, Naumann S, Kunstyr I, et al. Experimental viral pneumonia in guinea pigs: an ultrastructural study. Vet Pathol 1984;21(5):521–7.

104. Leyva-Grado VH, Mubareka S, Krammer F, et al. Influenza virus infection in guinea pigs raised as livestock, Ecuador. Emerg Infect Dis 2012;18(7):1135–8.

105. Lowen AC, Mubareka S, Tumpey TM, et al. The guinea pig as a transmission model for human influenza viruses. Proc Natl Acad Sci U S A 2006;103(26):9988–92.

106. Mubareka S, Lowen AC, Steel J, et al. Transmission of influenza virus via aerosols and fomites in the guinea pig model. J Infect Dis 2009;199(6):858–65.

107. Giebink GS. Otitis media: the chinchilla model. Microb Drug Resist 1999;5(1):57–72.

108. Decaro N, Lorusso A. Novel human coronavirus (SARS-CoV-2): a lesson from animal coronaviruses. Vet Microbiol 2020;244:108693.

109. Ruiz-Arrondo I, Portillo A, Palomar AM, et al. Detection of SARS-CoV-2 in pets living with COVID-19 owners diagnosed during the COVID-19 lockdown in Spain: a case of an asymptomatic cat with SARS-CoV-2 in Europe. medRxiv 2020;14:20101444.

110. Abdel-Moneim AS, Abdelwhab EM. Evidence for SARS-COV-2 infection of animal hosts. Pathogens 2020;9(7):1–27.

111. Brooke GN, Prischi F. Structural and functional modelling of SARS-CoV-2 entry in animal models. Sci Rep 2020;10(1):15917.

112. Smith TRF, Patel A, Ramos S, et al. Immunogenicity of a DNA vaccine candidate for COVID-19. Nat Commun 2020;11(1):1–13.

113. Vannevel J, Wilcock B. Bile duct carcinoma and nasal adenocarcinoma in a guinea pig. Can Vet J 2005;46(1):72–3. Available at: pmc/articles/PMC1082860/?report=abstract. Accessed September 1, 2020.

114. Konell AL, Gonçalves KA, de Sousa RS, et al. Mammary adenocarcinoma with pulmonary, hepatic and renal metastasis in a chinchilla (Chinchilla laniger). Acta Sci Vet. 2018;46. Available at: https://www.researchgate.net/publication/327968542_Mammary_Adenocarcinoma_with_Pulmonary_Hepatic_and_Renal_Metastasis_in_a_Chinchilla_Chinchilla_laniger. Accessed September 2, 2020.

115. Gallego Agundez M, Villaluenga Rodriguez J, Cassez Porquet N, et al. Niveles plasmáticos de vitamina c en cobayas mascota sugieren hipovitaminosis C subclínica en todos los individuos que acuden a la clínica diaria en un centro veterinario de Madrid. In: XXXIII congreso anual de La asociación madrileña de Veterinarios de Animales de Compañía. AMVAC. Madrid, Spain. 2016.

116. Betancourt SL, Martinez-Jimenez S, Rossi SE, et al. Lipoid pneumonia: spectrum of clinical and radiologic manifestations. Am J Roentgenol 2010;194(1): 103–9.

117. Lichtenberger M, Richardson JA. Emergency care and managing toxicoses in the exotic animal patient. Veterinary Clin North Am Exot Anim Pract 2008; 11(2):211–28.

118. Ojewole J, Kamadyaapa DR, Gondwe MM, et al. Cardiovascular effects of Persea americana Mill (Lauraceae) (avocado) aqueous leaf extract in experimental animals. Cardiovasc J S Afr 2007;18(2):69–76. Available at: https://www.researchgate.net/publication/6335066_Cardiovascular_effects_of_Persea_americana_Mill_Lauraceae_avocado_aqueous_leaf_extract_in_experimental_animals. Accessed October 18, 2020.

Respiratory Disorders in Rabbits

Vladimír Jekl, DVM, PhD, DCZM (Small Mammal)[a,b,*]

KEYWORDS

- Rabbit • Pasteurella • Dyspnea • Rhinitis • Sinusitis • Pneumonia • Lung tumor
- Thymoma

KEY POINTS

- Respiratory disorders are very common in rabbits.
- Rabbits are obligate nasal breathers, so any nasal airway obstruction (even "simple" rhinitis) can cause severe respiratory distress.
- Diagnosis is based on the combination of clinical examination (thoracic auscultation), imaging methods and pathogen isolation.
- Long -term use of antibiotics is advocated only in rare cases.
- Computed tomography and endoscopy will allow to identify the aetiology in chronic sneezing rabbits and allow targeted treatment.

ANATOMY AND PHYSIOLOGY

Several features of the rabbit nose anatomy have been claimed in regulating the inhaled airflows, thus adjusting the exchanges of air, heat, moisture, and inspired chemicals to the nasal mucosa.[1,2] These features include the alar fold that partially occludes the nose inlet and forms a comma-shaped naris, the spiral (or helical) nasal vestibule that splits the inhaled air into different flow streams, the swell body that causes the nasal cycle, and the dorsal meatus that leads directly to the olfactory region, among others.[3]

The nostrils of rabbits contain sensory pads, and at the tip of the nose is also a "blind spot," which makes this region very sensitive to the touch. Rabbits are obligate nasal breathers, which means that the normal anatomic position of the epiglottis causes it to be engaged over the caudal rim of the soft palate, sealing the oral pharynx from the lower airways. Therefore, rabbits with advanced upper airway disease will attempt

[a] Jekl & Hauptman Veterinary Clinic, Focused on Exotic Companion Mammal Care, Mojmirovo namesti 3105/6a, Brno 61200, Czech Republic; [b] Department of Pharmacology and Pharmacy, Faculty of Veterinary Medicine, University of Veterinary and Pharmaceutical Sciences Brno, Brno 61242, Czech Republic
* Jekl & Hauptman Veterinary Clinic, Focused on Exotic Companion Mammal Care, Mojmirovo namesti 3105/6a, Brno 61200, Czech Republic.
E-mail address: VladimirJekl@gmail.com

Vet Clin Exot Anim 24 (2021) 459–482
https://doi.org/10.1016/j.cvex.2021.01.006
1094-9194/21/© 2021 Elsevier Inc. All rights reserved.

to breathe through their mouths, which prevents feeding and drinking and could be quickly fatal. Also, inadvertent occlusion of the nasal passages during any procedure, including oral cavity examination, can lead to respiratory compromise because of the ineffectiveness of mouth breathing.

The *nasal cavity* is demarcated by paired nasal, incisive, maxillary, sphenoidal, presphenoidal, and ethmoid bones and by unpaired vomer. The long and flat nasal bones extend caudally and articulate with the frontal bone at the frontonasal suture, forming the nasal dorsum.[4] Dorsocaudally, the nasal septum articulates with the bony perpendicular plate of the ethmoid and caudoventrally with the presphenoid bone. Ventrally, the cartilaginous septum communicates with the vomer via the septovomeral joint. Cranially, the vomeronasal organ sits along the ventral midline margin supported by the dorsal surface of the palatine processes of the maxilla. The floor of the nasal fossae is formed primarily from the palatine process of the maxilla, which also forms the roof of the hard palate, with a central bony deficit in the midline anterior to the molars. This area is known as the *palatine fissure*, which provides a soft tissue window to enter the nasal fossae from the oral cavity.[4]

The nasal cavity is divided by the nasal septum into 2 equal passages, each comprising 4 anatomic regions (**Fig. 1**): nasal vestibule, maxilloturbinate region, nasomaxillary region, and ethmoturbinate region.[2] Maxilloturbinates has branching structures, and the ethmoidal region is scroll-like in architecture. The nasomaxillary region serves as a morphologic transition from between these 2 types of turbinates. The nasal septum supports a plate of hyaline cartilage, which extends dorsally and then laterally, supporting the outer surface of the nostrils, and medially, as the cartilage of nasoturbinates.[5]

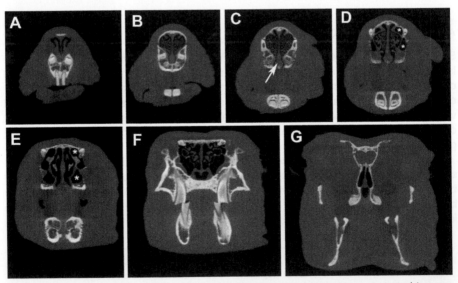

Fig. 1. CT scan of a rabbit with healthy nasal passages. Axial images are arranged in a rostrocaudal direction (*A–G*). Nasal cavity is divided by the nasal septum in the nasal vestibule (*A*), maxilloturbinate region (*B–D*), nasomaxillary region (*E*), and ethmoturbinate region (*F*). (*A*) Maxillary first incisors reserve crowns and clinical crowns of maxillary second incisors (peg teeth) are seen. (*B*) Maxillary first and second incisors reserve crowns and clinical crowns of peg teeth. (*C*) Apices of maxillary first incisors are seen; arrows pointed to the vomeronasal organ. (*D, E*) Paranasal cavity is visualized with asterisk. (*F*) Maxillary first molars are seen, (*G*) Nasopharynx. (*Courtesy of* Vladimir Jekl and Karel Hauptman.)

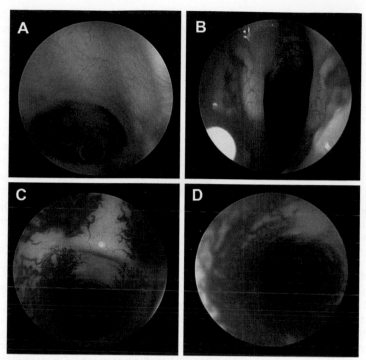

Fig. 2. Endoscopic images of a healthy rabbit (*A–D*). (*A*) Glottis is located caudally due to the long oral cavity and can be visualized when soft palate is gently pushed dorsally. (*B*) Detailed view of the rima tracheitis, which is demarcated by arytenoid cartilages. (*C, D*) Tracheoscopy, the "hypervascular" mucosa is a normal finding in a rabbit. In some cases, rigid endoscopy also allows visualization of tracheal bifurcation (*D*). (*Courtesy of* Vladimir Jekl.)

Rabbits have paired symmetric *paranasal processes*: the dorsal conchal sinus, the large maxillary sinus consisting of a dorsal and a ventral recess, and the sphenoidal sinus. A large connection is present between the dorsal conchal sinus and the maxillary sinus, resulting in 1 large conchomaxillary cavity (lateral paranasal process). The sphenoidal sinus lies most caudal and is surrounded by the presphenoid bone.[6] The paranasal cavities communicate with the main respiratory passages only via the small ostium located in the cranial part of the lateral paranasal process.

In the normal physiologic state, the epiglottis is engaged over the caudal margin of the soft palate, allowing air to only pass from the nasal cavity into the lungs. To see into the tracheal opening, the soft palate will need to be elevated to drop the epiglottis into view (**Fig. 2**). The larynx is formed by thyroid cartilage, which forms most of the ventral wall of the larynx; cricoid cartilage, which forms a complete ring extending around larynx caudally to thyroid cartilage; and arytenoid cartilages, which are obliquely situated cartilages on the dorsal surface of the larynx. Vocal cords are rudimentary and are attached to the arytenoids.[7]

The *trachea* is made of incomplete C-shaped cartilaginous rings held together by connective tissues (see **Fig. 2**). The tracheal cartilages exhibit a random pattern of anastomoses between adjacent rings.[8] The lumen is oval.[8,9] The trachea is bifurcated into the right and left principal bronchi.

The right *lung* has 4 lobes (cranial, caudal, medial, accessory), whereas the left lung has only 2 lobes (**Fig. 3**). Rabbit lungs have no small septa (lungs are not lobulated),

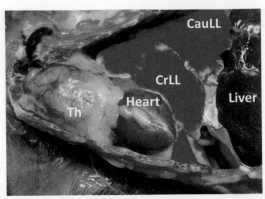

Fig. 3. Postmortem image of a rabbit thorax, lateral view. See left cranial (CrLL) and caudal (CauLL) lung lobes and heart, which are dislocated caudally by the cranial mediastinal mass (Th, thymoma). (*Courtesy of* Vladimir Jekl and Karel Hauptman.)

and airflow volume is higher in the left lung. The cranial lung lobes are small and are commonly superimposed with mediastinal fat. The caudal lung lobes have a pronounced vasculature. Pneumonia is always lobar, so clear determination whether the infection is bronchogenic or hematogenic is not possible in rabbits.

Rabbits have a relatively small thoracic cavity and at rest breathe mostly through the activity of diaphragm, showing minimal movement of the chest wall when breathing. The normal respiratory rate at rest is 30 to 60 breaths per minute. On auscultation, rabbits have more pronounced upper airway and bronchial sounds and may sound somewhat harsh. Significant respiratory compromise may occur if a rabbit is placed in dorsal recumbency for surgery when the gastrointestinal tract is distended or in obese animals, so elevating the thorax above the abdomen is recommended.[10]

The pleura is thin.

The cranial border of the heart, which is localized between 2(3)nd to 5(6)th intercostal spaces, is less distinct because of the presence of thymus and fat. Cardiac size is evaluated based on vertebral heart score.[11]

The thymus persists through the life of the rabbit.

HISTORY AND CLINICAL SIGNS

A thorough history of patients with respiratory disease (RD) can be challenging to obtain, as some owners can have a difficult time recognizing any abnormalities. Any stridor, presence of nasal discharge, or recent onset of snuffling might indicate nasopharyngeal disease. Weight loss, anorexia, and the presence and rate of progression of respiratory distress or exercise intolerance should be ascertained.

Rabbits are obligatory nasal breathers, so any obstructive disease of the nasal cavity could be life threatening. It is imperative that animals with severe respiratory distress must be stabilized before time is taken to obtain a thorough history. Stabilization may include oxygen therapy, appropriate medications (diuretics), and then a brief history.

CAUSE AND PATHOPHYSIOLOGY

Causes of dyspnea could be of primary origin or secondary, whereby diseases primarily affecting other organs can result in respiratory distress even if the respiratory system is healthy (eg, anemia, cardiac disease, metabolic acidosis, hyperthermia). Pathophysiology of dyspnea originates from lack of oxygen or excess of carbon dioxide in the body. The animal tries to resolve the problem with either increased ventilatory rate or increased ventilatory depth or both.

RD could be associated with restrictive or obstructive pattern. Determination, which pattern the animal exhibiting, can help to narrow the list of differential diagnoses.

Because of the small thoracic cavity, rabbits are predisposed to *restrictive diseases*, which prevent the lungs expanding, and lead to short, rapid, and shallow breaths. These signs could be associated with pneumonia, lung edema, pleural effusion, pneumothorax, mediastinal and lung tumors, or abscesses or because of increased pressure of abdominal organs into the diaphragm (eg, obstructive ileus). *Obstructive disease*, which is present in cases of narrowing of the airway passages, leads to slower and deeper breaths. Upper obstructive RD is associated with increased inspiratory effort, whereas in lower RD with increased expiratory effort, inspiratory problems could be also seen. Wheezes are usually heard on expiration and indicate obstruction or narrowing of small airways. Crackles are caused by the opening of small airways during inspiration and are heard with bronchial inflammation and pneumonia. A list of differential diagnoses for nasal discharge and dyspnea is given in **Table 1**.[10]

DIAGNOSTICS

The *clinical examination* is extremely important in assessing respiratory health. Even before approaching the animal, an attempt should be made to observe the animal while talking to the owner.

The mucous membranes should be checked for any indication of cyanosis or pallor. Both nostrils should be checked for airflow and signs of discharge (**Fig. 4**). Unilateral nasal discharge is usually indicative for upper respiratory rather than lower respiratory or systemic disease.

Because of the rabbit's regular grooming, signs of discharge can be seen only as wet hair on the front paws. Facial symmetry should be evaluated. Oral cavity and all maxillary teeth should be evaluated for the presence of any associated pathologic condition within the nasal cavity. Palpation of the skull, cervical area, thorax, and abdomen could reveal tumors, skeletal injury, or enlargement/distension of abdominal organs.

A properly fitted and functioning stethoscope is of great importance in the thorough examination of the heart and lungs. Care must be taken to identify the origin of potentially confusing sounds that commonly arise as a result of shivering, twitching, or movements of the stethoscope against the body. During the auscultation, the entire thorax at different places should be examined even in small rabbits to exactly identify the source of abnormal sound. The author also auscultates the trachea, as it can help distinguish between lung and nasal origin of abnormal sounds. Wheezes (musical sounds) are generated primarily by airway narrowing, stenosis, or obstruction. Crackles (short, explosive, nonmusical sounds) are typically produced by a delayed opening of small airways attributable to an abnormal fluid-air interface (pneumonia, pulmonary edema). Knowledge of the timing (systolic, diastolic) and location of abnormal heart sounds (murmurs, arrhythmias) allows the practitioner to rapidly establish a differential diagnosis. In rabbits, the arterial pulse is evaluated bilaterally to assess heart rate, rhythm, and arterial pulse quality. However, heart disease can be present without auscultable abnormalities, and not all murmurs are associated with heart disease (most commonly due to anemia).

Table 1
Possible causes of dyspnea in rabbits

Nasal discharge, upper airway disease	
Bacterial infection	P multocida
	S aureus
	B bronchiseptica
	Pseudomonas sp
	Mycobacterium sp
Viral infection	Myxomatosis, calicivirosis
Mycotic infection	Aspergillosis, candidosis
Parasitic	Pneumonyssus sp
Nasopharyngeal polyps	
Neoplasia	Osteoma, osteosarcoma, fibrosarcoma
Dental disease	Periapical infection
	Incisor malocclusion
	Elodontoma
Foreign bodies	Hay, seeds, prickles
Skull fractures	
Traumatic injury	
Lung edema	
Improper housing	Dust
	Improper humidity
	Nasal irritants
Lung disorders	
Aspiration	
Bacterial infection	P multocida
	S aureus
	B bronchiseptica
	K pneumonia
	M avium
	Chlamydophila sp, Mycoplasma sp
Viral infection	Myxomatosis
	Calicivirosis
Mycotic infection	Aspergillosis
Lung neoplasia	Mesothelioma
Metastases	Uterine adenocarcinoma
	Mammary gland neoplasia
	Lymphoma
Heart disease	
Cardiomyopathy	Idiopathic
Infectious	P multocida
	S aureus
	Salmonella sp
	Streptococcus viridans coronavirosis
Parasitic	E cuniculi
Degenerative	Valvular disease
Pleural disease	
Pneumothorax	
Chylothorax	

(continued on next page)

Table 1 *(continued)*	
Pyothorax	
Neoplasia	Uterine adenocarcinoma
	Lymphoma
Mediastinal disease	
Lymphoma	
Thymoma	
Uterine adenocarcinoma	
Systemic disease	
Gastric dilatation	
Cecal distension	
Hepatomegaly, liver failure	
Brain disease	Encephalitis (herpesvirus, *E cuniculi*, larva migrans *Bayliscaris procyonis*)
	Neoplasia
Kidney failure	
Anemia	Fleas
	Bleeding: trauma, urogenital tract
	Lead poisoning
Hyperthermia	
Lymphoma/leukemia	
Metabolic acidosis	
Stress, shock, pain	
Skeletal injury	
Acute smoke inhalation	
Status ante finem	

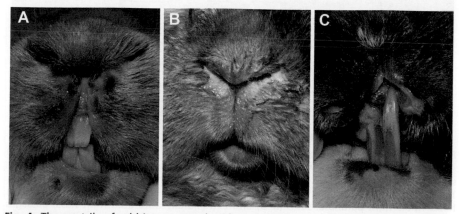

Fig. 4. The nostrils of rabbits presented with sneezing or dyspnea. (*A*) Petechial hemorrhages were associated with myxomatosis. (*B*) Bilateral purulent discharge associated with *P multocida* and *S aureus* infection; (*C*) Mucosal injury of the nostrils and the upper lips of a rabbit with maloccluded mandibular incisors. (*Courtesy of* Vladimir Jekl and Karel Hauptman.)

Many diagnostic methods are available to the clinician to help identify and describe the type of RD. It is imperative with small mammals that the potential hazard of any test be considered, because minor stress can lead to collapse of these patients. *Hematology and plasma chemistry* are often unremarkable; however, the most important contribution is to uncover systemic diseases that might be affecting the respiratory system, such as anemia, leukemia/lymphoma, or presence of liver and kidney failure. Urinalysis and analysis of acid base balance blood parameters show metabolic disturbances. *Enzyme-linked immunosorbent assay (ELISA) tests* are available for the antibody detection for *Pasteurella multocida* in rabbits; however, a paired blood sample examination is necessary to evaluate an increase in particular antibody titers.

Although our ability to closely describe patterns and abnormalities in the rabbit thorax is limited compared with our abilities in ferrets, *radiography* is still a very important imaging method for the evaluation of a patient with RD. It is preferable to ensure that the patient is in most cases under sedation or anesthesia when performing radiography because of proper positioning. It is preferable to use benzodiazepines, opioids, propofol, and isoflurane anesthesia. The author prefers to use a combination of midazolam 0.2 to 0.5 mg/kg intramuscularly (IM), ketamine 1 to 3 mg/kg IM, and isoflurane anesthesia. The optimal views for thoracic examination are dorsoventral (ventrodorsal) and right and left lateral view. For nasal cavity examination, dorsoventral, right lateral, and 2 lateral oblique views and rostrocaudal view are recommended. Intraoral radiograph of the nasal cavity is helpful in the evaluation of the nasal cavities and incisor and molar apices, without mandibular superposition. Cranial cardiac borders are often indistinct, and cranial mediastinum is opaque, especially if a large amount of fat is present. In some rabbits with chronic RD, one could identify indistinct bronchial pulmonary pattern throughout the lungs. In a more severe case of chronic RD, focal areas

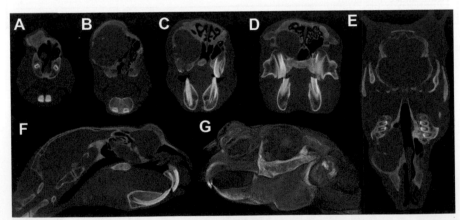

Fig. 5. CT images of a rabbit presented for progressive dyspnea and facial mass (*A–G*). (*A–D*) Axial images. (*E*) Coronal view. (*F*) Sagittal view. (*G*) 3D superficial reconstruction. Note absent conchal structures (*A–C*) and new bone formation at the area of inflammation (*A–G*). The clinical crown of the right maxillary second premolar is missing (*C, E*). Extensive mass filled whole right paranasal sinus (*B–D*) and extramurally obturated right nasal passages (*B–D*); rostral atrophic rhinitis was also present (*A*). Final diagnosis was unilateral rhinitis and paranasal cavity inflammation due to the odontogenic abscess. Bacteriology revealed infection with *Fusobacterium canifelinum, F nucleatum, Bacteroides ovatus, Atopobium parvulum,* and *Proteus mirabilis.* Surgery was performed, and the patient recovered uneventfully. (*Courtesy of* Vladimir Jekl and Karel Hauptman.)

of pulmonary consolidation could be seen. In cases of caudal lung lobe pathologic condition and some systemic diseases (eg, that causes anemia), cranial parts of the lungs are extremely aerated because of overinflation. It is important to remember that radiography should not be performed before basic patient stabilization. Interpretation of radiographs may document the presence of cardiomegaly, pulmonary edema, pleural effusion, or prominent pathologic lung patterns.

Both computed tomography (CT) and MRI provide tomographic images of the skull that allow improved anatomic information concerning many regions difficult to assess with conventional radiography. Nasal cavity, tympanic bulla, and pleural cavity disorders, particularly, are seen in detail on CT, so this examination is preferred by the author, especially in the case of sneezing rabbits (**Fig. 5**).

Endoscopy of the respiratory tract is indicated in cases of unilateral nasal discharge or other respiratory pathologic conditions, rhinoliths, nasal or tracheal foreign bodies, chronic RDs, or respiratory neoplasia. Rhinoscopy allows easy direct access to the nasal cavity for examination, biopsy collection, or exact determination of the follow-up surgical approach. A complete diagnostic approach to nasal diseases is required, and optimal diagnostic work up should be established. CT examination of the head is the optimal method for preoperative nasal cavity evaluation. Rigid endoscopes used for rhinoscopy include 1.0-, 1.9-, and 2.7-mm-diameter telescopes. The patient is intubated and placed in dorsal or lateral recumbency based on the preferences of the examiner. As the endoscope passes the external nares, irrigation with warm saline is started to achieve an optimal view of an examined region. Then, the telescope is slowly advanced caudally; all accessible structures should be examined (**Fig. 6**). Nasopharynx evaluation should be included in a complete nasal cavity evaluation. Bleeding could occur during rhinoscopy, so increasing the rate of irrigation is recommended. Endoscopy is a useful tool not only for direct pathologic condition visualization but also for guided biopsy or treatment (foreign body removal).

Otoscopy is also useful, as many rabbits have asymptomatic otitis media.

Echocardiography and electrocardiography are necessary to document cardiac function and to assess mediastinal masses. Echocardiography should not be performed if a patient has marked respiratory distress. Cardiac measurements and optimal treatment of particular cardiac diseases are similar to those in dogs and cats.

Cytology (nasal swab, bronchoalveolar lavage, fine needle aspiration, effusion determination) and bacteriology/mycology are important from the point of diagnosis, treatment, and prognosis. In the case of biopsy or any mass removal, histopathological examination should be made in all cases.

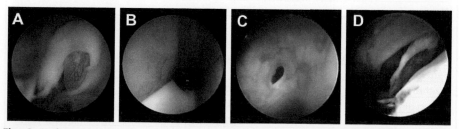

Fig. 6. Endoscopic images of rabbits presented for sneezing (A–D). (A) Presence of pus around medial concha. (B) Presence of pus in the ventral nasal meatus. (C) Normal opening of the paranasal cavities into the nasal cavity is very delicate. (D) Foreign body (hay) lodged in the caudal part of the nasal cavity. (Courtesy of Vladimir Jekl and Karel Hauptman.)

Thoracocentesis is performed with a rabbit in lateral recumbency, with hair shaved and surgically prepared. Thoracocentesis in rabbits involves placing a needle (21–23 gauge) or intravenous (IV) catheter (23–25 gauge) in the seventh to ninth intercostal space along the cranial border of the rib to avoid laceration of intercostal vessels and nerve. The needle or catheter should be placed along the body wall to minimize the risk of lung puncture. Fluid is aspirated directly via a syringe attached to the needle or through the 3-way stopcock. The rest of the approach is similar as was described in ferrets.[12] A sample is obtained to cytology, chemistry, and bacteriology if needed. For therapeutic purposes, fluid is aspirated until clinical signs resolve or negative pressure is reached. Clinical must be aware to not leave the needle or catheter "open," as pneumothorax can develop quickly.

THERAPY

Several challenges arise when evaluating a rabbit with RD. The respiratory system does not have such a high degree of ventilatory reserve as dogs and cats, which can make RDs difficult to treat. Once the diagnosis has been complete, treatment options should be discussed with the owner, as patients with respiratory distress are at increased risk of collapse. The primary goal is initially stabilizing the patient and restoring the normal breathing pattern as soon as possible. Rabbits with RD are at increased risk of collapse, even those with rhinitis, and the animal may require close monitoring and supportive care during first attempts of therapy.

Frequently, after evaluation of the historical and physical examination findings, laboratory examination, and interpretation of the thoracic radiographs, it is possible to determine whether heart or lung disease or other disease is the most likely cause for the respiratory distress.

If pulmonary infiltrates compatible with edema are present on thoracic radiographs, the rabbit should be treated with diuretics, oxygen, cage rest, and possibly, vasodilators. In the author's practice, furosemide (1–6 mg/kg IM or IV every 2–6 hours) is frequently used. Placement of an IV catheter in rabbits is essential and commonly is placed with minimal restraint into the cephalic or marginal ear vein.

Table 2
Common drugs used for respiratory tract infection in rabbits

Drug	Dosage	Frequency
Bacitracin	Local therapy, drops	q6h
Neomycin	Local therapy, drops	q6h
F10 (dilution 1:250)	Local therapy, nebulization	q8–12h
Gentamicin	Local therapy, nebulization	q8–12h
Ofloxacin, levofloxacin	Local therapy, drops	q6h
Systemic therapy		
Azithromycin	15–30 mg/kg orally	q24h
Doxycycline	2.5–5 mg/kg orally, IM	q12h
Enrofloxacin	10–15 mg/kg orally, IM	q12h
Marbofloxacin	5–10 mg/kg orally, IM	q24h
Penicillin G	40,000–60,000 Iu/kg IM	q12h
Trimethoprim sulpha drugs	20–30 mg/kg orally, subcutaneously	q8–12h

Oxygen delivery and air humidification are an important part of symptomatic therapy in rabbits. Oxygen is most easily administered by placing the animal within the oxygen cage.

If a moderate to large volume of pleural effusion is present, it should be removed under ultrasound guidance in order to improve the stability of the patient as well as to help aid in reaching the final diagnosis.

Antibiotics or other drugs should be administered systemically or topically based on the disease severity and exact cause (**Table 2**).

For nebulization, it is preferable to use disinfectants (eg, diluted F10), aminoglycosides alone or in combination with bronchodilators. Moreover, nebulization itself keeps mucosal membranes "hydrated" and acts as an excellent expectorant.

In chronic cases of nasal disease or in the case of periapical infections, rhinotomy, sinusotomy, tooth/teeth extraction, or affected bone removal is indicated.

Surgical treatment of the respiratory tract infection or neoplasia consists of rhinotomy, sinusotomy, and thoracotomy. The surgical approach is best established on CT imaging.[13,14]

Rhinotomy/Rhinostomy

The intubated rabbit is placed in dorsal or lateral recumbency with skin shaved and aseptically prepared. A local anesthetic block is injected along the incision sites and into the periosteum, after which a longitudinal incision is made through the skin and subcutaneous tissue. Blunt dissection of the subcutaneous tissue reveals the periosteum. The thin periosteum layer is gently incised with a scalpel blade and detached from the nasal bone with a periosteal elevator. An osteotomy of the nasal bone or maxilla is performed with a small cone or round rotating dental burr.[13] In the case of midline rhinotomy/rhinostomy, the osteotomy involves both nasal bones allowing nasal septum visualization and inspection of both nasal cavities. The exact place for sinusotomy or rhinotomy, which can be unilateral or bilateral, depends on CT findings. The sample is obtained for bacteriology, and the affected nasal/paranasal cavity is debrided; affected turbinates are excised, and the cavity is then carefully flushed with a sterile fluid (saline, Ringer) with the nostrils directed down to facilitate egress of fluid and to prevent fluid aspiration. If a foreign body or rhinolith is present, it should be removed. When performing a simple rhinotomy procedure, suture can be used to close the periosteum and skin over the surgical site.[13] Another option is to perform a small temporary rhinostomy site, and suturing the skin around the stoma or implantation of a fenestrated urethral catheter, which facilitates local therapy and flushing.[13] The author prefers removing a larger amount of bone, creating a temporary rhinostomy/sinusotomy in a larger extent (1 × 2 cm). The wound is then marsupialized and left open for at least 7 to 10 days. After 7 to 10 days, skin sutures are removed, and the wound is left to heal by secondary intention. The animal is reanesthetized in usually in a 3- to 4-day interval to facilitate optimal wound debridement. Careful patient monitoring, wound debridement, and wound flushing are essential to gain optimal results. In the case of sinusitis and/or rhinitis associated with periapical dental infection, affected bone and teeth need to be removed or extracted.

VACCINATION

Recommended vaccinations for pet rabbits include vaccination against myxoma virus, rabbit hemorrhagic disease virus 1, and rabbit hemorrhagic disease virus 2. In some European countries, vaccination against *P multocida* serotype A and D is also available. In larger rabbitries or rabbit farms, autologous vaccine against particular pathogens can be prepared.

OVERVIEW OF SELECTED RESPIRATORY DISORDERS IN RABBITS
Viral Infections

Rabbit hemorrhagic disease can be caused simultaneously or by both types of RHDV1 and RHDV2.[15,16] These caliciviruses are transmitted via air (short distances), via direct contact with an infected rabbit, via insect, or indirectly with the contaminated environment. The incubation period is 1 to 2 (RHDV1) to 2 to 9 days (RHDV2). Main clinical signs and histopathological findings are associated with liver failure (hepatocyte necropsy). In the case of respiratory tract, epistaxis, hyperemic tracheal mucosa, fluid in the trachea, and/or congested or hemorrhagic lungs can be found. Both diseases are mostly fatal. Diagnosis is based on reverse transcription polymerase chain reaction (PCR) of liver tissue (different RHDV genotypes can be diagnosed); serologic tests can be also used.[17] Prevention of these diseases is possible using vaccination against RHDV1 and RHDV2. Depending on the vaccine type, young rabbits can be vaccinated already from the age 5 or 6 weeks with or without booster at 10 weeks of age (please see particular vaccine leaflet recommendation, as many vaccines exist, especially in European countries). The vaccine is usually given every 12 months or twice yearly.

Myxomatosis

Myxomatosis is caused by leporipoxvirus and is transmitted via direct contact (oculonasal secretion, eroded skin lesions), via biting insects (fleas) or arthropods, or indirectly with the contaminated environment. Clinical signs may vary because of several field viruses with different virulency and are associated with acute death, the classic mucocutaneous form (eg, myxomatous/subcutaneous nodules at the eyelids, ear base, ear pinna, perianal region, mucopurulent keratoconjunctivitis, and blepharitis) and the amyxomatous form.[18,19] Myxoma virus causes immunosuppression, so other clinical signs or death is commonly associated with secondary bacterial infection. The respiratory tract can be affected by skin changes at the nostril area (see **Fig. 4**A) and by lung edema. Diagnosis is made based on typical clinical signs or by histopathology; serologic tests or cultivation is also possible. Prevention consists of vaccination from the age of 4 or 5 weeks of age with or without booster at 10 weeks of age (please see particular vaccine leaflet recommendation as many vaccines exists, especially in European countries). The vaccine is usually given every 6 or 12 months.

Other Viruses

Leporid-4 herpes virus infection was described in Alaska and Canada and was detected in commercial rabbitries. Rabbits developed conjunctivitis, weakness, anorexia, ulcerative dermatitis, respiratory distress, and abortion. Diagnosis is based on PCR of affected tissue. No treatment is yet described. Other viruses causing possible respiratory disorders are only used in laboratory rabbits (eg, *vaccinia virus*, orthopoxvirus).[20]

Under experimental conditions, the rabbits are susceptible to severe acute respiratory syndrome coronavirus 2 (SARS-CoV-2).[21] The infection was asymptomatic, but the infectious virus with peak titers corresponding to $\sim 10^3$ TCID$_{50}$ could be detected up to day 7 postinoculation in the nose. The minimum dose to establish productive infection was 10^5 TCID$_{50}$, indicating that virus transmission between rabbits may be less efficient compared with ferrets and hamsters. The use of young, immunocompetent, and healthy New Zealand white rabbits in the study, however, may not reflect virus shedding and disease in other rabbit breeds or rabbits at different ages. Thus, surveillance studies, including serologic testing, may be needed to assess the presence of SARS-CoV-2 in farmed rabbits.[21] Up until January 15, 2021, no information exists for the presence of spontaneous or transmitted SARS-Cov-2 infection to humans in pet rabbits.

BACTERIAL INFECTIONS
Pasteurella multocida

Pasteurellosis of rabbits is one of the most significant bacterial diseases throughout the world. *P multocida* is a gram-negative, nonmotile coccobacillus, and it is classified into several serotypes, based on 5 capsular antigens (A, B, D, E, and F) and 16 serovars (formerly serotypes) based on lipopolysaccharide antigens.[22–24] To date, pasteurellosis in rabbits is mainly caused by serogroup A, and to a lesser extent, by serogroup D and F strains. Patterns of disease include purulent rhinitis, atrophic rhinitis, otitis media/interna, conjunctivitis, bronchopneumonia, abscessation, genital tract infections, abortions, neonatal mortality, and septicemia.[25] The primary area of infection is a nasal cavity.[25] Cause of rabbit rhinitis and respiratory tract infection is complex, and also other bacteria are involved, *Staphylococcus aureus*, *Moraxella catarrhalis*, *Bordetella bronchiseptica*, *Mycoplasma* sp, and *Klebsiella pneumoniae*. Breeders and owners have named this multifactorial disease "snuffling rabbit or snuffles," as it is associated with nasal discharge and sneezing (see **Figs. 4**B and 6A, B).

The organism is transmitted through aerosol or direct contact with animals shedding the organism from nasal or vaginal secretions. *P multocida* is then spread to other tissues: to the lower respiratory tract by aerogenous route; to the middle ear via the Eustachian tube; hematogenously to other parts of the body; by local extension; and to the genital tract by venereal route. Chronic asymptomatic carriers exist, and the organism can be harbored in the middle ear cavity or nasopharynx.[25] In 1 study in 67 rabbits, 27% of rabbits had subclinical middle ear abnormalities detected using CT imaging; however, no bacterial cause was given, so not all cases may be assigned to Pasteurella infection.[26] Pasteurella is often recoverable from the watering nipples

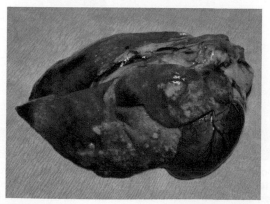

Fig. 7. Rabbit lungs of a pet rabbit infected with *P multocida*. Note multiple miliary and larger abscesses of yellowish color within the lung parenchyma. (*Courtesy of* Vladimir Jekl and Karel Hauptman.)

used by infected rabbits,[25] so disinfection of nipple-drinkers, if they are used, is also of great importance to prevent disease transmission.

Common clinical signs include mucopurulent nasal discharge, epiphora, sneezing, and dyspnea, which are associated with rhinitis/sinusitis, conjunctivitis, dacryocystitis, and, in the case of dyspnea, lower respiratory tract infection. As rabbits are obligate nasal breathers, obstruction of the nasal cavity with pus and mucosal edema associated with bacterial infection can led to cyanosis and open mouth breathing, which is a life-threatening condition preventing food and water intake and is quickly followed by the animal collapse and death. Other forms of the disease are pneumonia (**Fig. 7**), pleuritis, otitis media, meningitis, perioophoritis, salpingitis, pyometra, orchitis, and septicemia. Bronchopneumonia may vary from localized cranioventral involvement to acute necrotizing fibrinopurulent or fibrinohemorrhagic bronchopneumonia.[25] Chronic disease may encompass an entire lung lobe, with fibrinopurulent pleuritis, pericarditis, and empyema. In some cases, the disease can be localized only in 1 lung lobe or abscess/abscesses are formed. Abscesses, which contain white to yellowish pasty exudate, can involve subcutaneous space, mammary gland tissue, and various organs in the body (**Fig. 8**). Facial abscesses, however, are caused primarily by other bacteria than Pasteurella.[27]

The diagnosis is based on clinical signs, thoracic and tracheal auscultation, radiography, rhinoscopy, and bacterial culture. CT imaging is particularly useful in identifying nasal cavity disease (rhinitis, sinusitis), otitis media, and lung lesions. Sampling for bacterial culture consists of deep nasal swab or bronchoalveolar lavage; see the same technique in Maria Ardiaca García and colleagues' article, "Respiratory Diseases in Guinea Pigs, Chinchillas and Degus," in this issue. Nasal swabs, although useful in identifying carriers/shedders of the organism, will not necessarily detect all infected animals.[25] ELISA tests are available, but paired samples need to be examined to prove the increase of antibody titers. PCR can be used for bacteria detection, but molecular methods are more useful for characterizing isolates.

Therapy includes supportive care, nebulization (F10, aminoglycosides, oxymetazoline), and antibiotic treatment (local or systemic). Generally, *P multocida* strains isolated from rabbits are sensitive to chloramphenicol, novobiocin, oxytetracycline,

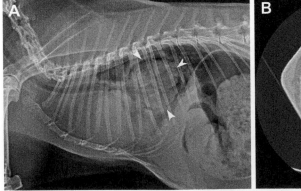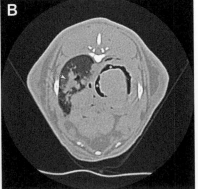

Fig. 8. Lateral radiograph (*A*) and CT axial view (*B*) of a rabbit with intrathoracic abscess. Large nodular pattern was obvious on radiograph and was surrounded with radiolucent halo (*A, arrowheads*) and mixed pattern, also seen on CT (*B; asterisk*). Left lung was consolidated, and no aerated area was detected on CT. Right lung was also affected with inflammatory changes (*B;* note hyperdense area within the parenchyma, *arrowheads*). Fine needle biopsy and cultivation revealed infection with *P multocida.*

penicillin G, nitrofurazone, fluoroquinolones, azithromycin, and trimethoprim-sulfa-methoxazole.[28] Local therapy may include oxymetazoline and local antibiotics (fluoroquinolones, sulfonamides, bacitracin, neomycin) in drops. In the case of rabbits, *P multocida* antibiotic resistance in farm rabbits is relatively low.[29,30] There is a report that enrofloxacin at the dosage of 5 mg/kg given subcutaneously twice a day for 10 days did not clear the infection, even though in vitro testing showed very good results.[31] This antibiotic sensitivity can be true for all antibiotic treatments, as the infection can be present also in the paranasal sinuses, Eustachian tube, and the middle ear cavity, where sufficient antibiotic concentration cannot be achieved, so reinfection of nasal cavity is common. Therefore, endoscopy and CT scan are of high diagnostic value and are important for the targeted treatment, especially for the upper respiratory tract infection. Nasal and ocular discharge cleaning with moistened gauze can help to remove irritant material from the nostrils and skin. Side-stream capnography done using a face mask may be clinically helpful to determine extant oxygenation/CO_2 levels. SpO_2 levels with pulse oximetry may also help evaluate response to treatment.[28]

In some European countries, a vaccine against most common Pasteurella serotypes (A, D) is available. Rabbits are vaccinated at the age of 4 weeks, with boosters at 7 and 10 weeks of age. Then, the rabbit should be vaccinated every 6 months. In the case of older rabbits, the vaccination protocol consists of primo-vaccination with 1 booster 3 weeks apart and then in 6-month interval.

Bordetella bronchiseptica and *Staphylococcus aureus* Infections

B bronchiseptica can be cultivated from the nasal cavity in both clinically normal and ill rabbits. B *bronchiseptica* is an opportunistic pathogen, especially in the case of P multocida infection and impair clearance mechanism by ciliostasis and thus facilitate lower respiratory tract infection with other bacteria. Lesions associated with *B bronchiseptica* infections, when present, are fibrinopurulent bronchopneumonia and interstitial pneumonia.[25] S *aureus* can cause mucopurulent rhinitis, bronchopneumonia, and/or lung abscessation. For diagnosis and therapy, see earlier discussion.

Cilia-Associated Respiratory Bacillus Infection

Colonization of the apices of ciliated epithelial cells lining the larynx, trachea, and bronchi with cilia-associated respiratory (CAR) bacillus has been observed in laboratory and farm rabbits. CAR bacillus was different than the rat isolate, causing rhinitis and mild to moderate inflammatory lesions in the respiratory tract, particularly bronchi.[25]

Streptococcus spp Infection

Streptococcus agalactiae caused acute respiratory distress, fever, and convulsions in farm rabbits. Necropsy revealed congestion and hemorrhage in multiple organs, particularly the lungs.[32] In pet rabbits at the author clinic, *Streptococcus intermedius* is relatively commonly associated with odontogenic abscesses and sinusitis in rabbits.

Treponematosis

Treponema paraluis cuniculi is a spirochete that causes ulcerative to crusty skin lesions at the nostrils and surrounding skin, which may influence both inspiration and expiration. Similar skin lesions can be seen at the anogenital area. Diagnosis is made with wet mount preparation and dark-field examination of the deep skin craping or using silver staining on histopathology. Serology and PCR confirm the presence of antigen. Treatment consists of a 5-day course of penicillin G IM administration (40–60,000 IU/kg every 12 hours).

MYCOBACTERIAL INFECTIONS

Mycobacterial infection of the respiratory tract of pet rabbits is extremely rare.[33,34] *Mycobacterium avium* and *Mycobacterium caprae* were identified mostly in farm rabbits.[35,36] Rabbits were cachectic. On postmortem examination, white nodules with a caseous necrotic center can be seen on serosal surfaces and within the parenchyma of lungs, liver, kidney, and in the mesentery, brain, and all layers of the intestine. Histopathology revealed acid-fast bacilli stained with Ziehl-Neelsen. Other specifications are possible with agglutination tests and PCR.

In pet rabbits, *Mycobacterium genavense* was diagnosed on postmortem examination of a pet rabbit with granulomatous pneumonia.[37] The organism was identified by PCR and 16S ribosomal RNA gene sequencing. In another 2 pet rabbits, *M avium* subsp *hominissuis* was diagnosed postmortem in 2 rabbits,[38,39] but lung granulomatous lesions were described only in one of them.[39]

Zoonotic potential should be considered because of the close contact between pets and their owners; however, as the rabbits are commonly asymptomatic, the pathologist or practitioner who is performing postmortem examination is in the closest contact with the mycobacteria, so protective and hygiene measures should be on high level (eg, using mouth drapes).

MYCOTIC INFECTION

Aspergillosis spp infection occurs only sporadically in rabbits. Infection is often subclinical with granulomatous lung lesions found during necropsy.[40]

PARASITIC DISEASE

Pneumonia of parasitic origin in pet rabbits is extremely rare. Cases of aberrant larva migrans (*Cuterebra* sp)[41] and verminous pneumonia (*Protostrongylus* sp)[42] were described.

NEOPLASTIC AND PSEUDONEOPLASTIC LESIONS

Intranasal adenocarcinoma was diagnosed in two 6- and 8-year-old pet rabbits presenting with dyspnea nonresponsive to antibiotic therapy.[43,44] Diagnosis was based on CT and histopathological examination after mass surgical excision. In 1 case, the patient was euthanized 3 days later because of only temporary improvement. In the other case, the surgery was complemented with radiotherapy and consisted of 8 fractions of 6 Gy administered once a week. After the completion of radiation therapy, the soft tissue density in the right nasal cavity, as detected by CT, significantly decreased. The prognosis has remained good for over 3 years after treatment.[44]

Various *oral cavity and dental tumors* present in rabbits. If they are growing near the nostrils or in the maxillary bone, they can affect breathing.[45]

Laryngeal and Tracheal Tumors

Progressive dyspnea was encountered in 2 rabbits suffering from intraluminal laryngeal osteochondrosarcoma and tracheal adenocarcinoma. No treatment was described as in 1 case the client elected euthanasia and in another rabbit the tumor was diagnosed postmortem.[46]

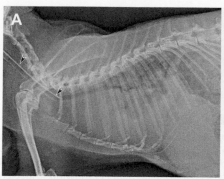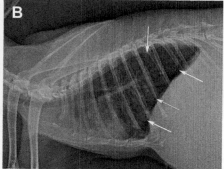

Fig. 9. Lateral radiographs of rabbit, which were presented with dyspnea (*A, B*). Note multiple lung nodules in both radiographs (*B; arrows*). (*A*) Metastases of uterine adenocarcinoma into the lung parenchyma; also thoracic effusion and lung edema are present. Metastases were also present in the cranial lung lobes, but they are not visualized because of superposition of the lungs with mediastinum, and thoracic effusion. Arrowheads showing the tracheal tube in the tracheal lumen. (*B*) Intrapulmonary metastases of the mammary gland adenocarcinoma.

Lung Tumors

Primary lung tumors are rare, and apart from others, papillary adenoma and adenocarcinoma were described. Most commonly, metastases of uterine carcinoma, mammary gland adenocarcinoma, or lymphoma are seen (**Figs. 9** and **10**).[47,48] Diagnosis is based on adspection, mammary gland and abdominal palpation, hematology, radiography, and abdominal ultrasound (**Fig. 9**). Metastatic lesions are seen on radiographs as a nodular pattern. Even though the metastases are not seen on the radiograph at the time of diagnosis, the patient should be monitored for a long term after surgery, and thoracic radiographs should be repeated in 3 to 69 months. The treatment of choice of uterine and mammary gland carcinoma is ovariohysterectomy and affected mammary gland excision. If the metastases are already present, euthanasia should be considered (**Fig. 10**). Prevention can be best achieved by preventative ovariohysterectomy or ovariectomy from 5 to 6 months of age.

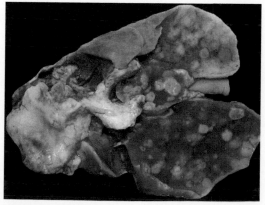

Fig. 10. Multiple pulmonary metastases of the uterine carcinoma in a rabbit presented with dyspnea. (*Courtesy of* Vladimir Jekl and Karel Hauptman.)

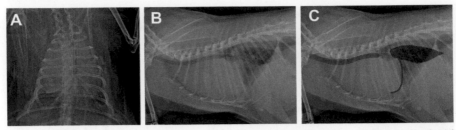

Fig. 11. Dorsoventral (*A*) and lateral (*B, C*) thoracic radiographs of a rabbit presented with progressive dyspnea and exophthalmos. Cranial mediastinal mass dislocated trachea dorsally (*B, C; blue*) and heart caudodorsally (*A–C; red line* on panel C showing caudal pericardial border). Caudal lung lobes were relatively easily seen (*purple* on panel C) showing suspected thoracic effusion. (*Courtesy of* Vladimir Jekl and Karel Hauptman.)

Thymoma is the most common mediastinal mass in the rabbit.[47,49] Apart from thymomas, thymic lymphomas, thymic carcinomas, and mediastinal abscesses should also be considered as possible causes of mediastinal masses in rabbits.[48,50,51] Rabbits with thymomas show clinical signs of dyspnea, exercise intolerance, bilateral exophthalmos, bilateral prolapse of the third eyelid, and anorexia. Some rabbits are asymptomatic. Reported paraneoplastic syndromes in rabbits with thymoma include anemia, hypercalcemia, systemic immune disorders, and dermatoses (eg, sebaceous adenitis).[48,49]

Diagnosis is based on thoracic radiography, thoracic ultrasound, or CT scan with subsequent tumor identification using fine needle aspiration biopsy or histology (**Fig. 11**).

Therapy includes medical therapy, radiation therapy, or surgical mediastinal mass removal. In the case of the presence of thymic cysts filled with fluid, this fluid can be aspirated to partially release the pressure on the lungs; however, this treatment is only temporary. Medical treatment includes administration of oral prednisone 0.5 to 1 mg/kg twice a day long term.[52] Surgical therapy consists of cranial thoracotomy and mass blunt and sharp dissection, vessel ligation, and excision (**Fig. 12**). Because of a high rate of perioperative mortality, intensive perioperative care, the provision of a low-stress environment, and analgesia (eg, methadone 0.5 mg/kg IM every 4 hours and meloxicam 1 mg/kg subcutaneously every 12 hours) are recommended for a successful outcome. Radiation therapy was used in rabbits with thymoma using intensity-

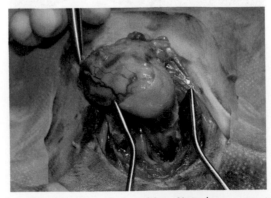

Fig. 12. Perioperative view of a thymoma excision. Note large mass evacuated from the thoracic cavity using cranial sternotomy and midline approach.

modulated radiotherapy of 42 to 48 Gy and hypofractionated radiotherapy of 24 to 32 Gy.[53,54] Described postradiation adverse effects were associated with acute death within a few days after radiation, anemia, cardiac failure, and suspected hypotrichosis. Thymoma size decreased to at least 30% of its original size. Median survival time was more than 700 days. Hypofractionated radiotherapy seems to be more promising as less adverse effects were seen; however, more studies need to be done to prove this hypothesis.[49]

OTHER DISEASES

Foreign body can be present in the nasal cavity (see **Fig. 6D**) or trachea and may cause mild to severe respiratory compromise. Most commonly, the foreign nasal body causes unilateral rhinitis with serous to mucopurulent discharge. Foreign bodies (particles of hay or grass) can be as long as 3 to 6 cm. Foreign body calcification can be seen as a radiopaque/dense small oval to rounded object in the nasal cavity. Diagnosis is made on radiography, endoscopy, or CT. The foreign body can be removed using endoscopy or via rhinotomy.

Nasal septum deformation was diagnosed in several animals at the author's clinic, which was asymptomatic or was associated with silent wheezing sounds.

Laryngeal paralysis was described in forums in several rabbits associated with abnormal respiratory sounds. Arytenoid cartilage was mostly affected. Laryngeal paralysis can be treated similarly as in dogs using nonsteroidal anti-inflammatory drugs or arytenoid lateralization by tie-back.[55,56]

Tracheal stenosis was described in rabbits in association with intubation.[57] Dyspnea was present 17 to 21 days after the procedure. At necropsy examination, focal chronic inflammation and significant localized narrowing of the tracheal lumen were found in all cases. The affected sites corresponded to the position of the bevel of the endotracheal tube during anesthesia. In another case, tracheal stenosis, which developed 12 days after intubation, was managed using a tracheal stent.[58] Although routine endotracheal intubation always carries the risk of secondary complications, such as tracheal stricture formation, factors such as excessive patient movement or movement of the endotracheal tube during intubation, aggressive intubation, cuff overinflation, or dehumidified air can contribute to increased risk of tracheal injury and subsequent stricture formation.[57] Therefore, care should be taken by clinicians to eliminate or minimize these risk factors.

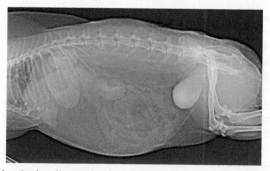

Fig. 13. Lateral abdominal radiograph of a rabbit with very subtle dyspnea. Diaphragmatic hernia of the right kidney and surrounding fat were diagnosed based on pyelography and confirmed on surgery.

ORGANOMEGALY, ABDOMINAL DISTENSION

Because of the small thoracic cavity, significant enlargement of abdominal organs (eg, gastric dilatation) or ascites can cause respiratory distress.[59] Also, during surgery with a rabbit in dorsal recumbency, slight thoracic elevation is recommended to not compromise spontaneous respiration or assisted ventilation. Diaphragmatic hernia (**Fig. 13**) is a very rare condition and is commonly associated with trauma.

PLEURAL EFFUSIONS

The total surface area of the visceral pleura (both cavities) is approximately 220 cm^2 in 2-kg rabbits.[60,61] The pleurae comprise a layer of mesothelial cells and the underlying connective tissue. The visceral pleura is thin ($\sim$ 15–35 μm) in rabbits and supplied by pulmonary arteries.[62] The total volume of liquid contained in both pleural spaces is approximately 1 mL (0.45 mL/kg).[60] Pleural fluid can be divided into the fluid which cannot be collected, because it adheres to the walls of the space (0.30–0.52 mL) and the liquid that can be collected (0.13–0.20 mL/kg) in rabbits. The pleural liquid in rabbits and dogs contains 1500 to 2500 cells·mm^3: mesothelial cells (9%–30%), monocytes/macrophages (61%–77%), lymphocytes (7%–11%), and neutrophils (<2%).[61,63]

Pleural effusions are commonly associated with congestive heart failure and cytologically characterized as *transudate or modified transudate*. Pleural effusions are present mostly together with lung edema, splenomegaly, and hepatomegaly. Animals are presented with exercise intolerance and dyspnea or tachypnea in the absence of signs of rhinitis. Diagnosis is based on radiography, echocardiography, electrocardiography, and cytologic evaluation of fluid aspirated from the thorax. Initial treatment consists of IV or IM furosemide administration (4–6 mg/kg) to support fluid absorption from the thorax while monitoring kidney function and patient hydration using IV fluid therapy. Further treatment depends on the particular cardiac disease.[11]

Inflammatory cells and the presence of bacteria in macrophages or neutrophiles (*pyothorax*) can be found in cases of pleuritis associated with severe respiratory bacterial infections (*P multocida, S aureus*, Streptococci, *Escherichia coli* infection).

Chylothorax is the accumulation of chyle (lymph) within the pleural cavity. Chylothorax occurs when a disruption occurs to normal lymphatic flow from the abdominal viscera to the vena cava via the thoracic duct.[64] Chylothorax was described in pet rabbits as idiopathic or in association with thymoma.[65,66] A pseudochylous effusion was described in another pet rabbit with intrathoracic malignant lymphoma.[51] Rabbits were presented with respiratory distress characterized by increased respiratory rate and effort. Diagnosis was made by radiography, ultrasound, and analyses of the aspirated sample of thoracic fluid. Chylous effusions are characterized by cholesterol concentrations that are decreased or within the reference range and an elevated triglyceride concentration when compared with plasma. Triglyceride concentrations may be markedly increased in chylous effusions. In contrast, pseudochylous effusions have elevated cholesterol concentrations, whereas triglyceride concentrations are equal to or lower than those of plasma. Cholesterol-to-triglyceride ratios in chylous effusions are generally less than 1. Fluid-to-plasma triglyceride ratios greater than 2 to 3:1 is diagnostic for a chylous effusion.[65,66]

ALLERGY/HYPERSENSITIVITY

Spontaneous allergic rhinitis in pet rabbits was not yet described in the literature. In the author's clinic, a referred rabbit with chronic sneezing had positive skin allergic testing to the meadow grasses. However, the final diagnosis was a foreign body (4-cm-long grass; see **Fig. 6**D) in the nasal cavity. After endoscopic foreign body removal and secondary bacterial infection treatment, the rabbit recovered uneventfully.

"Hay allergy," which is described by some owners, is when the rabbit is heard sneezing when is eating hay. Commonly, this sneezing is associated with dusty hay (dust inhalation and nasal irritation), so removal of dust or buying commercial hay without the dust is recommended.

CLINICS CARE POINTS

- Rabbits are obligate nasal breathers, and nasal cavity obstruction is a life-threatening condition.

- Rabbits at rest breathe mostly through the activity of diaphragm, showing minimal movement of the chest wall.

- Open mouth breathing is a life-threatening condition and must be addressed and treated immediately.

- The most common respiratory pathogen is *Pasteurella multocida*.

- Chronic rhinitis unresponsive to medical treatment can be associated with otitis media and paranasal cavity/sinuses infection.

- Diagnostic imaging, especially radiography, endoscopy and computed tomography, is extremely useful when evaluating rabbit nasal passages, tympanic bulla, and lungs.

- Therapy includes medical treatment, and in the case of nasal cavity disease, also rhinotomy/sinusotomy or rhinostomy/sinusotomy.

DISCLOSURE

The article was supported by internal agency of the University of Veterinary and Pharmaceutical Sciences Brno (ITA FVL 2020).

REFERENCES

1. Mlynski G, Grützenmacher S, Plontke S, et al. Correlation of nasal morphology and respiratory function. Rhinology 2001;39(4):197–201.
2. Xi J, Si XA, Kim J, et al. Anatomical details of the rabbit nasal passages and their implications in breathing, air conditioning, and olfaction. Anat Rec 2016;299(7): 853–68.
3. Churchill SE, Shackelford LL, Georgi JN, et al. Morphological variation and airflow dynamics in the human nose. Am J Hum Biol 2004;16:625–38.
4. Badran KW, Chang JC, Kuan EC, et al. Anatomy and surgical approaches to the rabbit nasal septum. JAMA Facial Plast Surg 2017;19(5):386–91.
5. Pereira ME, Macri NP, Creasy DM. Evaluation of the rabbit nasal cavity in inhalation studies and a comparison with other common laboratory species and man. Toxicol Pathol 2011;9(5):893–900.
6. Casteleyn C, Cornillie P, Hermens A, et al. Topography of the rabbit paranasal sinuses as a prerequisite to model human sinusitis. Rhinology 2010;48(3): 300–4.
7. Chin E Jr. The rabbit: an illustrated anatomical guide. Stockton, california, USA: University of the Pacific; 1957. Thesis. Available at: https://scholarlycommons. pacific.edu/uop_etds/1366.

8. Autifi MAH, EL-Banna AK, Ebaid AES. Morphological study of rabbit lung bronchial tree and pulmonary vessels using corrosion-cast technique. Al-Azhar Assiut Med J 2015;13(3 supl 1):41–51.
9. Loewen MS, Walner DL. Dimensions of rabbit subglottis and trachea. Lab Anim 2001;35:253–6.
10. Jekl V, Hauptman K, Knotek Z. Respiratory problems in rabbits and rats. Slov Vet Res 2011;(48 Suppl.13):143–5.
11. Orcutt C, Malakoff R L. Cardiovascular disease. In: Quesenberry KE, Orcutt C, Mans Ch, et al, editors. Ferrets, rabbits, and rodents. Clinical medicine and surgery. 4th edition. Amsterdam, Netherlands: Elsevier; 2020. p. 250–7.
12. Wyre NR, Hess L. Clinical technique: ferret thoracocentesis. Sem Avian Exot Pet Med 2005;14(1):22–5.
13. Lennox AM. Rhinotomy and rhinostomy for surgical treatment of chronic rhinitis in two rabbits. J Exot Pet Med 2013;22(4):383–92.
14. Capello V. Rhinostomy as surgical treatment of odontogenic rhinitis in three pet rabbits. J Exot Pet Med 2014;23(2):172–87.
15. Abrantes J, van der Loo W, Le Pendu J, et al. Rabbit haemorrhagic disease (RHD) and rabbit haemorrhagic disease virus (RHDV): a review. Vet Res 2012; 43(1):12.
16. Rouco C, Aguayo-Adán JA, Santoro S, et al. Worldwide rapid spread of the novel rabbit haemorrhagic disease virus (GI.2/RHDV2/b). Transbound Emerg Dis 2019; 66(4):1762–4.
17. Harcourt-Brown FM, Harcourt-Brown N, Joudou LM. RHDV2 epidemic in UK pet rabbits. Part 2: PCR results and correlation with vaccination status. J Small Anim Pract 2020;61(8):487–93.
18. Stanford MM, Werden SJ, McFadden G. Myxoma virus in the European rabbit: interactions between the virus and its susceptible host. Vet Res 2007;38(2): 299–318.
19. Rosell JM, de la Fuente LF, Francisco P, et al. Myxomatosis and rabbit haemorrhagic disease: a 30-year study of the occurrence on commercial farms in Spain. Animals (Basel) 2019;9(10):780.
20. Kerr PJ, Donnelly TM. Viral infections in rabbits. Vet Clin North Am Exot Anim Pract 2013;16:437–68.
21. Mykytyn AZ, Lamers MM, Okba NMA, et al. Susceptibility of rabbits to SARS-CoV-2. Emerg Microbes Infect 2020. https://doi.org/10.1080/22221751.2020. 1868951.
22. Deeb BJ, DiGiacomo RF, Bernard BL, et al. Pasteurella multocida and Bordetella bronchiseptica infections in rabbits. J Clin Microbiol 1990;28(1):70–5.
23. Jaglic Z, Jeklova E, Leva L, et al. Experimental study of pathogenicity of Pasteurella multocida serogroup F in rabbits. Vet Microbiol 2008;126:168–77.
24. Massacci FR, Magistrali CF, Cucco L, et al. Characterization of Pasteurella multocida involved in rabbit infections. Vet Microbiol 2018;213:66–72.
25. Barthold SW, Griffey SM, Percy DH. Rabbit. In: Pathology of laboratory rodents and rabbits. 4th edition. Oxford, UK: Wiley Blackwell; 2016. p. 253–324. https://doi.org/10.1002/9781118924051.ch06.
26. de Matos R, Ruby J, Van Hatten RA, et al. Computed tomographic features of clinical and subclinical middle ear disease in domestic rabbits (Oryctolagus cuniculus): 88 cases (2007-2014). J Am Vet Med Assoc 2015;246(3):336–43.
27. Gardhouse S, Sanchez-Migallon Guzman D, Paul-Murphy J, et al. Bacterial isolates and antimicrobial susceptibilities from odontogenic abscesses in rabbits: 48 cases. Vet Rec 2017;181(20):538.

28. Johnson-Delaney CA, Orosz SE. Rabbit respiratory system: clinical anatomy, physiology and disease. Vet Clin North Am Exot Anim Pract 2011;14(2):257–66.
29. Ferreira TSP, Moreno LZ, Felizardo MR, et al. Pheno- and genotypic characterization of Pasteurella multocida isolated from cats, dogs and rabbits from Brazil. Comp Immunol Microbiol Infect Dis 2016;45:48–52.
30. Bourély C, Cazeau G, Jouy E, et al. Antimicrobial resistance of Pasteurella multocida isolated from diseased food-producing animals and pets. Vet Microbiol 2019;235:280–4.
31. Mähler M, Stünkel S, Ziegowski C, et al. Inefficacy of enrofloxacin in the elimination of Pasteurella multocida in rabbits. Lab Anim 1995;29(2):192–9.
32. Ren SY, Geng Y, Wang KY, et al. Streptococcus agalactiae infection in domestic rabbits, Oryctolagus cuniculus. Transbound Emerg Dis 2014;61:e92–5.
33. McClure DE. Mycobacteriosis in the rabbit and rodent. Vet Clin North Am Exot Anim Pract 2012;15(1):85–99.
34. Gleeson M, Petritz OA. Emerging infectious diseases of rabbits. Vet Clin North Am Exot Anim Pract 2020;23(2):249–61.
35. Himes EH, Miller S, Miller LD, et al. Mycobacterium avium isolated from a domestic rabbit with lesions in the central nervous system. J Vet Diagn Invest 1989; 1:76–8.
36. Sevilla IA, Arnal MC, Fuertes M, et al. Tuberculosis outbreak caused by Mycobacterium caprae in a rabbit farm in Spain. Transbound Emerg Dis 2020;67(1): 431–41.
37. Ludwig E, Reischl U, Janik D, et al. Granulomatous pneumonia caused by Mycobacterium genavense in a dwarf rabbit (Oryctolagus cuniculus). Vet Pathol 2009; 46:1000–2.
38. Klotz D, Barth SA, Baumgärtner W, et al. Mycobacterium avium subsp. hominissuis infection in a domestic rabbit, Germany. Emerg Infect Dis 2018;24(3):596–8.
39. Bertram CA, Barth SA, Glöckner B, et al. Intestinal Mycobacterium avium infection in pet dwarf rabbits (Oryctolagus cuniculus). J Comp Pathol 2020;180:73–8.
40. Matsui T, Taguchi-Ochi S, Takano M, et al. Pulmonary aspergillosis in apparently healthy young rabbits. Vet Pathol 1985;22(3):200–5.
41. Sutherland M, Higbie CT, Crossland NA, et al. Aberrant migration of Cuterebra larvae in 2 domestic rabbits (Oryctolagus cuniculus). J Exot Pet Med 2017; 26(1):57–62.
42. Sharma R, Kapoor D, Kumar R. A rare case of verminous pneumonia in domestic rabbit. J Parasit Dis 2017;41(3):716–7.
43. Lennox AM, Reavill D. Nasal mucosal adenocarcinoma in a pet rabbit. J Exot Pet Med 2014;23(4):397–402.
44. Nakata M, Miwa Y, Tsuboi M, et al. Surgical and localized radiation therapy for an intranasal adenocarcinoma in a rabbit. J Vet Med Sci 2014;76(12):1659–62.
45. Miwa Y, Nakata M, Takimoto H, et al. Spontaneous oral tumours in 18 rabbits (2005–2015). J Small Anim Pract 2019. https://doi.org/10.1111/jsap.13082.
46. Bertram CA, Klopfleisch R, Muller K. Tracheal and laryngeal tumors in two domestic rabbits (Oryctolagus cuniculus). J Exot Pet Med 2019;29:142–6.
47. Bertram CA, Bertram B, Bartel A, et al. Neoplasia and tumor-like lesions in pet rabbits (Oryctolagus cuniculus): a retrospective analysis of cases between 1995 and 2019. Vet Pathol 2020. https://doi.org/10.1177/0300985820973460.
48. van Zeeland Y. Rabbit oncology: diseases, diagnostics, and therapeutics. Vet Clin North Am Exot Anim Pract 2017 Jan;20(1):135–82.
49. Summa NM, Brandão J. Evidence-based advances in rabbit medicine. Vet Clin North Am Exot Anim Pract 2017;20(3):749–71.

50. Wagner F, Beinecke A, Fehr M, et al. Recurrent bilateral exophthalmos associated with metastatic thymic carcinoma in a pet rabbit. J Small Anim Pract 2005;46(8): 393–7.
51. Weber KO, Willimzik HF. Intrathoracic malignant lymphoma and pseudochylothorax in a pet rabbit. Kleintierpraxis 1998;43(8):617–26.
52. Künzel F, Hittmair KM, Hassan J, et al. Thymomas in rabbits: clinical evaluation, diagnosis, and treatment. J Am Anim Hosp Assoc 2012;48(2):97–104.
53. Andres KM, Kent M, Siedlecki CT, et al. The use of megavoltage radiation therapy in the treatment of thymomas in rabbits: 19 cases. Vet Comp Oncol 2012;10(2): 82–94.
54. Dolera M, Malfassi L, Mazza G, et al. Feasibility for using hypofractionated stereotactic volumetric modulated arc radiotherapy (VMAT) with adaptive planning for treatment of thymoma in rabbits: 15 cases. Vet Radiol Ultrasound 2016;57(3): 313–20.
55. Lee S, Seon S, Park K, et al. Vocal fold reconstruction using an autologous pedicled fat flap in a rabbit model. Laryngoscope 2020;130(7):1770–4.
56. MacPhail CM. Laryngeal disease in dogs and cats: an update. Vet Clin North Am Small Anim Pract 2020;50(2):295–310.
57. Grint NJ, Sayers IR, Cecchi R, et al. Postanaesthetic tracheal strictures in three rabbits. Lab Anim 2006;40(3):301–8.
58. Ferris RL, Quesenberry KE, Weisse CW. Outcome of intraluminal tracheal stent placement for tracheal stenosis in a rabbit (Oryctolagus cuniculus). J Exot Pet Med 2019;31:23–7.
59. D'Angelo E, Pecchiari M, Acocella F, et al. Effects of abdominal distension on breathing pattern and respiratory mechanics in rabbits. Respir Physiol Neurobiol 2002;130(3):293–304.
60. Miserocchi G, Agostoni E. Contents of the pleural space. J Appl Physiol 1971;30: 208–13.
61. Zocchi L. Physiology and pathophysiology of pleural fluid turnover. Eur Respir J 2002;20(6):1545–58.
62. Bernaudin J-F, Fleury J. Anatomy of the blood and lymphatic circulation of the pleural serosa. In: Chrétien J, Bignon J, Hirsch A, editors. The pleura in Health and disease. New York: Dekker; 1985. p. 23–42.
63. Sahn SA, Willcox ML, Good JT Jr, et al. Characteristics of normal rabbit pleural fluid: physiologic and biochemical implications. Lung 1979;156(1):63–9.
64. Levshin S, Eshar D, Naor A. Idiopathic chylothorax in a pet rabbit (Oryctolagus cuniculus). Companion Anim 2016;21(9):534–7.
65. Pilny AA, Reavill D. Chylothorax and thymic lymphoma in a pet rabbit (Oryctolagus cuniculus). J Exot Pet Med 2008;17(4):295–9.
66. Fossum TW, Jacobs RM, Birchard SJ. Evaluation of cholesterol and triglyceride concentrations in differentiating chylous and nonchylous pleural effusions in dogs and cats. J Am Vet Med Assoc 1986;188:49–51.

Respiratory Disorders in Ferrets

Angela M. Lennox, DVM, DABVP-Avian, ECM, DECZM-Small Mammal

KEYWORDS

- Ferret • Respiratory • Pulmonary

KEY POINTS

- Ferrets are a model for many respiratory diseases in humans, in particular viral diseases such as influenza and SARS-CoV-2.
- Beyond viral diseases, ferrets are susceptible to many disorders affecting other mammal species, including bacteria, parasites, fungal organisms, and neoplasia.
- A thorough workup is important to identify important conditions that may directly or indirectly affect the respiratory tract.

Ferrets are susceptible to many disorders affecting the respiratory tract including both primary diseases and diseases of other body systems secondarily affecting the respiratory tract. Some primary respiratory diseases are shared with other mammal species including humans.

Infectious diseases include bacterial, fungal, parasitic, and viral.

RESPIRATORY TRACT ANATOMY

Anatomy is similar to that of other mammalian species and has been thoroughly described.[1]

The nasal cavity is divided by the nasal septum, both of which connect via the nasopharyngeal orifice to the pharynx. The Eustachian tubes connect the pharynx to the middle ear.

Lungs are made up of 2 left lobes (apical and diaphragmatic) and 4 right lobes (apical, middle, diaphragmatic, and accessory). Because the thorax is longer than in most mammals, the lungs occupy an area from the intercostal space 1 to 10–11.[2]

Ferrets share similarities with humans, including susceptibility for certain respiratory pathogens. For this reason, ferrets are often laboratory models for investigation of respiratory disease in humans.[3–5]

A few features of the respiratory tract are important and have clinical significance.

The author is a veterinary advisor for Oxbow Animal Health and Jurox Company.
Avian and Exotic Animal Clinic, 9330 Waldemar Road, Indianapolis, IN 46268, USA
E-mail address: alennox@exoticvetclinic.com

Vet Clin Exot Anim 24 (2021) 483–493
https://doi.org/10.1016/j.cvex.2021.02.002

The length of the trachea is relatively longer than that in dogs and cats, which reduces risk of passing an endotracheal tube into a single primary bronchus. The thoracic inlet is narrow compared with other similar carnivores and contains the trachea, esophagus, major blood vessels, and cranial mediastinal lymph nodes. Enlargement of the esophagus or mediastinal lymph nodes may have more severe consequences.[1,6] The thorax is long and cone shaped, and is highly compressible and compliant, allowing ferrets to fit into tight spaces and turn completely around.[2]

RESPIRATORY TRACT PHYSIOLOGY

Respiratory rate in the normal relaxed ferret is 33 to 36 breaths per minute. Ferrets do not pant as a physiologic mechanism to maintain body temperature. Panting is usually a sign of marked respiratory distress. Total lung capacity is about 3 times higher than what would be expected from an animal of this size.[2]

PREDISPOSING FACTORS

Any condition affecting the immune system can predispose to respiratory disease. Although some diseases may be more common in older animals (cardiac disease and failure), some neoplasms that can affect the respiratory tract such as lymphoma are reported in any age ferret.

CLINICAL SIGNS

Ferrets with symptoms related to the respiratory tract can present similarly to other traditional pet species and range from mild to severe dyspnea. All patients with suspected respiratory disease should be evaluated at rest from a distance before handling.

Upper respiratory signs can include ocular and nasal discharge (**Fig. 1**), audible wheeze, cough, and variable levels of respiratory distress, including increased inspiratory effort. Lower respiratory signs can include cough and variable levels of respiratory distress including increased expiratory effort. Disease in any portion of the

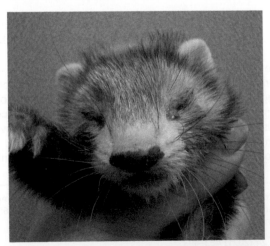

Fig. 1. Severe conjunctivitis and nasal discharge in a young ferret exposed to a human with influenza. (Used with permission Dr. Cathy Johnson-Delaney.)

respiratory tract can produce auscultable abnormalities consistent with those encountered in other mammal species. Reduced thoracic compliance and abnormalities on percussion of the thorax can suggest lung consolidation or a mass. Some respiratory diseases, in particular infectious diseases, may produce a fever.

Pulse oximetry and capnography have been investigated in ferrets; pulse oximetry was found to correlate well with oxygen saturation measured by blood gas analysis. Capnography was useful for measuring respiratory rate and pattern, but actual $Paco_2$ values were found to be less reliable.[7] Values are similar to those expected in traditional pet species with an ideal 98% to 100%. Both rectal and clamp-type capnography probes can be used in ferrets (**Fig. 2**).

DIAGNOSTICS

Although the primary goal of workup is to identify the cause of respiratory disease, sick ferrets benefit from general diagnostic testing as well (complete blood count, biochemistry panel). Some respiratory pathogens such as bacterial or fungal infections may cause changes in the hemogram. Venipuncture is well described in ferrets, and sites include the cranial vena cava, jugular, and tail veins and can usually be obtained in the conscious patient, providing restraint does not worsen respiratory symptoms. Workup should be thorough to distinguish causes that may produce similar clinical signs.

Some ferrets with severe symptoms require sedation. Drugs for sedation protocols are chosen based on patient condition; these typically include midazolam and an opioid. Butorphanol is particularly sedating in ferrets and may be adequate as a sole agent in very calm or ill patients.

For the stable patient, the author prefers midazolam, 0.25 to 0.5 mg/kg intramuscularly (IM), and butorphanol, 0.1 to 0.2 mg/kg IM, for initial sedation; if sedation is

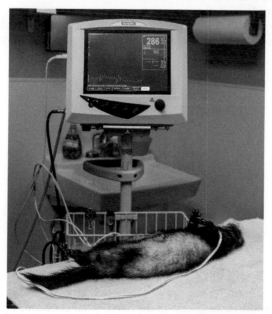

Fig. 2. Assessment of oxygen saturation with pulse oximetry using a clamp style probe on the left front paw of a sedated ferret. (Interpretation courtesy Dr. Kyle Vititoe.)

inadequate, alfaxalone can be added at 1 mg/kg IM and can be safely repeated. The author prefers to administer sedation drugs combined into a single syringe delivered IM or subcutaneously using low-stress handling techniques. All sedated ferrets should be offered oxygen and thermal support.

Immobilizing ferrets with inhalant agents alone is stressful, and cardiorespiratory depression may be dangerous in very sick patients, especially those with severe cardiovascular or pulmonary disease.

Infectious disease testing ideally results in identification of the organism and can include culture and sensitivity, molecular diagnostics (polymerase chain reaction [PCR]), and biopsy. Other infectious organisms can be inferred using serology. Direct sampling (culture and sensitivity, PCR) for specific respiratory pathogens can be challenging. Collection of deep nasal specimens is difficult in this species due to the size of the nares and nasal cavity.

Bronchoalveolar lavage is extremely useful for diagnosis of lower respiratory disease. In the anesthetized ferret a sterile urinary catheter is passed through the endotracheal tube, and 1 mL/kg of saline is introduced and immediately suctioned (**Fig. 3**). Bronchoscopy-guided bronchoalveolar lavage was described in ferrets using 1.5 mL/kg saline.[8]

Thoracocentesis is performed as for other small traditional pet species; target anatomic location is between the 6th and 10th ribs.[6]

Many reference ranges offer basic diagnostic and even specific pathogen testing for ferrets. At the time of writing, many individual states' Board of Animal Health were accepting animal specimens for testing for COVID-19.

Diagnostic imaging is used routinely in ferrets and includes radiology (**Fig. 4**), computed tomography, MRI, and ultrasound. Of these, ultrasound is easily accomplished by scruffing and distracting the ferret. However, sedation and in some cases anesthesia may be required to reduce struggling and obtain ideal positioning for diagnostic imaging. Normal radiographic appearance of the thorax of the ferret is well described (see **Fig. 4**).

A full cardiac evaluation, including echocardiography and electrocardiography, provides valuable information to rule out cardiac disease, which can produce respiratory symptoms.

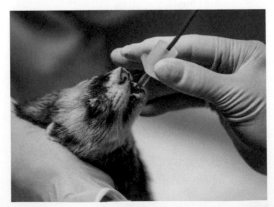

Fig. 3. Simple procedure for lung wash in the ferret. After anesthetizing, place an endotracheal tube. Feed a sterile urinary catheter through the endotracheal tube; suggested fluid volume for infusion is 1 mL/kg.[6]

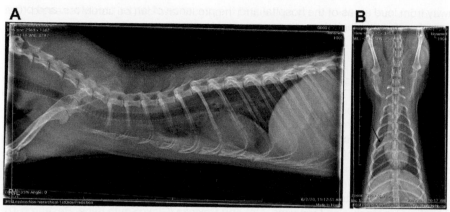

Fig. 4. (*A, B*) Right lateral and ventrodorsal (VD) thoracic radiographs of a 1-year-old male ferret. Of note is the large amount of intrathoracic mediastinal fat opacity causing widening of the cranial mediastinum and a diverging wedge-shaped fat opacity between the right lung lobes on the VD image (*black arrow*). On the lateral image the fat opacity between the diaphragm and heart can be easily discerned from soft tissue/fluid by the difference in opacity of the fat and adjacent heart. This is an incidental finding and should not be confused with mediastinal or pulmonary disease. (Interpretation courtesy Dr. Kyle Vititoe.)

THERAPY
General Supportive Care

Patients in respiratory distress should be offered oxygen either as flow-by or in an oxygen chamber. Conscious ferrets usually do not tolerate a face mask. Anxious ferrets with severe respiratory distress may benefit from low-dose sedation (discussed earlier).

Correct fluid deficits using protocols that are used in traditional pet species, for example, treatment of hypovolemic shock with 10 mL/kg boluses intravenously or intraosseously (IO) with a balanced electrolyte solution until normovolemia is restored.[9] Vascular access is relatively easy in the ferret, with the cephalic veins most commonly used; an alternative in severely hypovolemic ferrets is an IO catheter placed in the tibia. Blood pressure is monitored using a pediatric cuff and Doppler. Hydration is estimated as in other mammal species and calculated at % dehydration x body weight in kg x 1000. Maintenance fluids are added (estimated at x mL/kg/h) and corrected for ongoing losses.[9]

It should be noted that severe respiratory disease or any disease producing decreased appetite may result in decompensation of concurrent insulinoma. Insulinoma previously managed with diet alone may not require therapy with prednisone, or increases in dosages, which may be contraindicated in the face of an infectious cause. Rapid control of symptoms and frequent hand feeding of high-protein meals may help restore control of hypoglycemia.

The ferret is an obligate carnivore, and feeding products should be meat based without significant carbohydrates. Oxbow Carnivore Care (Oxbow Animal Health, Murdoch NE) is supplied in powder form for reconstitution and is easily administered by oral feeding syringe.

Some conditions may produce discomfort. Doses of commonly used analgesics are available in exotic animal formularies.[10] As mentioned earlier, butorphanol is a commonly used opioid analgesic but is very sedating in many ferrets.

Treatment and hospitalization are stressful, and care must be taken to optimize the entire hospital experience. This can include hospitalization with a bonded companion, away from loud areas of the hospital and the presence of larger predators, and provision of preferred blankets or sleep sacs and toys from home.

MEDICAL THERAPY

Beyond supportive care, medical therapy is designed based on the underlying cause. Dosages for many drugs have been suggested; some are based on research, but many are extrapolated from doses used in other species and some are anecdotally reported.[10]

Antibiotics are commonly used for bacterial respiratory disease and should be chosen based on results of culture and sensitivity. Broad-spectrum antibiotics, including amoxicillin and enrofloxacin, are well tolerated. Common formulations of metronidazole often result in marked stress reactions during administration, even when masked with flavorings or syringe fed with food.[10]

Antiviral treatments may be helpful in ferrets with influenza; these include oseltamivir (Tamiflu, Genetech, San Francisco, CA) and Relenza (GlaxoSmith Kline, Research Triangle Park, NC) alone or combined with amantadine.[1] Dosages for ferrets have been suggested.[10] Some antiviral medications may be in short supply during human influenza outbreaks and should not be used. Most ferrets respond well to general supportive care and do not require antiviral treatment.

Drugs for treatment of cardiac disease and neoplasia in ferrets are reported.[10]

Ferrets generally tolerate oral medication well, which is facilitated by scruffing and introducing medication into the side of the mouth. Medications can be flavored for better compliance; interestingly enough, some ferrets prefer sweet fruit flavors to meat or fish flavors.

Medications can also be delivered by nebulization, including antimicrobials, mucolytics, and bronchodilators. The ability of powdered and liquid markers to reach various areas of the ferret respiratory tract has been investigated.[11] The author has nebulized ferrets with enrofloxacin 10 mg/mL saline and N-acetyl L-cysteine 10% to 20% at 22 mg/mL saline q8–12 h prn. Other drugs may be considered at dosages extrapolated from dogs or other species.

SURGICAL THERAPY

Both invasive and noninvasive surgery may be indicated for some respiratory diseases, including tracheal foreign bodies and thoracic trauma.

Premedication, induction, intubation, and maintenance in the ferret are well described. Intubation is performed as in a cat using a 2.5 mm endotracheal tube via direct visualization, similar as to performed in cats. For smaller patients, an endoscope using an over-the-top endotracheal tube can be beneficial.

SPECIFIC DISEASES

Infectious (parasitic, viral, bacterial, fungal)

Parasitic

Dirofilariasis is well described in ferrets. Cases are commonly reported in heartworm endemic areas but rarely seen in mid- to Northern regions of the United States. Because ferrets are relatively small, the presence of even a single worm can produce severe disease.[6] Symptoms are similar to those seen in other susceptible animals and include cough, lower respiratory signs, and occasionally sudden death.[6] Worm burden is typically low and often single-sex infections. For this reason, ferrets do not always show microfilaria, and direct testing (Knott test) is not recommended. Serologic tests to identify adult worms are available, but sensitivity and specificity in the ferret are uncertain. Some tests depend on detection of female heartworm protein, decreasing usefulness. Echocardiography may be the best choice for identification of disease and determination of worm burden.[6]

The most common treatment recommendation is adulticide drugs with concurrent systemic steroids. Drugs reported include melarsomine, ivermectin, and moxidectin (**Table 1**).[6]

Transvenous heartworm extraction has been reported in a ferret; in a single published case, 3 heartworms were removed, but 1 remained in the right ventricle. Clinical signs of heartworm infection included generalized weakness and resolved postextraction. Medical management posttreatment included prednisolone, 0.3 mg/kg, PO q12 h for 2 months and ivermectin, 55 mcg, PO monthly.[12]

Viral

Several viruses infect ferrets; among these the most common affecting the respiratory tract in clinical practice are canine distemper and influenza. In many cases diagnosis is achieved post mortem.

At the time of writing (January 2021) a novel, coronavirus outbreak (COVID-19/SARS-CoV-2) had produced a human global pandemic. Two studies from China and Korea demonstrated ferrets are susceptible to SARS-CoV-2; most affected animals become febrile (up to104.50), and viral replication was confirmed and found in nasal washes, saliva, urine, and feces. Noninfected indirect contact ferrets also demonstrated virus within their respiratory traits, confirming airborne transmission. No ferrets succumbed to the virus.[4,5]

It is currently unknown if humans can transmit the virus to ferrets; early results from the Coronavirus Epidemiologic Response and Surveillance (CoVERS) Study at Cummings School of Veterinary Medicine at Tufts University suggest transmission between humans and ferrets may not readily occur. Thirty-seven swabs (shallow nasal, buccal, or rectal) were collected from 32 domestic ferrets. Of these, 29 ferrets were living in a home with at least one confirmed COVID-19 positive adult who was their primary caretaker. Of the remaining ferrets tested, one was euthanized with serious respiratory disease, one was euthanized for unrelated reasons, and one had unrelated symptoms. All swabs tested negative by real-time PCR for SARS-CoV-2 nucleocapsid (N), envelope (E),

Table 1
Selected medications used for treatment of specific respiratory conditions in ferrets[10]

Drug	Indication	Dosage mg/kg	Dosing Interval	Comments
Ivermectin	Heartworm treatment	0.05 PO	q30 d until negative testing	Give with prednisone 1 mg/kg q24 h concurrently
	Heartworm prevention	0.2 PO/SC	q30 d	
Melarsomine dihydrochloride	Heartworm treatment	2.5 IM	Once, repeat in 30d, 24h apart	Give with prednisone 1 mg/kg q24 h × 4 mo Less commonly used
Moxidectin	Heartworm treatment	0.17 mg SC	Once	Adulticide
Aminophylline	Bronchodilator	4–6.6 PO/IM/IV	q12 h	
Terbutaline	Bronchodilator	2.5–5	q12–24 h	
Theophylline	Bronchodilator	4.25	q8–12 h	

RNA-dependent RNA polymerase (RdRp), and polyprotein ORF1 genes. These preliminary data suggest a low rate of human to ferret transmission in a domestic setting (personal communication, Kaitlin Sawatzki, Department of Infectious Disease and Global Health, Cummings School of Veterinary Medicine at Tufts University, May 2020).

Canine distemper can produce respiratory disease, and severity often depends on strain of the virus. Although the neurologic form of this disease is usually fatal, a milder strain may produce pneumonia, and mortality rates are lower.[6,13]

Diagnosis can be supported by vaccine history and evidence of exposure to the virus. Antemortem testing traditionally includes fluorescent antibody (FA) of conjunctival smears, mucous membranes, or blood smears. PCR, immunohistochemistry and serology are also available.[13]

Influenza A has been identified in pet ferrets; in several documented cases the source was proved to be ill humans.[3,14] There are unsubstantiated reports of ferrets transmitting the disease to humans. Many cases feature fever, sneezing, and oculonasal discharge, but some strains may produce severe disease of the lower respiratory system (**Fig. 5**) and even neurologic symptoms.[6] Secondary bacterial pneumonia is common, especially in young stressed and likely immunocompromised ferrets. In adult, otherwise healthy ferrets, disease is often mild with a 5- to 7-day course.[15] Immunohistochemistry and PCR are available for antemortem diagnosis of influenza in ferrets.[13]

Lesions produced by ferret systemic coronavirus may be detected in the lung.[16]

Bacterial

Ferrets are susceptible to bacterial rhinitis, tracheitis, and pneumonia but in many cases is not a single or primary pathogen.[15] Multiple pathogens have been isolated, including *Pseudomonas (Chryseomonas) luteola*, *Pseudomonas sp.*, *Bordetella bronchiseptica*, and *Escherichia coli*.[15]

Mycobacteriosis has been documented in ferrets, including a report of 17 cases in ferrets in France between 2005 and 2013. Diagnosis was based on histopathology and special staining or PCR. All organisms were atypical and nontuberculous.[17] Many cases presented as eyelid lesions. Conjunctival lesions were a feature of other reported cases as well.[18] Culture of specimens from suspected mycobacterial cases is available from Michigan State University and other laboratories.[1] Mycobacterial species are potentially zoonotic; atypical nontuberculous species are generally a risk to immunocompromised humans.

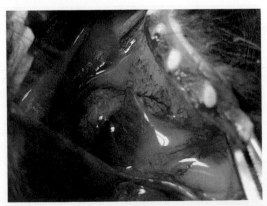

Fig. 5. Post mortem image of the heart and lungs of a young ferret with severe upper airway disease and pyothorax; influenza was suspected and *Staphylococcus aureus* cultured. (Used with permission Dr. Cathy Johnson-Delaney.)

A novel mycoplasma species was associated with an outbreak of both severe upper and lower respiratory disease in more than 8000 ferrets between 2009 and 2012. Ferrets were imported from a breeding facility in Canada; morbidity was high with very little mortality.[19] Culture and PCR for mycoplasmosis in other species can be considered for suspected cases. Mycoplasma species are difficult to culture, and consultation with a reference laboratory is recommended before submission. For this reason, PCR is more commonly used.

Fungal

Sporadic cases of systemic fungus infections occur and include blastomycosis and cryptococcosis.[20,21] These typically produce nasal cavity disease or pneumonia. In immunocompromised ferrets disseminated cryptococcus can affect multiple organs.[6] Histoplasmosis was identified post mortem in a ferret with gastrointestinal and central nervous system symptoms. In most cases, diagnosis is via identification of the organisms in specific samples.[22]

Diagnosis is generally via cytology, culture, or histopathologic evaluation.

Cardiac Disease

Cardiac disease, including cardiomyopathy and heart failure, and conduction disturbances have been described in ferrets. As in other species, left-sided heart failure can result in pulmonary edema and pleural effusion.[6]

Trauma

Any portion of the respiratory tract can be traumatized. Sources of injury include other pets, compression injuries, and falls from heights. Pneumothorax was noted in a ferret after a fall from a height.[23] Another ferret demonstrated bilateral rib fractures and possible pulmonary contusions or hemorrhage due to trauma.[23]

Bleeding and swelling (nasal cavity, trachea, thorax) cause respiratory compromise. Trauma may produce increased respiratory rate due to pain and anxiety as well.

Metabolic

As in other species, respiratory acidosis and alkalosis can occur with derangements of carbon dioxide from various respiratory abnormalities such as edema or pneumonia.

Neoplasia

Lymphoma is commonly reported in the ferret and can occur anywhere in the body, including the mediastinum. Mediastinal lymphoma is often recognized radiographically. Some cases produce marked pleural effusion.[23]

Treatment of lymphoma has been attempted but comparison of outcomes and selection of the ideal protocol is hampered by inability to accurate stage the disease.[24] A review of the evidence for type, treatment, and outcomes for lymphoma in ferrets has been presented.[25]

Pulmonary neoplasia can be chemically induced in the ferret[26]; spontaneous tumors, however, seem uncommon.

SECONDARY DISEASES

Anaphylaxis may produce dyspnea; this is most commonly seen postvaccination for distemper and rabies.[6] Acetaminophen toxicity can produce symptoms referred to the respiratory tract.[6] Hyperestrogenism (seen in intact female ferrets) can produce severe anemia and increased respiratory rate due to decreased oxygen carrying capacity.[6]

Dental disease and periapical abscess may extend via a fistula into the nasal cavity and may present as chronic nasal discharge.[6] Treatment is similar to that in canine and feline patients with antibiotics based on culture and sensitivity and in some cases surgical management. A case report in a ferret was treated with dental extractions, debridement of the fistula, and placement of medicated gauze, along with supportive care.[27]

HYPERTHERMIA

Hyperthermia can be due to overheating or severe infectious diseases, in particular viruses. Ferrets present with increased respiratory rate and seem uncomfortable. A recent study on comparison of body temperature in ferrets acquired via rectal and auricular methods showed auricular measurements using multiple devices to vary from rectal methods by as much as 1.8° F. In this study, normal body temperature using rectal methods with glass and digital thermometers was 98.6 to 103.2°F.[28]

MISCELLANEOUS/IDIOPATHIC

Megaesophagus has been reported to produce respiratory signs associated with aspiration pneumonia[6]; however, one case seen by the author did not produce any respiratory symptoms.[23]

Endogenous lipid pneumonia was described in a ferret with severe respiratory disease; cause was not determined.[29]

Two cases of chylous ascites were reported in ferrets. One was secondary to lymphatic drainage obstruction, and one was a postoperative complication of adrenal carcinoma and metastases. Neither ferret survived long term.[30]

Asthma or other inhalant allergies have not been well documented in the ferret. Ferrets would be expected to be susceptible to airborne toxins similar to that in other pet species.

REFERENCES

1. Johnson-Delaney C, Orosz S. Ferret respiratory system: clinical anatomy, physiology and disease. Vet Clin N Am Exot Pet Prac 2011;14(2):357–67.
2. Applied clinical anatomy and physiology. In: Johnson-Delaney C, editor. Ferret medicine and surgery. Boca Raton (FL): CRC Press; 2017. p. 13–29.
3. Belser JA, Katz JM, Tumpey TM. The ferret as a model organism to study influenza A virus infection. Dis Model Mech 2011;4(5):575–9.
4. Kim Y-I, Kim S-G, Kim S-M, et al. Infection and rapid transmission of SARS-CoV-2 in Ferrets. Cell 2020;27(5):704–9.
5. Shi J, Wen Z, Zhong G, et al. Susceptibility of ferrets, cats, dogs and different domestic animals to SARS-coronavirus-2. Science 2020;368(6494):1016–20.
6. Disorders of the respiratory tract. In: Johnson-Delaney C, editor. Ferret medicine and surgery. Boca Raton (FL): CRC Press; 2017. p. 311–23.
7. Olin JM, Smith TJ, Talcott MR. Evaluation of noninvasive monitoring techniques in domestic ferrets (Muystela putorius furo). Am J Vet Res 1997;58(10):1065.
8. Bercier M, Langlois I, Dunn M, et al. Cytological analysis of bronchoalveolar lavage fluid acquired by bronchoscopy in healthy ferrets: a pilot study. Can J Vet Res 2016;80(1):74–80.

9. Gladden J, Lennox AM. Emergency and critical care of small mammals. In: Quesenberry Q, Orcutt C, Mans C, et al, editors. Ferrets, rabbits and rodents clinical medicine and surgery. 4th edition. St Louis (MO): Elsevier; 2021. p. 595–608.
10. Morrisey JK, Johnston MS. Ferrets. In: Carpenter JW, editor. Exotic animal formulary. 5th edition. St Louis (M)O: Elsevier; 2019. p. 532–57.
11. Kuehl PJ, Chand R, McDonald JD, et al. Pulmonary and regional deposition of nebulized and dry powder aerosols in ferrets. Pharm Sci Tech 2019;20(6):242.
12. Bradbury C, Saunders AB, Heatley JJ, et al. Transvenous heart worm extraction in a ferret with caval syndrome. J Am Anim Hosp Assoc 2010;46:31–5.
13. Ferrets. In: Mayer J, Donnelly T, editors. Clinical veterinary advisor Birds and exotic pets. St Louis (MO): Elsevier; 2013. p. 430–501.
14. Lin H, Wang C. Natural A(H1N1) pdm09 influenza virus infection case in a pet ferret in Taiwan. Jap J Vet Res 2014;62(4):181–5.
15. Perpinan D. Respiratory diseases of ferrets. In: Quesenberry Q, Orcutt C, Mans C, et al, editors. Ferrets, rabbits and rodents clinical medicine and surgery. St Louis (MO): Elsevier; 2021. p. 595–608.
16. Autieri CR, Miller CL, Scott KE, et al. Systemic coronaviral disease in 5 ferrets. Comp Med 2015;65(6):508–16.
17. Mentre V, Bulliot C. A retrospective study of 17 cases of mycobacteriosis in domestic ferrets (Mustela putorius furo) between 2005 and 2013. J Exot Pet Med 2015;24:340–9.
18. Lucas A, Furber H, James G, et al. Mycobacterium genavense infection in two aged ferrets with conjunctival lesions. Aust Vet J 2000;78(10):685–9.
19. Kiupel M, Desjardins DR, Lim A, et al. Mycoplasmosis in ferrets. Emerg Infect Dis 2012;18(11):1763–70.
20. Darrow BG, Mans C, Drees R, et al. Pulmonary blastomycosis in a domestic ferret. J Eotic Pet Mod 2014;23(2):158–64.
21. Le K, Beaufrere H, Laniesse D, et al. Diagnosis and long-term management of blastomycosis in two ferrets (Mustela putorius furo). J Exot Pet Med 2019;31:39–44.
22. Greenacre C, Dowling M, Nobrega-Lee M. Diagnosis and treatment of histoplasmosis in a groups of four domestic ferrets (Mustela putorius furo) and a review of histoplasmosis. J Exot Pet Med 2019;29:194–201.
23. Capello V, Lennox AM. Ferrets. In: Clinical radiology of exotic companion mammals. Ames (IO): Wiley-Blackwell; 2018. p. 358–409.
24. Huynh M, Chassang L, Zoller G. Evidence-based advances in ferret medicine. Veterinary Clin North Am Exot Anim Pract 2017;20(3):773–803.
25. Webb J, Graham JE, Burgess KE, et al. Presentation and survival time of domestic ferrets (Mustela putorius furo) with lymphoma treated with single and multi-agent protocols: 44 cases *(1998-2016). J Exot Pet Med 2019;31:64–7.
26. Kim Y, Xiaolone L, Liu C, et al. Induction of pulmonary neoplasia in the smoke-exposed ferret by 4-methylnitrosamino)-1-(3-pyridyl)-1-butanone (NNK): A model for human lung. Cancer Lett 2006;234(2):209–19.
27. Thas I. Acquired oronasal fistula in a domestic ferret (Mustela putorius furo). J Exot Pet Med 2014;23(4):409–14.
28. Aguilar LAB, Chavez JO, Ducoing-Watty A. Comparison of body temperature acquired via auricular and rectal methods in ferrets. J Exot Pet Med 2019;28:148–53.
29. Perpinan D, Ramis A. Endogenous lipid pneumonia in a ferret. J Exot Pet Med 2011;20(1):51–5.
30. Vilalta L, Altuzarra R, Molina J, et al. Chylous ascites in two ferret. J Exot Pet Med 2017;26(2):150–5.

Moving?

Make sure your subscription moves with you!

To notify us of your new address, find your **Clinics Account Number** (located on your mailing label above your name), and contact customer service at:

Email: journalscustomerservice-usa@elsevier.com

800-654-2452 (subscribers in the U.S. & Canada)
314-447-8871 (subscribers outside of the U.S. & Canada)

Fax number: 314-447-8029

Elsevier Health Sciences Division
Subscription Customer Service
3251 Riverport Lane
Maryland Heights, MO 63043

*To ensure uninterrupted delivery of your subscription, please notify us at least 4 weeks in advance of move.

Printed and bound by CPI Group (UK) Ltd, Croydon, CR0 4YY

24/10/2024

01778553-0003